Visit our website

to find out about other books from Churchill Livingstone
and our sister imprints in Harcourt Health Sciences

Register free at
www.harcourt-international.com

and you will get

- **the latest information on new books, journals and electronic products in your chosen subject areas**

- **the choice of e-mail or post alerts or both, when there are any new books in your chosen areas**

- **news of special offers and promotions**

- **information about products from all Harcourt Health Sciences imprints including W. B. Saunders, Churchill Livingstone, and Mosby**

You will also find an easily searchable catalogue, online ordering,
information on our extensive list of journals...and much more!

Visit the Harcourt Health Sciences website today!

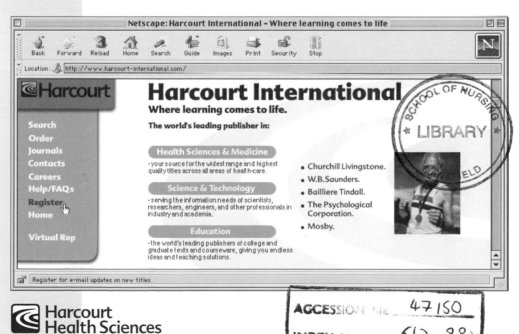

Pain Management

An Interdisciplinary Approach

For Churchill Livingstone:

Editorial Director, Health Professions: Mary Law
Head of Project Management: Ewan Halley
Project Development Manager: Katrina Mather
Designer: George Ajayi

Pain Management

An Interdisciplinary Approach

Chris J. Main PhD FBPsS
Consultant Clinical Psychologist, Head of Department of Behavioural Medicine, Hope Hospital,
Salford and Honorary Professor, University of Manchester, Manchester, UK

Chris C. Spanswick MB ChB FRCA
Consultant in Pain Management and Anaesthesia, Manchester and Salford Pain Centre, Hope Hospital,
Salford and Honorary Clinical Lecturer in Anaesthesia, University of Manchester, Manchester, UK

Associate Editors

Helen Parker
Paul Watson

With contributions by

Serena Bartys
C. K. Booker
A. K. Burton
Wolfgang Dumat
Raymond Million
George Peat

FOREWORD BY

Professor Sir Michael Bond
Vice Principal, Faculty of Medicine, University of Glasgow, Glasgow, UK

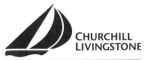

CHURCHILL
LIVINGSTONE

EDINBURGH LONDON NEW YORK PHILADELPHIA ST LOUIS SYDNEY TORONTO 2000

CHURCHILL LIVINGSTONE

An imprint of Harcourt Publishers Limited

© Harcourt Publishers Limited 2000.

 is a registered trademark of Harcourt Publishers Limited

First published 2000

ISBN 0 443 05683 8

British Library Cataloguing in Publication Data
A catalogue record for this book is available from the British Library

Library of Congress Cataloging in Publication Data
A catalog record for this book is available from the Library of
Congress

Note
Medical knowledge is constantly changing. As new information
becomes available, changes in treatment, procedures, equipment and
the use of drugs become necessary. The authors, contributors and the
publishers have taken care to ensure that the information given in this
text is accurate and up to date. However, readers are strongly advised
to confirm that the information, especially with regard to drug usage,
complies with the latest legislation and standards of practice.

The
publisher's
policy is to use
**paper manufactured
from sustainable forests**

Printed in China

Contents

Contributors

Serena Bartys
Research Psychologist, Department of Behavioural Medicine, Hope Hospital, Manchester, UK

C. K. Booker
Consultant Clinical Psychologist, Head of Speciality, c/o The Manchester and Salford Pain Centre, Hope Hosptial, Salford, UK

A. K. Burton
Director, Spinal Research Unit, University of Huddersfield, Huddersfield, UK

Wolfgang Dumat
Head of Pain Psychology, Medizinisch-Psychosomatische Klinik, Bad Bramstedt, Germany

Raymond Million
Consultant Rheumatologist, Oaklands Hospital, Salford, UK

Helen Parker
Consultant Clinical Neuropsychologist, 25 St John's Street, Manchester, UK

George Peat
Research Fellow, Primary Care Sciences Research Centre, Keele University, Staffordshire, UK

Paul Watson
Research Fellow, Department of Behavioural Medicine, University of Manchester, Manchester, UK

Foreword

In the past 35 years and since the publication of *The Gate Theory of Pain* in particular, the fields of pain research and clinical practice have been developed very substantially. With those developments has come a huge outpouring of books dealing with pain and its management from many different aspects and they can be grouped broadly under the headings of basic neurological sciences, psychological & social sciences and clinical management methods. This reflects the development of a wide range of specific interests but nevertheless there remains a great deal of general interest in pain. It is after all a problem at a clinical level which demands input from several different professional groups and especially when pain is chronic. Therefore, there is a continuing need for books which give broad coverage, although relatively few are written now which can be read by all the various groups involved in pain research and pain management.

This book provides just that blend of basic sciences and clinical management methods that is needed by those wishing to encompass the topic. In order to be a fully competent manager of people in pain it is necessary to have good understanding of the basic sciences and the information needed is supplied in some detail but in a readily digestible form for those reading outside their specialist area. The authors point out that psychological and social factors are often more important than knowledge of physical treatments in individuals with chronic pain with which this book is primarily concerned. As a result, there is an emphasis in it on psychological and social concepts necessary to the understanding of pain and associated behaviour, to forgetting the important role of family and cultural influences upon each person's attitudes and behaviour.

Often patients' complaints of pain and their levels of disability are out of proportion to the original injury or disease process and therefore it is vital not only to recognise this fact and so avoid unnecessary physical investigations and treatments, but also to understand the psychological and social processes that lead ultimately to chronic disability and the inability of individuals to resume their former roles and activities at home, at work and in society at large. The text includes excellent models to illustrate those processes and there are case histories that give a clear view of the various clinical presentations to which the models apply.

In order to steer a path through the varied symptoms and signs, including behaviours of individuals with chronic pain, a carefully constructed series of questions is needed backed by questionnaires designed to address specific aspects of emotion, for instance anxiety, depression and fear and to measure disability in its different forms. The authors have provided a section dealing with these issues in which they have covered the much neglected topic of the assessment of outcome in the short and longer term using reliable and valid measures. The current emphasis upon evidence-based medicine is now an aspect of management. The tools to which this eduction refer will facilitate the development of much needed information about the outcome of a range of treatments for chronic pain disorders attending strength to the emerging evidence that cognitive and behavioural techniques have a significant role to play in pain management.

It will be evident to the reader as the complexities of chronic pain unfold before them in the text, that the personnel needed will include a range of professionals including medical doctors, psychologists, nurses and phsiotherapists as a basic core with the possibility of others being needed from time to time for example, pharmacists. The authors make it clear that chronic pain is a problem for which the term 'cure' is seldom applied. What is required is that the person in pain learns to take control of their problem rather than remaining in the dependency role so often promoted by medical care. This represents a fundamental change in attitude for many professionals coming to grips with chronic pain management for the first time and with it comes the realisation that the solution does not lie in the hands of a single professional but in the inter-professional team mentioned earlier.

Therefore, questions of status, leadership and others that have kept the professions apart for so long have to be addressed if the team is to be effective. The provision for the development of such teams in the NHS is well below what is needed. Recently (April 2000), a Government appointed Clinical Standards Advisory Group (CSAG) produced a report entitled 'Services for Patients with Pain'. It identifies the need for improved pain management services particularly in the field of chronic pain where there is a signifcant shortfall.

This book should be on the shelves of all professionals who deal with chronic pain sufferers. Pain and chronic pain in particular is a vast drain on human and economic resources. Further improvement in knowledge and services will help to reduce these costs to society and, with this in mind, it is hoped that readers will use the information given here and their experiences from clinical practice to exert pressure for better services for chronic pain sufferers.

Professor Sir Michael Bond

Preface

During the last 30 years there has been a progressive increase in the number of pain management programmes. They have varied in sophistication from little more than modality clinics to sophisticated multidisciplinary programmes with a wide range of staff. The term 'pain management' itself has come to include a wide range of therapeutic interventions from specific pain relief procedures such as nerve blocks to multifaceted in-patient rehabilitation programmes lasting for 3 or 4 weeks. Any treatment approach is based on assumptions about the nature of the problem. In the field of chronic pain treatment the narrow medical model has become replaced by the wider biopsychosocial model. This change in perspective has allowed a much wider range of therapeutic options, incorporating behavioural and cognitive aspects of care along with physiotherapeutic activation and medical interventions. There have been many attempts to distil the essence of pain management. In truth, it can be viewed from a wide variety of angles and from varying distances.

In attempting to produce a textbook on such a rich and diverse subject, it is important that we attempt to define our assumptions (or biases). We view pain management essentially as based on self-control and consider that, above all, our principal objective in engaging patients in pain management is to assist them in the re-establishment of a degree of control over their pain and its effects. We do of course 'do things' to patients, and at times are directive and specific in our recommendations, but in the last analysis we are attempting to help patients understand their pain, understand themselves and acquire the necessary skills and confidence to instigate and sustain therapeutic change in order to maximise their own management of their pain.

The difference between 'multidisciplinary' and 'interdisciplinary' pain management is more than pedantic or even political. It is our firm conviction that a large contributing factor to unnecessary disability is poor management by health-care professionals. It could be argued of course that working in pain management programmes leads to a jaundiced view of the quality and efficacy of health care. It is our view none the less that as professionals we have to take at least some responsibility for some of the distress and dysfunction that are clearly evident in many chronic pain patients. The term 'interdisciplinary' stresses the important aspect of working as a professional team, giving patients a consistent message about the nature of their condition and what might be done about it.

Since the development of the first Salford pain management programme in 1983, we have often been asked what on earth we do. We attempted some years ago to explain it to patients, and developed a patient manual that we eventually turned into a small book (Parker & Main 1993). We have run a number of training courses and have in consequence developed a range of teaching materials. Eventually we decided we would have to try to systematise our thinking. This textbook is the result of our endeavours. There are of course already impressive books addressing various aspects of pain management on the market. We have attempted to do something slightly different with this book. Our focus has been not only on what should be done, but also on whether it is done, and why it is done. That is, we have tried to communicate our understanding not only of the *content* of interdisciplinary pain management, but also of the *process*. We have also, however, attempted to consider aspects of pain management in terms of our theoretical understanding of the nature of the processes involved in the hope that increased understanding may assist the development of a more patient-centred approach to pain management, with improved outcome as a consequence.

In the first section of the book we attempt to give an overview of the theoretical foundations of pain management, and offer some suggestions about how the various factors combine within individuals who become chronically disabled. In the second section of the book we address the various facets of assessment and how these influence interdisciplinary decision making. In the third section of the book we offer a description of some of the content of our programme, at the time of writing (in truth it is a stage of continuing evolution). In the fourth section we also address some of the logistic problems in establishing and maintaining pain management programmes (including the need to recognise the requirement for training to competency amongst the staff), and the assessment of outcome. Finally, we take the principles of pain management and consider their extension into the fast developing areas of secondary prevention (in both health and occupational settings). Please note that on several occasions throughout the text, we have used 'doctor' where we wish to refer to 'healthcare professionals'.

During the gestation of this book our ideas have changed about what we were attempting to do. As can be seen from the authorship of the various chapters, many different people have contributed to the final product. We have not attempted to constrain the various contributions to precisely the same format. Many of the chapters can be read on their own, although we have attempted to provide both 'vertical links' to other chapters in the same section, and also 'horizontal links' joining theoretical considerations with implications for both assessment and intervention.

REFERENCE

Parker H, Main C J 1993 Living with back pain. Manchester University Press, Manchester

Manchester 2000

Chris J. Main
Chris C. Spanswick

Acknowledgements

It is always difficult to recognise adequately the contribution of others, both directly and indirectly, in the gestation of a book such as this. We would like to acknowledge a massive debt to the pioneers of pain management such as John Bonica, Wilbert Fordyce and John Loeser. The focused perspectives of Robert Gatchel, Francis Keefe, Ronald Melzack, Dennis Turk and Patrick Wall in particular have inspired a generation. On a more direct personal level, we should like to acknowledge a major contribution also to our close friend and colleague Gordon Waddell, whose systematic analysis of the nature of back pain and back-associated disability has had a worldwide influence and changed the way people think about illness. Similarly, our long term working relationship with Kim Burton has been both inspiring and enjoyable. To our many friends and colleagues in the 'pain management industry' we also owe a huge debt for both their inspiration and friendship. It seems inappropriate perhaps to single any out, but we should like especially to thank Amanda Williams and Charles Pither (of the St Thomas's Hospital Pain Management Programme) and of course our colleagues in the Manchester and Salford Pain Centre particularly Lorraine Moores for her contribution to the appendix in Chapter 13 part 3.

The book would have been immeasurably poorer without the contributions of the other authors in the book, but our greatest professional debts are undoubtedly to our associate editors (Helen Parker and Paul Watson) for not only their professional skill but also their forbearance; and also to our publishers, particularly Mary Law and Katrina Mather, for remarkable courtesy and patience as well as technical help. Finally, of course, we owe an embarrassingly large debt to our neglected wives and families for allowing us to indulge ourselves in this venture.

If we have contributed in some small way to encouraging our colleagues to develop a sustained interest in biopsychosocial pain management then our effort will have been worth while.

Introduction to pain management

The theoretical foundations of modern interdisciplinary pain management are presented. The influence of Melzack and Wall's gate control theory of pain on the interaction between physiological and psychological processes cannot be overstated. In Chapter 2 the nature of psychological factors is considered. An understanding of behavioural and cognitive factors is at the heart of modern pain management. In Chapter 3, the influence of cultural, subcultural and social factors on the perception of pain, treatment seeking and response to treatment are considered. The role of social learning mechanisms is also discussed. In Chapter 4, the influence of economic and occupational factors on pain and disability is viewed from the standpoints of treatment seeking and as potential obstacles to recovery. In Chapter 5, biomedical, psychological and socioeconomic factors, in conjunction with the important influence of iatrogenic misunderstandings and distress, are integrated into a model of disability. Finally, in chapter 6 the historical origins of pain management are traced.

1

Models of pain

Chris J. Main   Chris C. Spanswick

INTRODUCTION: THE NATURE OF PAIN—A PERPETUAL PUZZLE

The nature of pain has puzzled humanity for centuries. As a personal experience pain has an immediacy and impact. This experience seems difficult to capture in words, yet such is the power of its impact that it could be considered that pain can be described adequately only in picture or metaphor. For centuries there has been a sustained attempt to develop a philosophical and scientific understanding of it. Many different models of pain have been offered and it is sometimes difficult to appreciate the extent to which our thinking is constrained by the prevailing conceptual models, or Zeitgeist. In this chapter an attempt will be made to view the nature of pain from a historical perspective through the eyes of influential thinkers from a variety of disciplines. Interestingly, although theoretical models are a product of their time, they can cast a long shadow. Contemporary conceptualisations about the nature of pain echo thinking from the past.

Any scientific understanding of the nature of pain requires consideration of fundamental physiology, psychology and the relationship between mind and body. Such an analysis requires consideration also of the use of language and the nature of scientific discourse. An overview of earlier theories about pain is offered to identify their influences on contemporary thinking. We are indebted to Bonica (1990) for much of the historical source material.

Table 1.1   Models of pain and their origins I: pre-Cartesian

Epoch	Key figures	Pain sources and mechanisms
Primitive		Magical fluids; exorcism; sorcery; women healers; medicine men
Ancient Egyptian		Influences of gods; spirits of dead; network of 'metu'; object intrusion
Ancient India		Frustration of desires; all joy/pain in heart
Ancient China		Yin–Yang balance; vital energy (Qi); network of 14 meridians; acupuncture
Ancient Greece (6th–4th BC)	Alcmaeon	Brain centre of sensation
	Anaxagoras	All sensations associated with pain
	Hippocrates	Four humours; pain as deficit/excess
	Plato	Pain from both peripheral sensation and heart; pain/pleasure affect whole body; pain as a 'passion of the soul'
	Aristotle	Five senses; brain no direct function in sensation; pain as increased sensitivity of every sensation; caused by vital heat
Ancient Rome (3rd BC)	Galen	Central and peripheral nervous system; brain as centre of sensibility Three classes: soft nerves with 'psychic pneuma' (sensory), hard nerves (motor) and pain nerves
Middle Ages (10th AD)	Avicenna	Five 'external' and five 'internal' senses (in brain); 15 different types of pain (due to humoral changes)
	Magnus	Sensation in anterior cerebral ventricle
	Mondino	Brain seat of sensation with power to cool heart
	da Vinci	Brain centre of sensation; nerves tubular; spinal cord as a conductor

Abstracted from Bonica J J 1990, pp. 2–17, with permission.

THEORIES OF PAIN

Pre-Cartesian

Although any contemporary model of pain will include both physiological and psychological factors, early theories of pain were very different (Table 1.1). Early civilisations offered a variety of explanations for pain and attributed it to such factors as religious influences of gods, the intrusion of magical fluids, the frustration of desires and deficiency or excess in the circulation of Qi.

The early Greeks gave more specific consideration to the nature of pain. Plato believed that the heart and liver were the centres for appreciation of all sensation, and that pain arose not only from peripheral sensation but as an emotional response in the soul, which resided in the heart.

Aristotle believed that the brain had no direct function in sensory processes. This view was not universally held. Nerves had been described during the Renaissance and, indeed, there was an understanding that these were connected to the brain and spinal cord. They were thought to be responsible for other sensations that were felt in the brain and not associated with pain at all. Pain due to external injuries was thought to be due to the entry of evil spirits. There was even less understanding of pain from internal or visceral causes. It was frequently attributed to the influence of evil spirits or the gods.

Hippocrates considered that pain was a consequence of deficiencies or excesses in the flow of one of the four fluids or humours (blood, phlegm, yellow bile or black bile). Galen in contrast clearly established the anatomy of the cranial and spinal nerves. He distinguished three types of nerve: 'soft' nerves, 'hard' nerves and pain nerves. He also considered that the centre of sensibility was the brain.

Nonetheless Aristotle's theories still had considerable influence. For a long time pain was still considered to be an emotion or sensation experienced in the heart or an effect possibly of the entry of evil spirits. The brain was thought to play no part in the experience of pain. Indeed, the controversy over whether pain should be regarded as a sensation or as an emotion has continued to the present day and led to an over-stated dichotomy between sensory and emotional factors. Descartes' new theory was, therefore, a massive leap in the understanding of the mechanism of pain, and drew significant criticism from his contemporaries at the time.

Cartesian model

Descartes' explanation of pain (Descartes 1664) needs to be understood against the background of his philosophy. He attempted to show that humans consisted of an earthly machine (*machine de terre*) inhabited by and governed by a rational soul (*ame raissonnable*). He tried to explain how blood, itself derived from food, gave rise to animal spirits by means of which the special earthly machine, the brain with its nerves, carried out the behests of the rational soul. The spirits dilated the brain, thus enabling it to receive the impressions of external objects, and flowed from the brain along the nerves into the muscles, thus enabling the nerves to serve as 'the organs of the external senses'. Thus animal spirits constituted a very subtle fluid amenable to the physical laws governing fluids, and the nerves were hollow tubes along which the spirits flowed in a wholly mechanical manner (Foster 1901). The nerves were not merely hollow tubes, however, but contained also delicate threads which spread all over the body from their origins at the internal surface of the brain and served as organs of sense. These threads were easily set in motion by the objects of the senses and at the same instant pulled upon the parts of the brain from which they originated.

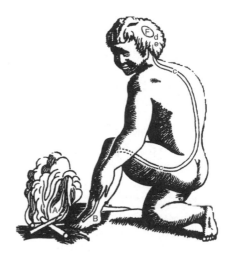

Figure 1.1   Descartes' model of pain From Waddell The Back Pain Revolution 1998, reproduced with permission.

Descartes offered the example of a foot coming into contact with fire (Fig. 1.1):

If for example the fire comes near the foot, the minute particles of this fire, which as you know have a great velocity, have the power to set in motion the spot of skin of the foot which they touch, and by this means pulling upon the delicate thread which is attached to the spot of the skin, they open up at the same instant the pore against which the delicate thread ends, just as pulling at one end of a rope one makes to strike at the same instant a bell which hangs on the other end. (Descartes 1664, translated by Foster 1901, p. 265).

As Foster points out, Descartes' theory required these nerves to have physical properties for which he had no evidence.

Descartes offered a dualistic view of mind and body. The body essentially was a machine whose workings could be explained by the laws of nature. The 'rational soul' was the 'conductor of the orchestra'. Descartes never really satisfactorily resolved the relationship between the two. There certainly does not seem to be any central 'processing' of the information, although it is consistent with the notion of summation.

The Cartesian legacy

In understanding pain mechanisms, there have been two major assumptions that have been inherited from Descartes: first that of a one-to-one relationship between the amount of damage (or nociception) and the pain experienced, and secondly the separation of mind and body.

The model of a one-to-one relationship between the amount of tissue damage and the amount of pain experienced has attractiveness, in that it seems to be consistent with the everyday experience of acute pain. It has to be remembered of course that pain is first and foremost a biological warning signal. Pain is necessary to protect us from damage. There are well-recorded instances of children with an insensibility to pain who unknowingly injure themselves. They are unable, for example, to experience pain from internal disease and need to have their temperature monitored regularly in order to alert their carers to the possibility of internal pathology. They do not have a normal life expectancy. Thus the function of pain in alerting us to actual or potential tissue damage is extremely important. We are programmed to react rapidly to pain. Sudden pain produces an instinctive withdrawal response. We attend immediately to it. We attempt to escape from the source of pain and we try to protect the injured tissue from further damage. The pain is giving us important information about the source, nature and intensity of the pain. On occasions, such information may be of life-threatening importance. Avoidance of further painful experiences will necessarily avoid damage, aid healing and return to the 'normal' state. The assumption that a higher level of pain is indicative of more serious physical damage (Fig. 1.2) is therefore useful, but an *accurate* appraisal of the pain is not necessary.

Most patients have little understanding of the complexity of the neurophysiology and anatomy of nociceptive pathways and pain experience and indeed do not require such knowledge. They are unlikely to have experienced pain in the past without some injury or cause. The concept of pain experience as *not* directly associated with the amount of tissue damage is alien and illogical to them. Perhaps we should not be surprised. For unless the pain persists there is usually no need for a patient to understand pain mechanisms. Furthermore, the medical profession and allied disciplines will, to a large extent, have reinforced

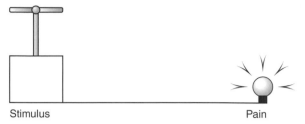

Stimulus   Pain

Figure 1.2 The patient's model of pain. This model of pain demonstrates a direct relationship between stimulus (the pressure on the T bar) and the amount of pain (the brightness of the electric bulb). It implies information travelling in one direction only, and does not allow for any modulation of the stimulus. This model implies: that a small stimulus may not cause pain, a large stimulus will always cause pain and when pain is sensed there is always damage causing it. Stopping the stimulus is the *way* of stopping the pain. Cutting the wire is the only other alternative.

this model of pain and damage. Rest is usually prescribed for any painful injury, along with pain killers and other treatments. Certainly patients are advised not to move something if it hurts. The message 'let the pain be your guide' is commonly given to patients recovering from an acute injury, reinforcing the notion of pain being a direct measure of tissue damage.

A legacy of the 'mind–body split' has been the conceptualisation of pain as being *either* physical *or* psychological. Patients' general defensiveness about considering anything from a psychological viewpoint has made contemporary pain management, which accepts an interaction between physical and psychological factors, difficult for patients to accept. (Many patients view discussions about 'non-physical' influences on pain with disbelief, suspicion and sometimes downright hostility.) Attribution to a psychological influence on the perception of pain by a professional may be taken by the patient as synonymous with an implication of some sort of mental illness, a suggestion that the pain is imaginary or even that the patient is malingering.

In conclusion, the Cartesian theory represented a significant advance on its predecessors, in postulating a mechanism of pain transmission from the periphery of the body to higher centres in the brain, but every theory has its limitations.

Table 1.2 Models of pain and their origins II: 17th–mid 20th century

Epoch	Key figures	Pain sources and mechanisms
17th and 18th centuries		
1628	Harvey	Heart as site of pain
1664	Descartes	Body as a machine; nerves as tubes containing threads; pineal gland and ventricles as reservoirs of animal spirits; spirits flow along tubes; bell-rope mechanism
1794	Darwin (E.)	Pain as 'phase of unpleasantness'; intensity
19th century		
1827	Bell	Dorsal and ventral roots
1839	Muller	Special nerve energies
1859	Schiff	Specificity (sensory) theory
1894	von Frey	Pain as fourth cutaneous modality
1895	Erb	Intensity (summation) theory
1895	Goldscheider	Skin sensory input summated at dorsal horn; spinal 'summation path'
1895	Marshall	Pain as an affect
1895	Strong	Pain includes original sensation plus psychic reaction
20th century		
1900	Sherrington	Pain having both sensory and affective dimensions
1920	Head	Pain centre in the thalamus
1932	Nafe	Spatial and temporal patterning of impulses
1943	Livingston	Central summation theory; T cells critical
1951	Gerard	Nerve lesions and 'synchronously firing pools'
1952	Hardy	4th theory–primary perception and secondary reaction
1955	Sinclair	Peripheral pattern theory
1959	Nordenboos	Sensory interaction theory

Abstracted from Bonica J J 1990, pp. 2–17, with permission.

It was unable to explain clinical phenomena such as phantom pain (where pain is felt in a part of the body that has been amputated), the absence of pain in the presence of injury (such as battle wounds that are noticed only when the threat to life has passed), or the persistence of pain beyond tissue-healing time (as in chronic pain conditions). Finally it could be argued that its assumptions of a one-to-one relationship between nociception and pain experience, and its dualistic separation of mind and body, have been particular hindrances to the development of an adequate theory of pain.

Post-Cartesian developments

Two major physiological theories of pain became the object of research in the 19th century (Table 1.2). Descartes had developed the concept of a pain pathway linking the periphery of the body with higher centres in the brain. It led to the specificity theory, in which pain was considered to be a *specific sensation* independent of other sensations. According to the intensive (summation) theory, however, touch was experienced as a painful sensation only when it reached a certain threshold (following intense stimulation). Both these theories and their later derivatives were essentially physiological in nature and the *perception* of pain was not specifically addressed. They offered a relatively simple relationship between tissue damage and pain perception. The sensory system responsible for mediating pain was regarded as relatively rigid and straightforward in that any tissue damage initiated a sequence of neural events that inevitably produced pain. An unfortunate inference from this simplistic view was that pain was fixed solely by characteristics of the noxious stimulus and that the nociceptive system functioned primarily as a passive relay mechanism. Neither of the theories could explain either pain in the absence of tissue damage or variation in pain between individuals with (apparently) the same amount of tissue damage. The latter tended to be attributed to long term personality characteristics rather than be seen as a feature of the psychological impact of the pain itself.

We now know that pain perception depends on complex neural interactions where impulses generated by tissue damage are modified both by ascending systems activated by innocuous stimuli and by descending pain-suppressing systems activated by various environmental and psychological factors.

With the addition of the later sensory interaction theory (postulating a fast and a slow system of pain transmission), the foundation of the gate control theory (GCT) (Melzack & Wall 1965) was laid.

The gate control theory

In 1965 Melzack & Wall proposed the original gate theory of pain, or GCT-I (Fig. 1.3). This theory marked a turning point in our understanding of pain (Table 1.3). It was of landmark importance in two respects: first in terms of the mechanisms of the transmission and modulation of nociceptive signals, and secondly in terms of its recognition of pain as a psychophysiological phenomenon resulting from the interaction between physiological and psychological events.

The GCT incorporated physiological specialisation, central summation patterning and modulation of input by psychological and other factors into a new model that has formed much of the contemporary psychology of pain.

The GCT postulated spinal 'gates', in the dorsal horn at each segmental level in the spinal cord, determining which of the competing impulses (pain, heat or touch) was transmitted at any particular moment. Successful transmission through the gate was affected not only by the

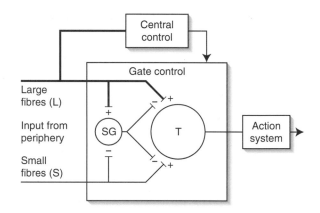

Figure 1.3 Gate control theory I (GCT-I). L, the large diameter fibres. S, the small diameter fibres. The fibres project to the substantia gelatinosa (SG) and first central transmission (T) cells. The inhibitory effect exerted by the SG on the afferent fibre terminals is increased by activity in L fibres and decreased by activity in S fibres. The central control trigger is represented by a line running from the large fibre system to the central control mechanisms; these mechanisms, in turn, project back to the gate control system. The T cells project to the action system. (+, excitation, −, inhibition.) From Melzack & Wall 1965, p. 971, reproduced with permission.

Table 1.3 Models of pain and their origins III: since the gate control theory

Epoch	Key figures	Pain sources & mechanisms
1962, 1965	Melzack & Wall	GCT-I: competition at dorsal horn for transmission
1966	Mendell	Wind-up
1968	Melzack & Casey	Ascending and descending influences; motivational, cognitive and behavioural aspects of pain experience
1983	Travell	Myogenic pain theory
1991	Jones	Limbic system mapping (PET)
1991	Dubner	Neuroplasticity
1994	Flor	Psychophysiological mechanisms
1996	Ohrbach	Stress–hyperactivity theory
1996	Melzack	Neuromatrix theory

intensity of the stimulation, and competing local stimuli, but also by descending impulses from the higher central nervous system. In contrast to the model of Descartes, the transmission of information about events in the periphery is not a simple one-way system. There is continual modulation of information from the periphery—in the gate theory's case, nociception.

Figure 1.3 is a schematic representation of the sensory input at each segmental level in the dorsal horn of the spinal cord. The large fibres (L) and the small fibres (S) project into the substantia gelatinosa (SG) and the first transmission cells (T). It can be seen from the figure that input from large fibres will *reduce* the amount of nociceptive traffic, whereas input from the smaller fibres will *increase* nociceptive traffic going further up to the action system.

The diagram also shows the influence of 'central control' (at the dorsal horn). This central control is initiated by input from the large fibres and feeds back into the 'gate control system'. These large fibres carry specific information about the nature and location of the stimulus. They conduct rapidly, not only potentially setting the sensitivity of the cortical neurons but

also influencing the sensory input in the gate itself. This may occur not only at the level of the original input but also at other levels.

This rapid transmission allows the brain to identify, evaluate and modulate input before the action system is activated by the T cells. The final common pathway is provided through the 'T' cell, which, when the output from this exceeds a critical level, sends information further on to the 'action system'. The 'action system' describes those areas of the brain responsible for the behavioural responses to pain and the 'experience' of pain itself.

Soon after the first publication the theory was expanded (Melzack & Casey 1968) to describe the neural system beyond the gate (Fig. 1.4). The expanded theory suggested different systems for the motivational, affective and cognitive aspects of pain experience. The neospinothalamic projection serves to process *sensory discriminative* information (location, intensity and duration). The information passing through the paleospinothalamic system activates the reticular and limbic areas, giving rise to the unpleasant affect and aversive (*motivational*) drive, which ultimately produces action. The higher centres in the brain

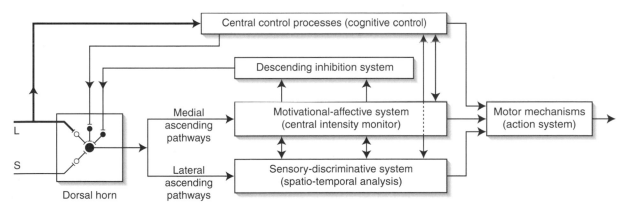

Figure 1.4 Gate control theory II (GCT-Ib). The output of the T cell in the dorsal horn projects to the sensory–discriminative system via the lateral ascending system and to the motivational–affective system via the medial ascending system. The central control 'trigger', composed of the dorsal column and the dorsolateral projection systems, is represented by a heavy line running from the large fibre system to the central control processes, which take place in the brain. These in turn project back to the dorsal horn as well as to the sensory–discriminative and motivational–affective systems. Added to the scheme of Melzack & Casey is the brainstem inhibitory control system activated by impulses in the medial descending system, and which provides descending control on the dorsal horn. Moreover, there is much interaction between the motivational–affective and the sensory–discriminative systems as indicated by the arrows. The net effect of all of these interacting systems is activation of the motor (action) system. Modified from Melzack & Casey, The Skin Senses edited by DR Kenshalo 1968. Courtesy of Charles C. Thomas, Publisher Ltd, Springfield, Illinois, USA.

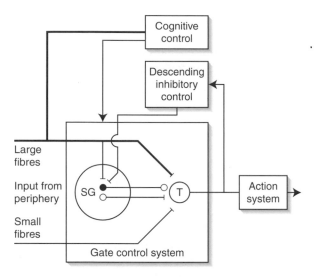

Figure 1.5 Gate control theory II (GCT-II). The new model includes excitatory (white circle) and inhibitory (black circle) links from the substantia gelatinosa (SG) to the transmission (T) cells as well as descending inhibitory control from brainstem systems. The round knob at the end of the inhibitory link implies that its actions may be presynaptic, postsynaptic, or both. All connections are excitatory, except the inhibitory link from SG to T cell. Modified from Melzack R & Wall PD 1983, reproduced with permission of Penguin Books Ltd.

(neocortical) influence the sensory–discriminative and the motivational–affective systems having evaluated the input in the light of past experience.

In 1983 Melzack & Wall modified the GCT model in the light of new information. The model retained the excitatory and inhibitory links from the substantia gelatinosa and added the expanded version of the central controls as described by Melzack & Casey (1968) (Fig. 1.5).

Further developments from the GCT

Much work has been done over the last 30 years to tease out the details of Melzack & Wall's theory. The general framework of the theory remains intact. Much more is now known about the complexity of the neurophysiology and neuroanatomy of the pain pathways, in particular the mechanisms of ongoing transmission of nociception that take place in the dorsal horn of the spinal cord. Anatomical pathways,

neurotransmitters and gene expression have all been described. Perhaps the most important discovery is the 'plasticity' of the nervous system by Dubner (1997)—in other words, the ability of the nervous system to change its sensitivity following tissue injury or nerve injury. Both central and peripheral sensitisation may occur following injury.

Peripheral sensitisation

Tissue injury is heralded by electrical activity of nociceptors. However, there is also evidence of increasing sensitivity of nociceptors at the site of injury, following injury. In addition there is also evidence of 'silent' nociceptors, which are normally dormant and become active only following tissue injury.

Central sensitisation

The increased neuronal barrage appears to lead to functional changes in the spinal cord and brain that contribute to hyperalgesia and spontaneous pain. This appears to be mediated by excitatory amino acids such as glutamate and aspartate at N-methyl-D-aspartate (NMDA) receptor sites. This in turn is enhanced by neuropeptides such as substance P (SP), calcitonin gene-related peptide (CGRP) and dynorphin.

In addition to sensitisation other changes occur in the spinal cord that lead to amplification of peripheral signals. There is an increase in the receptive field of wide dynamic response (WDR) cells in the dorsal horn following peripheral tissue injury. WDR neurons respond not only to input from primary nociceptive afferents but also to low threshold mechano receptive primary afferents (touch and other non-painful sensory input). The enlarged receptive field together with peripheral and central sensitisation may lead not only to amplification of nociception but also to potentially painful experience from non-nociceptive stimuli.

For a detailed exposition of recent advances in the understanding of pain physiology the reader is directed to other writings (Dubner 1997, Price, Mao & Mayer 1997).

Technological advances in brain imaging (Roland 1993) have permitted investigation into the relationship between regional cerebral blood flow (rCBF) and neuronal synaptic activity. Development of functional magnetic resonance imaging (fMRI) has allowed the rapid detection of magnetic field changes with spatial localisation using position emission tomography (PET) scanning. Recent research has identified differences in the extent to which parts of the limbic system are activated in different patients in response to the same experimental pain stimulus. Investigation of attentional mechanisms and the role of memory of pain are being actively researched. (It seems, for example, that painful memories can themselves act as pain stimuli and lead to the experience of pain in the absence of any new pain stimulus.)

In a sense much of the research into physiological and psychological factors has been developed along separate or parallel tracks. More recently, the development of pain-associated incapacity has been investigated from a *dynamic* point of view and can be viewed as an attempt to 'put the mind and the body back together again'.

The GCT has also been important from the *psychological* point of view. It has offered a testable model of how psychological factors could activate descending pain-inhibitory systems, influence nociceptive processing and thereby modulate pain. It offered a way of integrating concepts of pain behaviour, both as a *response* to pain and as behaviour that could come under environmental control. The theory has stimulated interest into beliefs, appraisal and fears about pain and pain-related coping strategies. It has encouraged the investigation of the nature of pain-associated disability and led to the development biopsychosocial models, which have attempted a wide integration of physical, psychological and social perspectives. The importance of psychological influences on the perception of pain has been increasingly recognised. Experimental studies into pain threshold and tolerance have highlighted the importance of fatigue, depression and fear. Several research groups are currently investigating the role of attentional mechanisms and memory. Studies

in phantom pain have led to the formulation of the recent neuromatrix theory (Melzack 1996), which has stimulated much debate into cognitive representation of sensation. Finally, the link between psychology and physiotherapy has led research away from the myogenic pain theory of Travell & Simons (1993) to the investigation of psychophysiological resonses to pain (Flor & Birbaumer 1994) and stress–hyperactivity theory (Ohrbach & McCall 1996).

MODELS OF PAIN AND MODELS OF ILLNESS

There are similarities between the Cartesian model of pain and the traditional disease model of illness in their assumption of a direct one-to-one relationship between physical signs of disease and accompanying symptoms.

In 1858 Virchow in his model of cellular pathology established the basis of the medical model of illness and disease that has influenced medical treatment for the last century. In arriving at a diagnosis and treatment, the physician proceeded through a number of stages. On the basis of the patient's presenting symptoms (complaints), the doctor investigated the presence of associated physical signs. Having identified treatable pathology and arrived at a diagnosis, treatment was then prescribed with the expectations that the disease would be cured, the physical signs would disappear and the patient would no longer be troubled by the presenting symptoms. Consider, for example, patients who present with ear pain. Doctors will inquire further about the nature of the ear pain and consider a range of possible causes for the pain. They will then examine the patient to confirm their provisional diagnosis. Doctors will see an inflamed ear drum and infer that the patient has an infection that is causing the pain. They will prescribe antibiotics to cure the infection and both doctors and patients expect the symptoms (the pain) and the signs (the redness of the ear drum) to improve. In other words, an explanation for the symptoms and signs has been found. By treating the cause of the symptoms and signs it is expected that they will be cured.

This model is dependent, however, on there being a close relationship between symptoms, signs and disease. It does not take into account the variability of the patient's response to illness and in the self-report of symptoms. Despite these shortcomings, the model works well for most acute medical and surgical conditions.

LIMITATIONS OF THE TRADITIONAL MEDICAL MODEL FOR THE TREATMENT OF PAIN

Syndromes and diagnoses

Medicine has categorised disease and illness in order to aid diagnosis and subsequent treatment. Textbooks abound with 'clinical syndromes'. These indicate a number of different symptoms and physical signs, which when present should lead the doctor to reach a specific diagnosis. The 'diagnosis' may then be further confirmed or refuted by performing specific tests. The results of these tests may be included in the description of the 'clinical syndrome'.

It is not necessary, usually, to have all the recognised symptoms, signs or test results to make a diagnosis of the clinical syndrome. The observations may be given different emphasis so that some features of the syndrome may be more heavily weighted than others with the result that sometimes patients may be given a diagnosis on very little evidence. Furthermore, many of the symptoms, signs and even test results may be found also in other 'clinical syndromes' (the diagnosis of 'complex regional pain syndrome' (CRPS) is a good example of this), thus making a specific diagnosis more difficult and highly subjective. In some cases it may not be considered possible to confirm the diagnosis until the response to treatment is known. In such situations it is difficult to have full confidence in the accuracy of the initial diagnostic process.

The variations detected in the types, number and severity of symptoms, signs, tests and even responses to treatment are usually attributed to variations in the disease process rather than in the patient. If the level of 'complaints' made by the patient is high, this is usually attributed to long term personality characteristics and is often ignored. Failure to respond to treatment following 'diagnosis' usually leads to re-evaluation to assess the diagnosis. This will usually entail at least further investigations in the hope of 'turning up something'. It may also lead to repeated attempts at treatment that unfortunately have a high chance of failure. This in turn may lead to different diagnoses from doctor to doctor, which is very confusing for patients.

If patients cannot be classified into a known syndrome or diagnosis and fail to improve following several trials of treatment, they may end up with the label of 'hysteria', 'hypochondriasis' or 'functional overlay'. The difficulty may be to do more with limitations of the classification system than with the nature of the patient's response to illness. Nonetheless, some patients are left with no clear diagnosis and, having failed to respond to treatment, are discharged without the prospect for any further treatment and told to 'learn to live with it'. It can be seen how strict adherence to the disease model of illness can leave patients without an adequate explanation for their pain, may offer no prospect of helpful treatment and may lead to the suggestion that their fundamental problem is one of mental attitude or psychiatric disorder.

Failure to recognise the importance of variability in response to pain

There is a large variation of self-report of symptoms with (apparently) the same pathology and recent research has demonstrated large variation in complaints of pain with specific pathology. In one study (Croft, personal communication) only 57% of patients with demonstrable major arthritis of the hip joint as identified by X-ray complained of pain. A recent magnetic resonance imaging (MRI) study of the lumbar spine found that 76% of asymptomatic volunteers demonstrated a disc herniation at one or more levels (Boos et al 1995). There is clearly no direct relationship between disc abnormalities and pain. The reasons for this are not fully understood, but the data suggest that the disc bulge is often not the pain source. Without doubt psychological factors are important influences on the perception of pain, decision to consult and response to treatment, but it is clear that the physical basis of pain is still inadequately understood. Recent research suggests that ascription of all patient variability to the 'mental realm', in the sense of discrediting it, would appear to be extremely unwise; yet this has been an inevitable consequence of overstrict adherence to the narrow medical model.

Reconceptualisation of reaction to pain and illness

Since the 1920s, and particularly between 1940 and 1960, psychologists have been developing a specific interest in the determinants of human behaviour. Experimental studies (initially on animals) have led to a science of human behaviour in which the *context* in which a behaviour is observed is considered to be of major importance. In understanding the behaviour, sociologists articulated concepts such as the 'sick role' to describe certain patterns of response to disease and incapacity. Terms such as 'consulting behaviour' (currently in vogue in the context of health economics) entered professional parlance. Studies of psychological disorder meanwhile identified functional and dysfunctional responses to the stresses and strains of life. A range of psychological features are associated with both the experience of pain and the reaction to it (Ch. 2). Recognition that understanding a patient's pain behaviour, thoughts and feelings are necessary to understand the patient's pain has led to a move from the disease model of pain to an illness model that recognises the importance of physical and psychological factors in pain. Further considerations of consulting behaviour, reaction to illness and socioeconomic factors have led to biopsychosocial models of disability (Ch. 5) (Waddell 1992) and multidimensional approaches to treatment (as evidenced by interdisciplinary pain management programmes).

Acceptance of the complexity of the nature of pain with adoption of newer theoretic models is of more than intellectual importance. Models affect clinical practice, as will be illustrated in the following three cases. Simply put, the bio-psychosocial model represents an alternative to the disease model of illness and pain.

FROM THEORETICAL MODELS TO CLINICAL PRACTICE

Patients demonstrate a wide range of responses to acute pain (ranging from the understated or stoical to the highly florid and dramatic). In most cases of acute pain, the cause of pain will be clear, the diagnosis is unambiguous and the only issue of concern will be matching up the analgesic strategy with the patient's particular response. Marked pain behaviour may or may not accompany the pain experience. Usually, particularly with episodes of acute pain, treating the cause of the pain successfully will also have a significant effect on the 'pain behaviour' and the latter becomes of little concern. Analgesia may be effective even when behaviour is quite bizarre. This may be taken to confirm the view that all pain behaviour, however bizarre, is secondary to nociception and consequently that targeting treatment solely at the nociceptive source is all that is required to manage both the pain and the consequent behaviour. If the treatment of the pain does not change the pain behaviour then the pain is often regarded as psychological or imagined. Although this may not be made explicit to the patient, the patient often picks up such implications from the behaviour and manner of the treating staff.

In order to emphasise the importance of the interpretation of pain behaviour, we have posed two theoretical questions about pain behaviour and offered some alternative answers, which are further illustrated by case examples.

Each strategy represents a way of understanding the patient's needs and reflects the model of pain adopted by the clinician.

Read Case studies 1.1–1.3. Which answer do you consider to be appropriate in each case? Consider each option in terms of its recognition of pain and distress and whether a narrow medical or a cognitive–behavioural approach is being adopted.

Case study 1.1   Straightforward case of uncontrollable pain behaviour that stops as soon as an epidural is working

Mrs G. was 32 years old and having her first baby. She had been admitted during the night having started in labour. Her contraction pains had increased steadily over the early morning, but she was still early on in labour. She became increasingly distressed by her pain and by mid morning was literally screaming with pain. She became very restless and difficult for the midwives to manage. Clinical examinations were virtually impossible and she began to become progressively agitated. She became abusive, shouting and swearing. She would not let anyone near her to perform a vaginal examination to assess progress. She started throwing the Entonox around saying it was useless but would not listen to any instructions that would enable her to use it more successfully.

With much difficulty an epidural was successfully given. Mrs G.'s behaviour changed rapidly as the epidural became effective. Assessment was completed and there appeared to be no obstetric problems or cause for alarm. She apologised for her outburst and her labour continued uneventfully.

Case study 1.1

Although pregnancy is not normally painful, delivery usually is. Large variation in the pain of labour is well recognised. Some mothers appear to experience little or no pain whereas others have a considerable amount of pain and require significant intervention with various analgesic techniques.

If there are problems with delivery, such as obstructed labour, most if not all clinicians would expect the mother to experience more pain than normal. In fact an increase in the complaint of pain is one of the features that is specifically observed as an indication of possible trouble. An increase in pain complaints and pain behaviour (rolling around, restlessness, etc.) will lead the carers to make further investigations.

Pain behaviour during delivery can be quite bizarre even if there are no major problems with delivery. Such behaviour can make the management of even the most straightforward delivery almost impossible. The mother may become so agitated and restless that it may be impossible to carry out a proper evaluation The marked pain behaviour is frequently attributed to culture, personality type, low pain threshold or anxiety.

However, it is well recognised that if the 'pain signals' are prevented from getting to the brain the bizarre behaviour as well as the pain will usually stop, rendering the patient much easier to assess and manage. Mothers certainly like epidural analgesia because it is generally effective and preferable to alternatives, but perhaps the most important reason for the rise of epidural analgesia is that the midwives like it. It not only makes even the most 'difficult' mother much more easy to deliver but more importantly it simplifies assessment and monitoring of progress. Any other complaints can be attributed to the patient's psyche rather than nociception.

This 'model' reinforces the idea that behavioural and other responses to pain are only secondary so that if the source of the pain is identified and isolated from the brain then not only should the pain get better but so also should the bizarre behaviour. All efforts should be directed towards identifying the source of pain and eliminating the pain. There is no need to tackle the pain behaviour directly. Both objectives may be reached simply by concentrating on finding and treating the cause of the pain.

Case study 1.2   Marked pain behaviour that is not helped by an epidural

Mrs H. was 28 years old and was making very slow progress in labour. Her previous labour had also been difficult. She complained of a lot of pain, but this had not responded well to the usual pethidine. The pain had reached unbearable levels and she pleaded for something to be done. An epidural was given. The siting of the epidural, however, was difficult and painful and Mrs H. asked for a consultant to be brought to complete it. Not only was a consultant not available but unfortunately the epidural did not work perfectly. She continued to complain, demanded to know why it hadn't worked and requested that something further be done.

Mrs H. became even more agitated and started to complain about the soreness of the drip site, the epidural catheter in her back and a number of other things. The staff gradually became disaffected with her and began to ignore her complaints, giving them progressively less credence.

Unfortunately, when Mrs H. later became extremely distressed, the staff dismissed her pain complaints as being 'rather exaggerated'. It transpired that she was in obstructed labour and in fact needed an emergency caesarean section.

Case study 1.2

This case illustrates that, even though some pain behaviour may be considered as not directly due to nociception, there is little doctors and others can do since the excessive pain behaviour is considered to result from factors outside their control (such as the patient's cultural background, pain threshold or mental make-up). Such ascriptions can of course simply illustrate prejudice on the part of the staff.

The treating doctors and nurses may become increasingly dismissive in their attitude to the patient's complaints and miss important organic causes of increased pain. Patients may feel the need to impress the doctor even more to take their pain complaints seriously. This may be reflected in more florid pain behaviour.

Case study 1.3   A patient with profound pain behaviour and little to find in the way of objective signs of nociception

Mr A. presented with chronic low back pain and a high level of disability. There were no positive neurological findings to suggest a prolapsed intervertebral disc or any major structural pathology. Apart from guarded movements and some behavioural responses to examination there was little else to find. Thorough physical examination and a review of health did not reveal any other problems. X-rays of lumbar spine were reviewed and a diagnosis of degenerative spinal disease was made. The degeneration was considered to be the principal cause of his pain.

Mr A. was very angry as he had been told in the past that there was nothing wrong with him. He was convinced that he had a serious problem with his back. He could walk only short distances with the aid of two walking sticks and spent most of his day resting because any activity caused intense pain. He had undergone a number of treatments without any relief. His doctors had given up on him.

Case study 1.3

The narrow medical model is particularly unhelpful in assisting the management of patients with pain that is persistent, intractable or unexplained. In such situations, there seems to be even less association between patients' complaints, their

behaviour and the level of 'nociceptive' input. However, doctors and others frequently persist none the less with the narrow medical model (whether out of prejudice, laziness or simply habit). Such patients are often treated by most doctors and therapists as if there is a nociceptive cause even if there is no evidence to support this. Treatment may be instigated on the basis that there *may be* a nociceptive source, however unlikely.

Despite the lack of evidence of a link between degenerative spine disease and pain (as reported above), patients are often told that their pain is due to degenerative disease or disc bulges. They are given an explanation that reinforces their view of a one-to-one relationship between physical damage and pain. (They may then be unreceptive to pain management with its emphasis on self-help.)

When no identifiable cause can be found, doctors may change the way in which they relate to the patient. Patients' behaviour may become the focus of attention. If there happens to be a compensation claim, then exaggeration, faking and malingering will be considered. If patients

Q   Why do some patients exhibit more pain behaviour than others?

A   1.   They may be frightened of the pain, and emphasise their discomfort lest it is underappreciated (and under treated).
2.   They may have suffered poorly controlled pain in the past.
3.   It may be part of their style.
4.   They may have learned to behave like this.

Q   How do clinicians respond to pain behaviour and why?

A   1.   They may disregard the behaviour as 'random noise', simply ignore it and continue to treat with analgesia.
2.   They may seek to alleviate the distress and ignore the requests for analgesia.
3.   They may seek to alleviate the distress as part of their overall management.
4.   They may give the patient inadequate treatment and reject them.

weep or intimate they cannot cope then psychiatric illness, depression or personal inadequacy are often inferred. The pain may be dismissed as unworthy of attention or even regarded as imaginary. Most patients will identify such changes in perspective even if it is not communicated directly to them by the way in which they are treated. As one might expect, this serves only to increase the level of distress. Patients may find themselves being discharged with little more in the way of help than being told that they 'will have to live with it'. Unfortunately they are frequently given little advice on *how* to 'live with it'.

DEVELOPMENT OF IATROGENIC DISTRESS AND DYSFUNCTION

Chronic pain and pain-associated incapacity can become progressively distressing for patients. The level of distress can be made even worse by the way in which they are managed by their doctor.

Influence of symptom presentation on the treating doctor

Without a definitive diagnosis it is difficult for doctors to form a clear treatment plan. Doctors often do not know what to do with the patient and this may lead them to adopt a number of strategies:

- further or repeated investigation on the assumption that something 'has been missed'
- referral to another/different pain specialist
- a trial of treatment on the 'assumed' best bet diagnosis
- communication in body language, if not explicitly, that the problem is psychiatric and possibly even referral to psychiatry
- no further offering of assistance.

The very fact that the patients' symptoms and signs do not match with the traditional model of the illness can have a subtle effect on the way

that doctors communicate with and manage them. Firstly it colours doctors' beliefs about the veracity of the complaints. Doctors will tend to be dismissive of 'non-organic' findings. They will tend to ignore them at best or regard them as signs of malingering, faking, secondary gain or psychiatric problems at worst. Such 'behavioural findings' are often described as 'bizarre'.

Doctors, having made certain judgements about patients and their illnesses, begin (unwittingly) to communicate this to the patient. This is done in the way they talk to the patient, their (the doctor's) non-verbal behaviour and sometimes what they explicitly say to the patient. Often doctors are not aware that they communicate anything to the patient, but our experience has shown that most patients who we have seen for assessment for pain management feel that it has been implied by their previous doctors that 'it is all in the mind'. This, of course, colours how patients interact with their doctors.

Effect on the patient of the doctor's 'difficulties'

The fact that the doctor appears not to make any sense of the physical findings is quickly perceived by the patient, who is then likely to lose confidence in the doctor. From the patient's point of view the doctor does not understand their problem or does not know enough about it. This in turn colours the way the patient communicates with the doctor. If patients suspect that their doctor do not believe them they may be reluctant to disclose more worrying symptoms. Furthermore, the patient will be less likely to accept the doctor's formulation or recommendations.

Unfortunately patients may have no one else to turn to. If doctors order some more physical tests in the unremitting search for a purely physical explanation of patients' problems, then they will tend to go along with it, hoping that something will be found. Usually such hopes are dashed, the patient becomes even more distressed and the doctor–patient relationship is significantly damaged. This experience may be repeated with other doctors until patients then begin to lose faith in all doctors. They have become damaged and distressed by the process of seeking treatment. Their pain persists and they may believe they have to try even harder to persuade specialists that their pain is not 'all in the mind'. Unfortunately, the attempt to convince them often enhances their pain behaviour and therefore makes it even more likely for other doctors to be dismissive, especially if the patient has been previously described in their case notes as showing 'functional overlay'.

It can be seen how an attempt to understand chronic pain in terms of the narrow medical model not only fails to do justice to the complexity of the problem, but can be harmful to the patient and, in many cases, is probably responsible for a considerable proportion of the distress associated with chronic pain problems.

CONCLUSION

In so far as we can tell, pain has always been an aspect of the human condition, but its precise characterisation has been elusive. It has been regarded both as a sense and as an emotion, but prior to the time of Descartes there does not seem to have been any clear recognition that there was central processing of pain signals in the brain. The role of sensory transmission and central registration in the brain of pain signals was recognised by Descartes, but the 'divorce' of the mind from the body, which was explicit in his Cartesian dualism, posed considerable difficulties in explaining the relationship between the experience of pain and underlying physiology. The advent of Melzack & Wall's gate control theory of pain in 1965, however, has led to developments in both the physiology and the psychology of pain such that modern pain management requires consideration not only of the perception of pain, but of the reaction to it (whether behaviourally, cognitively or emotionally). The move from unidimensional explanations to multidimensional perspectives offers not only a formidable intellectual challenge but also a wonderful opportunity to improve our understanding of chronic pain and its management.

KEY POINTS

- Chronic pain differs from acute pain and has to be understood in terms of a complex interplay between physical and psychological features.
- The narrow disease model needs to be replaced with a broader illness model.
- Decision making and management are coloured by the doctor's own implicit model of pain.
- Inconsistencies in diagnosis and prescription of ineffective or ineffectual treatments may profoundly distress patients, thereby confounding their management.
- Adequate formulation of the patient's problem requires a multidimensional perspective.
- Chronic pain patients require illness management not just disease management.
- Proper management of chronic pain requires recognition of the interplay between physical and psychological factors and the socioeconomic context in which the consultation occurs.

REFERENCES

Bonica J J 1990 History of pain concepts and therapies. In: Bonica J J (ed) The management of pain, 2nd edn. Lea & Febiger, New York, ch 1

Boos N, Rieder R, Schade V, Spratt K F, Semmer N, Aebi M 1995 The diagnostic accuracy of magnetic resonance imaging, work perception and psychosocial factors in identifying symptomatic disc herniations. Spine 20:2613–2625

Descartes R 1664 L'homme. E Angot, Paris

Dubner R 1997 Neural basis of persistent pain: sensory specialisation, sensory modulation and neuronal plasticity. In: Jensen T S, Turner J A, Wiesenfeld–Hallin Z (eds) Progress in pain research and management (Proceedings of the 8th World Congress on Pain) vol. 8. IASP Press, Seattle, pp 243–257

Flor H, Birbaumer N 1994 Focus article: acquisition of chronic pain. Psychophysiological mechanisms. APS Journal (Pain Forum) 3(2):119–127

Foster M 1901 Lectures on the history of physiology during the 16th, 17th and 18th centuries. Cambridge University Press, Cambridge

Melzack R 1996 Focus article: gate control theory: on the evolution of pain concepts. Pain Forum 5:128–138

Melzack R, Casey K L 1968 Sensory, motivational and central control determinants of pain. In: Kenshalo D R (ed). The skin senses. Charles C Thomas, Springfield IL, pp 423–439

Melzack R, Wall P D 1965 Pain mechanisms: a new theory. Science 150:971–979

Melzack R, Wall P D 1983 The challenge of pain. Basic Books, New York

Ohrbach R, McCall W D 1996 The stress–hyperactivity–pain theory of myogenic pain. Proposal for a revised theory. Pain Forum 5:51–66

Price D D, Mao J, Mayer D J 1997 Central consequences of persistent pain states. In: Jensen T S, Turner J A, Wiesenfeld-Hallin Z (eds) Progress in pain research and management (Proceedings of the 8th World Congress on Pain) vol 8. IASP Press, Seattle, pp. 155–184

Roland P E 1993 Brain activation. Wiley-Lass, New York

Travell J G, Symond D G 1993 Myofascial pain and dysfunction: the trigger point manual. Williams & Wilkins, Baltimore MD

Virchow R 1858 Cellular pathologie in ihrer Begrundurg auf physiologische und pathologische. A Hirschwald, Berlin

Waddell G 1992 Biopsychosocial analysis of low back pain. Clinics in Rheumatology 6:523–557

Waddell G 1998 The Back Pain Revolution. Churchill Livingstone, New York, USA

2

The nature of psychological factors

Chris J. Main   C. K. Booker

INTRODUCTION

Recent conceptualisations about the nature of pain (Ch. 1) and disability (Ch. 5) have emphasised the importance of understanding the psychological component of pain and disability. In this chapter, the nature of psychological factors will be addressed.

HISTORICAL FOUNDATIONS OF THE MODERN PSYCHOLOGY OF PAIN

During the last half-century theories of pain have gradually moved from simple single-cause explanations to more complex multicausal formulations. There has been a long tradition of the measurement of individual differences in psychology dating from the experimental psychophysics of the mid 19th century and the subsequent sensory psychology.

Developments in sensory psychology led to an improved understanding of the pain system and the perception of pain damage. Certain aspects of tissue damage (e.g. location and severity) are associated with some predictable and well-understood perceptual abilities (e.g. spatial extent and pain intensity), but individuals can experience pain without injury (or apparent injury) and they can also sustain injury without experiencing pain. Clinically it is well recognised that individuals report very different pains from (apparently) the same type and extent of tissue damage. Melzack & Wall's (1965) gate control theory of pain was the first theoretical model specifically attempting to integrate both nociceptive and perceptual factors in pain and offer an explanation for this 'plasticity' or variability in response. Much research has been conducted to try to identify the critical factors responsible for this plasticity and to elucidate the complex 'gating' mechanisms underlying pain perception. A diverse array of cognitive, behavioural, emotional and environmental factors have been identified as key components of a complex pain modulation system.

The study of individual differences in the clinical field, however, was dominated by three separate paradigms: the psychodynamic model (derived from psychosomatic theory), the personality model (derived from classical psychopathological theory) and the behavioural model (derived from the experimental analysis of behaviour). The psychodynamic model was heavily influenced by psychosomatic theories and purported to explain disease in terms of emotional mediation. According to classical psychoanalytical tradition, the psychological component was to be understood in terms of unconscious conflicts, established during childhood, 'reactivated' during situations of stress during adulthood and 'expressed' in a range of somatic symptoms that, if sufficiently severe, could lead to illness. Initially physicians believed that pain was caused by organic *or* psychological factors. Persistent pain that eluded diagnosis or treatment was labelled as hysterical or psychogenic and relegated to the psychiatric domain. Pain was explained as a defence against psychic conflict and psychoanalytic approaches were used in treatment. Typically, the patient continued to suffer pain while the psyche was examined and 'treated'.

In parallel with these developments, however, advances in statistical methodology in the field of education led to the construction of psychological tests. The same 'technology' was applied to the investigation of personality and led to the development of tests such as the Minnesota Multiphasic Personality Inventory, or MMPI, and its later derivative the MMPI-2 (Butcher et al 1989). The personality model with its understanding of individual differences in terms of

personality profiles seemed to offer an advance on the previously largely unsubstantiated clinical observations, or on the 'pseudo-objectivity' of projective tests such as the Rorschach ink-blot test. MMPI research in the late 1960s and 1970s led to the notion of a 'pain-prone personality' (Engel 1959).

Finally the behavioural model (Fordyce 1976) offered the most radical model to the disease model of illness. Pain *behaviour* became the focus of therapeutic investigation and intervention, and led to the development of behaviorally based rehabilitation programmes, the forerunners of modern interdisciplinary pain management programmes.

More recently, cognitive perspectives derived initially from the treatment of depression have offered a further conceptual basis for treatment. Since the 1980s, there has been increasing emphasis on cognitive factors and theorists have studied the influence of beliefs and coping styles on pain (Turk, Meichenbaum & Genest 1983). Factors such as attributions, expectations, self-efficacy, pain control, coping self-statements and imagery have all been investigated.

Finally recent research into psychobiology and psychophysiology has further illustrated the importance of psychological factors in pain and pain-associated incapacity (Flor & Turk 1989). (These recent developments will be discussed in the context of the development of disability in Ch. 5.)

The present chapter will consider the nature of psychological influences on pain in terms of presenting characteristics. Later chapters will describe the levels at which each of these factors can be addressed by an interdisciplinary pain management approach.

PSYCHOLOGICAL INFLUENCES ON PAIN AND INCAPACITY

Psychological factors have a wide-ranging effect of the perception of pain and its effects. These are summarised in Box 2.1.

As observed in the previous chapter, there is now convincing evidence that central mechanisms can influence the perception of nociceptive

Box 2.1 Influence of psychological factors on pain and incapacity

- Fundamental mechanisms
- Health-care seeking
- Response to treatment
- The family context
- Recovery from injury and development of chronic incapacity

Box 2.2 Influence of psychological factors on response to treatment

- Patient's expectation
- Non-specific (placebo) responses to treatment
- Compliance with treatment (including adherence to treatment protocols)
- Acceptance of appropriate responsibility for the management of their symptomatology

signals from the periphery of the body. The perception of pain is influenced both by sensory qualities and by the emotional impact. Recent research into experimental pain using PET scanning suggests that individuals may differ in how the brain first reacts to incoming pain signals and they perceive pain differently in terms of both intensity and aversiveness because of the way in which different parts of the brain are 'energised' (Derbyshire et al 1994). It is commonly observed clinically that pain 'feels worse' when patients are feeling tired or depressed. Pain often seems to feel worse during the night when the brain has 'less to do'. Attentional factors are also important (Eccleston 1995); some patients can be taught to distract themselves quite successfully from pain. Research has also shown that individuals differ not only in pain threshold but also in their ability to discriminate pain of different qualities and intensities. The reasons for this are not fully understood. Research into memory for pain, however, suggests that aversive pain memories may have a powerful influence on the perception of new pain stimuli (Bryant 1993). Psychobiological investigations have demonstrated a wide range of conditioned peripheral and central responses to pain involving both physiological and biochemical events (Flor & Turk 1989).

In conclusion, it would appear that the significance of fundamental psychological mechanisms in the perception of clinical pain may be of much more importance than has been recognised hitherto.

Psychological influences on health-care seeking are well recognised. Decisions to seek health care are dependent on perception of physiological functioning and interpretation of symptoms.

These in turn have to be understood in terms of the individual's 'model of illness'. Simply put, unless an individual perceives a symptomatic abnormality that is defined in health terms, the issue of consultation does not arise. The individual has to believe further, however, that it is *appropriate* to consult with the symptom: that the doctor or therapist is *likely* to be able to help and some good will result from the consultation. Of course these beliefs are themselves multiply determined and will have been influenced by the individual's sociocultural background, tolerance of symptoms and the impact of symptoms on quality of life and work (Skevington 1995).

Some of the more important psychological factors influencing response to treatment are shown in Box 2.2.

Patients attending pain clinics or pain management programmes have often seen several other professionals. Failed treatment can have a profoundly demoralising effect. The patient may have lost confidence in the likely benefit of *any* further treatment. They may be concerned that 'something has been missed' (e.g. cancer). They may be significantly disaffected with health-care professionals, particularly if they feel they have been misled in terms of likely benefit from treatment, if they feel that they have not been believed or it has been implied that the problem is 'all in their mind'. Such iatrogenic factors can have a significant influence both on a patient's decision to accept treatment or to comply with it.

At times it is helpful to consider the psychological influence on pain from a familial rather than an individual perspective. Individuals reactions to pain are heavily influenced by the limitations imposed by it. Inability to sustain the previous role in the family, whether as a breadwinner or as a care provider, can have a profound effect on morale. Changes in role necessitated by pain-associated incapacity may not only have practical and financial implications, but they may also have a significant effect on relationships within a family.

Pain affects families, not just patients. Sleep disturbance, depressed mood, increased irritability and disturbed sexual functioning can be difficult to tolerate by those living with the pain patient. This change in affairs may lead in turn to distress, disaffection and hostility directed towards the patient. Alternatively it may lead to oversolicitous behaviour and the reinforcement of maladaptive behaviours and (eventually) to chronic invalidism.

Several recent studies in back pain have demonstrated not only that psychological factors are predictive of a wide range of treatments, but also that they are more powerful predictors than demographic factors, clinical history or clinical examination findings. Their influence is seen in the treatment response not only of patients with chronic pain, but also of those with acute pain (Burton et al 1995). The implications of these findings are important and have led to a shift of emphasis from tertiary care to secondary prevention both in health care (Ch. 18) and in occupational settings (Ch. 19).

PSYCHOLOGICAL IMPACT OF DIFFERENT TYPES OF PAIN

Different sorts of pain may have widely differing psychological impacts, and different types of pain are perceived differently by doctors as well as by patients. Of general concern to patients is the cause of their pain, its likelihood of responding to treatment and what they can expect in the future. Pain associated with disease (such as rheumatoid arthritis) may have a predictable relationship with recurrence of inflammation. Such pain is not necessarily easier to tolerate, but it is more easily comprehended and consistently managed. Several of the special problems are shown in Box 2.3.

Box 2.3 Special problems in the psychological impact of pain
• Difficulties in diagnosis • Degree of successful pain control • Impact on everyday life • Likely future course

With acute pain, clear diagnosis often can be made with little disagreement amongst diagnosticians. With chronic pain problems, however, patients may have been offered a variety of diagnoses. Lack of consistency and clarity in diagnosis can be extremely distressing for patients because they may worry that the 'real' cause of their pain has not been established. Such diagnostic confusion in turn undermines their confidence in their treating doctors or therapists and can lead to the sort of iatrogenic distress described above.

Different pains are controllable to different extents. Neurogenic pain is particularly unresponsive to analgesics and can therefore be particularly distressing. Alternatively some types of pain may be responsive to analgesics or non-steroidal drugs but only in doses that produce significant side-effects that are difficult to tolerate. Radicular pain may be eased by resting and exacerbated by walking. Headache may be predominantly stress related, postural or cardiovascular in origin, and therefore manageable to different extents.

Pain differs not only in quality and severity but also in its impact on activities of daily living, quality of life and work. There is evidence that whether or not people become depressed with pain is dependent primarily, perhaps surprisingly, not on the severity of the pain but on the extent to which it interferes with their life. Depression reduces pain tolerance. The likely *effects* of the pain therefore have to be considered in evaluating the likely psychological impact of a particular pain condition.

The probable future course also varies amongst pain conditions. This is also unrelated to the severity of the pain. Patients are often able to muster resources to cope reasonably successfully with pain of short duration. Pain that is likely to become chronic requires a much wider range of coping skills and may require a range of alternative coping strategies.

In summary, although there are many similarities in the nature and management of chronic pain problems, it is important to allow for variations in the likely psychological impact of different sorts of pain.

THE INFLUENCE OF GENERAL PERSONALITY CHARACTERISTICS

The earliest systematic attempts to assess personality characteristics were focused on the identification of possible psychopathology, conceptualised principally in terms of psychiatric disorder. By far the most widely used psychometric measure has been the MMPI (Hathaway & McKinley 1967) and until the 1980s investigation of psychological factors in pain relied almost exclusively on this test. The original MMPI contained a large pool of individual items derived from psychiatric concepts and practice in the 1930s and 1940s. The 566 items yielded scores on 10 clinical and three validity scales. With the exception of some later scales that were derived using more complex methods, most of the scales relied principally on items that differentiated between psychiatric groups and patients or staff of the Mayo clinic. The MMPI focused specifically neither on pain perception nor on adjustment to pain-associated dysfunction or incapacity, but the test came to be used in the study of refractory pain patients because difficulties in the clinical management of such patients became increasingly recognised. The more recently developed MMPI-2 (Butcher et al 1989) is similarly reliant on concepts of psychopathology. The vast majority of items are unchanged, the same scale names have been retained as have the links with the original diagnostic system. Investigation of personality type has become almost synonymous with the investigation of MMPI profiles. The MMPI has been used in three distinct ways described in the following section.

The identification of personality disorder

In practice it is difficult to make a clear distinction between personality disorders and other formal mental disorders, and even more difficult to differentiate one personality from another reliably (Zimmerman 1994) The fourth revision of the Diagnostic and Statistical Manual (DSM-IV) (1994), which formed the basis of the studies reviewed, defines personality disorder as:

behaviours or traits that are characteristic of the individual's recent (past year) and long term functioning (generally since adolescence or early adulthood). The constellation of behaviours or traits causes either significant impairment in social or occupational functioning, or subjective distress.

It should be noted, however, that behaviours or traits limited to episodes of illness are not considered in making a diagnosis of personality disorder.

It may be important to identify certain types of personality disorder, such as alcohol abuse, substance abuse or pathological lying, which might confound assessment or serve as a contraindication to acceptance for treatment. This is particularly relevant within health systems offering direct access to care. Where the system requires a medical gatekeeper such as a general practitioner (GP) for referral, the need for a formal assessment may be unnecessary. A competent clinical history and review of medical notes should make MMPI screening unnecessary. Suspected personality disorder is perhaps better viewed along a series of dimensions rather than as distinct categories. Such characteristics are perhaps best considered as obstacles to rehabilitation (see below).

The identification of psychiatric illness

The MMPI was developed originally to assess the probability of unrecognised psychiatric disorder amongst medical and surgical patients presenting for treatment. Unfortunately a number of items that are taken as indicative of psychiatric difficulties may be a direct result of pain or pain-associated incapacities (such as changes to sleep, and social functioning). For the diagnosis of psychiatric illnesses, the MMPI has been superseded by more recently developed psychological instruments (Ch. 10).

The understanding of pain and pain-associated incapacity

In the field of pain, it has long been recognised that individuals differ in their reaction to pain and in their response to treatment. Early studies investigated whether personality factors might explain such differences. With pain patients, the MMPI has been used diagnostically in profile analysis and in the prediction of outcome. Early MMPI studies frequently attempted to differentiate 'organic' from 'psychogenic' pain. Such a differential diagnosis relies on a classification of pain that does not recognise the interaction between physical and psychological factors and is reliant on an outmoded conceptualisation of pain (Ch. 1). The use of the test for this purpose has been largely discredited.

Since development of the original test, a large number of alternative scales and associated personality profiles have been developed. There has remained some enthusiasm for profile analysis. The most frequently cited profiles in pain patients are the 'neurotic triad', identified by elevated scores on the hypochondriasis, depression and hysteria scales, and the related 'conversion-V' profile with elevated scores on the hypochondriasis and hysteria scales relative to depression. Wade et al (1992) compared pain patients on the MMPI and one of the most rigorously standardised measure of normal personality available (the NEO Personality Inventory or NEO-PI, Costa & McCrae 1985). They demonstrated that only emotionally overwhelmed patients (high scorers on NEO-PI neuroticism) could be differentiated by the MMPI neurotic triad; all other NEO-PI scale scores were within the range for the normal population. Neuroticism in personality assessment, otherwise referred to as 'negative affectivity', is most highly correlated with measures of anxiety and depression. The neurotic triad therefore is perhaps best understood as a measure of distress for the assessment of which simpler

symptomatic screeners may be more sensitive and practical (see Ch. 10).

There are, however, more serious problems of clinical validity of the more popular profiles. In a commentary on the 'conversion-V' profile, Main & Spanswick (1995) concluded: 'The Conversion-V profile is frequently found among pain patients, but is poorly defined, has poor discriminative validity, and, because of the nature of the items, may reflect the impact of disease or disability rather than specific psychological factors'.

The more recent MMPI-2 has been an attempt to address some of the acknowledged statistical shortcomings of individual scales, but its focus is still on the identification of psychopathology and therefore its relevance specifically to pain patients remains questionable.

Recent studies have tended to focus on MMPI scores as predictors of outcome. The hysteria scale was a significant predictor of non-return to work in Gatchel, Polatin & Kinney's study (1995) amongst patients with low back pain. However, the triad is not consistently predictive of poor outcome and there is a substantial overlap in profile amongst patients with good and poor outcome (Keller & Butcher 1991). Turk & Fernandez (1995), although acknowledging the replicability in clustering of individuals according to MMPI clinical scales, argued that at best particular profiles indicate an increased probability of poor outcome and are of use primarily for descriptive rather than prescriptive purposes. They comment further on the fact that patient profiles are subject to change following intervention, which disputes their claim of the test to measure personality (i.e. immutable dispositions).

Conclusion

Despite the clear limitations of personality trait measures such as the MMPI in evaluation of the psychological impact of pain, one would be ill advised to ignore the potential importance that enduring characteristics and propensities for response can have in tailoring treatment and predicting outcome. Much of the above critique of the 'personality trait' approach can be laid at the specific limitations of the MMPI in terms of its theoretical underpinning and statistical structure. Although much pain behaviour seems to be 'context dependent' (see below), various personality configurations may predispose individuals to respond in an idiosyncratic fashion, and this responsiveness is manifest in the mutual interaction of cognition, emotion, behaviour and physiology. Existing measures of personality seem somewhat blunt instruments with which to tap such a diverse and multifactorial phenomenon as the human response to pain. Models that employ personality as one component in a battery of psychosocial measures, and target more discrete cognitive styles and strategies as well as the behavioural and socioeconomic contexts within which the pain is expressed, seem to hold more promise for describing individuals and predicting treatment outcome. An unfortunate legacy from MMPI studies has been the promulgation of terms such as 'low back pain personality' and 'low back loser'. It is perhaps time to abandon such pejorative labels and re-evaluate the specific meaning of the pain to the pain patient.

PRESENTING PSYCHOLOGICAL CHARACTERISTICS

The principal psychological characteristics of patients presenting with pain are shown in Box 2.4.

Anxiety, depression and anger are the three emotions that best characterise the distress of chronic pain sufferers. Much of this is observed in the behaviour the patient displays or expresses. It is possible to consider these psychological phenomena from three distinct clinical perspectives in terms of:

1. psychiatric disorder
2. cognitive or behavioural dysfunction

3. psychobiological or psychophysiological substrates.

Since interdisciplinary pain management is derived principally from a cognitive–behavioural framework, this chapter will primarily address the second of these perspectives. Brief consideration will be given first, however, to the psychopathological perspective. The psychobiological bases of emotion and the role of emotion in psychophysiological responsiveness will be considered briefly in the context of the development of disability in Chapter 5.

Identification of psychiatric disorder

Chronic pain patients are frequently distressed, but the level of distress or manner of symptom presentation occasionally raises the question of a primary or coexistent psychiatric disorder requiring treatment in its own right. Some clinics include formal psychiatric assessment as part of their initial evaluation The psychiatric diagnoses more commonly ascribed to pain are shown in Box 2.5. The formal DSM-IV diagnostic criteria are presented in the appendix to Chapter 10, and they are discussed further in that chapter.

Consideration of psychiatric illness affects primarily *what* treatment is to be offered. Consideration of characterological disorder (such as personality disorder) is more important in the decision about *whether* to offer treatment. The utility of the psychiatric perspective in the context of interdisciplinary pain management is considered in more detail in Chapters 10 and 12. An excellent review of the relationship between emotion and pain is offered by Robinson & Riley (1999).

Box 2.4   Principal presenting psychological characteristics

- Anxiety
- Depression
- Anger and hostility
- Pain behaviour

Box 2.5   Psychiatric diagnoses most commonly ascribed to pain patients

- Generalised anxiety disorder
- Anxiety due to a general medical condition
- Adjustment disorders
- Somatiform disorders
- Conversion disorder
- Hypochondriasis
- Depression
- Pain disorder

Box 2.6 Aspects of anxiety and somatic concern

- The spectrum of anxiety
- The symptoms of anxiety
- Symptom perception and anxiety
- The interpretation of symptoms
- The focus of anxiety and somatic concern
- Influence on pain perception and response to treatment
- Implications for clinical management

The nature of anxiety

The summary of the major considerations in the evaluation of anxiety in pain management is shown in Box 2.6.

Anxiety can vary in its severity from little more than a mild irritation to an emotionally crippling psychiatric disorder. A certain degree of anxiety is normal in many aspects of everyday life. In small amounts it acts as a 'motivator', and is a component of enhanced performance in different sorts of tasks. Excessive anxiety in contrast leads to demoralisation, disturbed concentration and impaired performance.

High levels of anxiety are characterised by a range of symptoms such as impaired concentration, worry, irritability and disturbed sleep. The anxiety may be observed as excessive alertness, restlessness and disturbed thinking. The subjective and behavioural features may be accompanied by symptoms of physiological arousal such as sweating, nausea, dry mouth, tremor or palpitations. If the symptoms are sufficiently severe, it may constitute a psychiatric disorder ranging from a generalised anxiety state to more specific disorders such as phobias of various sorts, obsessive–compulsive disorders and panic disorders in which hyperventilation and avoidance behaviour may be clearly evident. It has been estimated about 7% of the population suffers from an anxiety state in any one month (Regier et al 1988) and that about one in four of patients consulting their general practitioner have some sort of anxiety state.

A degree of anxiety is a common feature of pain patients, particularly when they have not been given a clear explanation for their pain and its likelihood of responding to treatment. From the diagnostic point of view it is important to take a careful clinical history of the development of the anxiety. Widespread long-standing anxiety may require treatment in its own right.

Heightened awareness of all sorts of symptoms is characteristic of some pain patients (Main 1983). This heightened somatic awareness can be indicative of somatic anxiety. The process of somatisation has been defined in a number of ways but is perhaps best understood as a *normal* phenomenon rather than as a psychopathological one. According to Sullivan & Katon (1993, p. 141): 'A primary care perspective on somatization reveals it to be a ubiquitous and diverse process linking the physiology of distress and the psychology of symptom perception. Nearly all somatization is transient and treatable through modification of physician behavior and the proper application of psychiatric and psychological therapies.' If such concern is long standing and the focus has been on a wide range of different types of bodily symptoms, the patient may fulfil the criteria for a somatisation disorder; most pain patients, however, do not. The experience of somatically focused anxiety is, though, a common and apparently stable characteristic of pain sufferers and it is perhaps best understood as a cognitive distortion or misperception. A recent study of temporomandibular disorder (TMD) pain found that high somatisation patients were three times more likely than low somatisation patients to report pain in sites unrelated to the disorder (Wilson et al 1994).

Furthermore, patients differ in their *interpretation* of symptoms. In an exposition of the 'cognitive–perceptual model of somatic interpretation', Cioffi (1991) reviewed evidence supporting the view that the meaning patients assign to physical symptoms is profoundly influenced by their beliefs, assumptions and 'common-sense explanations' (causal attributions) and those of other influential individuals. These psychosocial processes and cognitive styles of thinking in turn guide behaviour. The primary task of the clinician is to determine the specific focus of the anxiety and determine whether patients' fears are based on misunderstandings about the nature of the pain or its future course. (Specific assessment of fear and anxiety will be discussed in Ch. 10.)

If the anxiety is sufficiently severe or widespread, it may preclude the patient's active engagement in a pain management programme. If it antedates the development of a pain condition, it may confuse and complicate assessment and make the identification of achievable goals of treatment difficult to attain. The diagnostic features of clinical anxiety are shown in Chapter 10.

If anxiety is primarily focused on the pain and its likely future course, however, the anxiety may be better understood as incapacitating fear based on mistaken beliefs. Diagnostically, the anxiety may be better viewed as a pain-associated psychological dysfunction rather than as a primary psychiatric disorder. To the non-specialist such distinctions may seem a little contrived (and indeed require careful assessment), but are highly significant as far as appraisal of suitability for pain management is concerned (this will be discussed further in Ch. 12).

In terms of clinical management, the therapeutic goal is to attempt to modify the way in which anxiety, heightened somatic concern or fear may have led to misinterpretation of patients' symptoms and subsequent *labelling* of relatively normal sensations as abnormal if not pathological. Frequently apparently unfocused anxiety is based on specific fears of hurting/harming or pain becoming uncontrollable or progressively increasing pain-associated incapacity. Individuals high in somatic anxiety have a strong propensity for catastrophic thinking (see p. 34) and, whereas post-treatment report of catastrophic thinking is significantly diminished, levels of somatic anxiety are little changed. It may be that in individuals who are somatically focused it is the degree of catastrophising that governs emotional and physiological arousal. Failure to 'correct' these distortions during the pain management process will prevent successful rehabilitation and perhaps reinforce further mistaken beliefs about symptoms and conviction of pathology or disease.

Box 2.7   Depression and pain
• Understandable emotion or psychiatric illness? • Characteristics of depression • Importance in pain patients • Relationship between depression and pain • Biological and psychosocial perspectives • Implications for clinical management

The nature of depression

The relationship between pain and depression is complex and has been the subject of much debate (Banks & Kerns 1996). A number of the key issues are shown in Box 2.7.

The term 'depression' can be misleading. In common parlance it is used to refer to a wide spectrum of emotions ranging from the slightly demoralised or fed-up to the suicidal. It can be considered on the one hand to be a normal human emotion of variable intensity, but if sufficiently severe may be better understood as a major mental illness (in which individuals may no longer be capable of taking charge of their own affairs).

Undoubtedly, pain patients frequently seem to be demoralised or depressed. The similarities between chronic pain patients and depressed patients have led to a vigorous debate about the nature of depression in pain patients. Widely varying reported estimates in rates of depression among pain patients illustrate differences in methods used to assess depression as well as differences across diagnostic groups and stage of chronicity. It is therefore important to distinguish dysphoric mood from depressive *illness*, for which there are clear diagnostic criteria (shown in Ch. 10). Diagnosis is not always straightforward. It is important to note that the somatic symptoms of depression (weight change, sleep disturbance and fatigue) may also be a function of the chronic pain state, and that cognitive intrusion is a common experience in both acute and chronic pain. Substance abuse and anxiety are also concomitants of depression.

There are various explanations for the development of depression. Depression can be viewed as a purely biological or biochemical phenomenon requiring pharmacological treatment. Recent research has demonstrated that, although a history of depressive illness increases the risk for the development of chronic pain, pain has a stronger influence as a *precursor* of depression (Magni et al 1994).

The initial reaction to a painful injury is usually recognised in terms of anxiety, shock and fear rather than depression. With the passage of time and the failure of treatment, however, a patient's coping skills can become exhausted and depression or anger can become evident. If it is possible to avoid painful activities or compensate successfully by changing activities and routines then patients are unlikely to become depressed (even with persistence of pain). If, however, the pain is sufficiently severe, cannot be controlled and as such has a widespread effect on a patient's life, then depression is much more likely.

Pain-associated depression can be described using traditional behavioural language in terms of either a reduced availability or impact of positive reinforcement from the environment or an increase in the frequency or impact of aversive events (i.e. punishment), or both. More simply, depression is often best viewed as a form of 'learned helplessness' that can develop after many different types of chronic unresolved stress, including health-related problems. In the context of chronic pain it is best understood as a psychological consequence of the persistence of pain and its incapacitating effects. If sufficiently severe it may merit pharmacological treatment in its own right (Ch. 13), but can usually best be treated using a cognitive–behavioural approach.

Pain-associated depression is relieved by returning to patients a measure of control over their pain and pain-associated incapacity. It may be appropriate to offer individual psychological therapy to patients with a significant level of pain-associated depression. The treatment strategy of choice, however, usually is an interdisciplinary pain management programme as the influence of other patients can be a key element in re-establishing self-confidence.

Box 2.8   Anger: most frequent themes

- Persistence of pain
- Failure of treatment
- Lack of clear and specific diagnosis
- Inconsistent diagnoses
- Perpetrator of injury
- Current/previous employer
- Benefit system
- Lawyers

Anger and hostility

Anger is commonly observed amongst pain patients and is a common feature of the chronic pain syndrome. According to Fernandez & Milburn (1994) anger, fear and sadness together are significant predictors of the affective component of pain, yet the literature examining the relationship between chronic pain and adjustment has focused primarily on the influence of anxiety and depression. Free-floating anger, like anxiety, is a mood disturbance and is not clearly focused. More commonly, anger has a declared focus. Some of the common themes are shown in Box 2.8.

Patients express anger in a number of ways. Anger is often self-evident from the manner and content of their communication. Patients may be disaffected with many aspects of their situation. They may be angry about how they have been treated in the past, or may believe that referral to a pain management programme may have been undertaken simply because their doctor could offer no better alternative. Emotional intensity may range from mild annoyance to hostility or even frank aggression.

Psychosomatic theorists have attempted to make a distinction between suppressed anger and expressed anger, but the distinction is of little value except in so far as it affects the decision whether or not to offer the patient assistance (Ch. 12) or compromises the patient's response to and compliance with treatment (Ch. 13). Provided that the patient has sufficient trust in the staff to enable participation in the programme, most of the issues of concern will be addressed during the group treatment programme.

The themes in Box 2.8 include both aspects of medical care and the socioeconomic consequences of pain-associated incapacity. During groups, individuals can be assisted to come to terms with their anger and disappointment, but adjustment to pain also seems affected by the responses of others such as family. Anger may be expressed as hostility to others although there appear to be gender differences in the interaction between response to pain, style of anger management, level of hostility and response of spouse (Burns et al 1996). In men with the highest ratings of anger expression, the degree of pain severity and activity interference was partly accounted for by the perceived negative responsiveness of their wives. This relationship between anger, hostility and adjustment remained even when the effects of depression had been taken into account.

According to Fernandez & Turk (1995) and Robinson & Riley (1999), the role of anger in chronic pain and the removal of anger as part of the healing process have not so far been investigated sufficiently. Anger has physiological effects and persistent anger clouds judgement. It would seem to merit much further investigation.

Pain behaviour

About a quarter of a century has passed since Fordyce (1976) advocated the application of behavioural principles to the formal analysis and modification of dysfunctional behaviour in patients suffering with pain. In his focus on pain *behaviour* he advocated an approach to the management of pain that was radically different from the traditional medical model. Pain behaviours may be verbal (e.g. complaints of pain and suffering, groans or sighs), postural and gestural (e.g. bracing, guarding, rubbing or grimacing) and are evident in patterns of behaviour that differ from the normal (e.g. excessive resting or reclining). The early behaviourally oriented pain management programmes applied experimental principles specifically to the analysis and modification of such behaviour and behaviour patterns.

Strictly controlled behavioural change programmes are difficult to deliver, but even in less strictly controlled programmes an understanding of the basic principles of learning theory can be of enormous help in recognising the patient's response to change and to professional guidance.

Respondent and operant conditioning

Respondent conditioning (or learning) refers to the learned association between a *neutral* stimulus and a *reflexive* response as a result of frequent co-occurrences. For example, when patients with temporomandibular joint (TMJ) pain experience a surge in nociceptive input they may wince. Chewing does not normally produce pain behaviour, but if, upon chewing, individuals expect *intense* pain they may emit learned responses in the form of pain behaviours such as grimacing, raising shoulders, or other signs of agitation. Thus pain behaviour that was previously produced by TMJ pain comes to be produced by chewing. This is an example of *classical conditioning* (like Pavlov's experiments on his dogs).

Pain behaviours can also come under the influence of environmental factors. If a pain patient receives sympathetic attention when they show signs of pain, a pattern of pain behaviour may become established (because of the sympathetic attention). In this example, the mechanism is one of *operant conditioning*. The pain behaviour can be understood not simply as a response to nociceptive input but also as a behaviour that is being operantly maintained. It is important to stress that couples are often completely unaware of the interrelationships amongst these behaviour patterns. With the passage of time, pain behaviours that were originally *responses* to nociception come to be *stimuli* for the behaviour for others, which thereby reinforce the behaviour.

Pain behaviour has to be understood in terms of its *social context*. Indeed pain has been defined as 'an interesting social communication the meaning of which has still to be determined' (Fordyce 1976). Chronic pain patients can display widespread changes in behaviour following injury. Pain may affect a wide range of activities, and displays of pain behaviour can produce marked and unpredictable reactions in others. This is particularly true in social situations, when the reaction of others to any display of incapacity can be unpredictable. The responses of others may range from displays of concern to downright unpleasantness. There may be no apparent reaction at all. In patients who lack confidence and self-assurance such unpredictabilities can be daunting.

Let us reconsider the TMJ patient once again from a social perspective.

TMJ disorder: the social context

In TMJ disorders:

- the patient has developed pain-associated difficulty in eating
- the patient feels pain when eating
- others may observe these difficulties in eating. They may notice *pain behaviours* such as wincing, laboured chewing or slowness in eating and comment adversely
- this may lead to distress and embarrassment for the patient
- the adverse comments act as a *negative reinforcer*
- the patient may develop reluctance to eat in public again
- the patient may refuse further social invitations involving eating in public
- escape from or avoidance of such encounters may produce relief of anxiety
- a pattern of avoidance may become established
- the sense of relief has acted as a *negative reinforcer*

Examination of such events from a behavioural perspective may not only clarify the nature of the problem but also offer specific remedies in terms of attempting to change the behavioural contingencies (interdependencies) concerned.

The influence of pain behaviour on families

Pain and pain-associated incapacity affect not only individuals but their families. In any relationship or family context a pattern of behaviours will have developed. This pattern contains an element of predictability so that mutual needs can be met. However, people behave and function differently when they are in pain, and the balance of relationships can be significantly changed. Behavioural changes include verbal and non-verbal expressions of pain (as previously discussed). Expressions of pain produce a variety of reaction in others, ranging from anxiety and solicitousness through indifference to anger and social distancing. Persistence of pain can produce helplessness in partners as well as patients. Interference with valued activities makes matters worse. There may be a major impact on both quality of life and financial stability of the family unit. Changes to quality of life can range from disruption of social activities to personal intimacies including sexual functioning. Distress amongst family members can produce further distress and helplessness and feelings of guilt in the pain patient. Most families can cope with transient crises, but continuing disruption to family life may require a degree of adaptation and adjustment that is not always possible. A major ingredient in all chronic pain management programmes is the impact on the patient's family. Quality of life for the family may be a legitimate concern in the planning of pain management, but behavioural analyses of such a complex interaction of behaviours can be a daunting task. The TMJ case may be considered also in terms of the patient's family.

TMJ disorder: the family context

The families of TMJ patients may react as follows:

- the patient's spouse has become noticeably more attentive and caring when they notice the patient in discomfort (displaying pain behaviour)
- the patient may feel better as a result of the additional concern demonstrated by their spouse
- the pain behaviour has been *positively reinforced* by the attention received

- the patient frequently breaks promises to the family when their pain is severe
- when the pain is severe they become irritable
- other family members may complain about the broken promises and displays of irritability (*positive punishment*)
- the patient appears gloomy and depressed at times
- when they are displaying such pain behaviours, other family members avoid eye contact and stop interacting with then (*negative punishment*)
- if not overcome, such changes in the reinforcement contingencies can lead to feelings of alienation, hostility or depression, and ultimately social withdrawal.

The influence of pain behaviour on the treatment process

Pain behaviour is evident not only in family situations, but also in treatment contexts. As aforementioned, the biopsychosocial model offers a broader understanding of pain than the traditional medical model. If consultation is considered as a pain behaviour, then it becomes possible to address the assessment, treatment and management of pain from a wide set of perspectives. Consideration of the psychosocial determinants of consultation opens access to an interlocking web of psychological mechanisms, affecting doctor-patient consultation, assessment of suitability for treatment, design of pain management and evaluation of outcome. It becomes possible to understand patients emotional response to pain and investigate the psychological impact of failed treatment.

Development of problems in doctor–patient communication following a road traffic accident (RTA)

The possible sequence of events is as follows:

- a patient has become injured in a RTA
- the pain persists and the patient becomes anxious
- an orthopaedic surgeon is consulted

- the patient appears anxious and presents their worries to the surgeon
- in the course of the physical examination the patient is required to bend forward as far as possible
- the patient finds this very painful and becomes frightened
- the patient requests reassurance but is told by the surgeon there is nothing wrong
- the patient become more upset and anxious about the nature of their pain
- the patient becomes apprehensive about further such 'encounters'
- later other doctors examining them find them difficult to interview and consider that they are 'overreacting to examination'
- the patient then believes that these doctors do not believe the severity of pain
- the patient worries that the doctors are implying that they are psychologically disturbed or even untruthful.

The above example is not analysed technically in behavioural terms as in the previous case, but illustrates how fears and anxieties can lead to altered patterns of pain behaviour and considerable distress following communications between doctor and patient. Repeated ineffective treatment, differences in diagnosis (as offered by different specialists) and involvement in adversarial legal proceedings can compound such problems significantly. When analysed from a *behavioural* perspective, the psychological impact of chronic pain can be more clearly understood. Any complex formulation must, however, be developed from careful behavioural observation. A number of specific tools have been developed specifically for the assessment of pain behaviour in clinical settings. They are described in Chapter 9.

The key features of pain behaviour are summarised in Box 2.9.

COGNITIVE FACTORS IN PAIN

The term 'cognitive' has come to refer to a wide range of factors influencing the perception of pain and response to treatment, but it is perhaps

---

Box 2.9   Important features of pain behaviour

- Observable
- May contain verbal, subverbal and non-verbal components
- May contain both respondent and operant features
- Often highly context dependent
- Patients not always aware of their own pain behaviour
- Can be influenced by cultural and social factors
- In treatment and familial contexts, best understood as a form of communication
- May be highly influential in clinical decision making

Box 2.10   The development of illness perception theory and measurement (Petrie & Weinman 1998)

- Parallel processing of health information
- Cognitive and emotional representation
- Cognitive representation of threat and resulting actions
- Attributes of illness representations:
  — identity
  — cause
  — time-line
  — consequences
  — controllability

---

helpful to think of these in terms of three distinct fields of enquiry: specific beliefs about pain and treatment, nature of cognitive processes and coping styles/strategies. It should be remembered, however, that even though it is possible to distinguish separate aspects of cognition each patient is characterised by an individual combination of cognitive features, which underpins the appraisal of pain and the response to treatment. The complexity of these interrelationships is indicated in the following quotation (Jensen et al 1991, p. 249): 'Patients who believe they can control their pain, who avoid catastrophising about their condition; and who believe they are not severely disabled appear to function better than those who do not. Such beliefs may mediate some of the relationships between pain severity and adjustment'.

Health beliefs models (HBMs)

Within the field of health psychology there have been a large number of theoretical models attempting to link thoughts, emotion and behaviour in health-care contexts. Indeed many of the theoretical constructs underpinning measurement instruments used in the pain field have their origins in other aspects of health care. Some of the key developments in illness perception theory and measurement are shown in Box 2.10.

Some of the earlier research into the influence of fear on health threats suggested that there was a parallel processing of health information and that beliefs or appraisals (cognitive representations) of events could be distinguished from the emotional representation in terms of fear or arousal. Furthermore, these cognitive representations of threats could be distinguished from resulting actions or action plans. It seemed helpful to distinguish five distinct features (as shown in Box 2.10).

According to Petrie & Weinman (1998, pp. 2–3) these attributes:

provided the basis for the coping responses or procedures for dealing with the health threat. Thus, in being faced with a situation such as the experience of an unusual symptom, or the provision of a diagnosis from a doctor, individuals will construct their own representation which, in turn, will determine the behaviour and other responses, including help-seeking and medicine-taking. In addition to their representations of the threat, the individual will also draw upon their expectations and beliefs about the different behavioural choices.

Although pain has certain distinct features that make it more puzzling and potentially problematic than other symptoms (Ch. 1), the representational perspective is helpful in offering a possible framework for understanding the response to pain. Recent interest in self-help approaches to health is based on the recognition that individuals can influence their own health and well-being in a wide variety of situations. Indeed the notion of self-help is fundamental to the philosophy of pain management (Ch. 6).

Social cognition models (SCM) are now widely employed in health psychology. According to Conner & Norman (1998) they can be divided into 'attribution models', focusing primarily on individuals' beliefs about cause (causal attributions) and a second more diverse set of models (of which the best known are probably the theory of planned behaviour, or TPB, and the theory of reasoned action, or TRA) invoked to try to predict future health-related behaviours and outcomes. There are three major concerns about the usefulness of these theoretical models. First, although conceptually illuminating, there is as yet little research on the predictive value of these models (Quine, Rutter & Arnold 1998). Secondly, there is controversy about the relative utility of beliefs 'supplied' by the models and individually generated beliefs (Agnew 1998). Finally, different cognitions may be important at different stages of the initiation and maintenance of health behaviour.

There has been little research specifically into the utility of HBMs to either the treatment of rehabilitation in general or pain in particular, although Kerns et al (1997) have recently tried to apply the transtheoretical model of change (Prochaska & Diclemente 1982) to pain patients.

In conclusion, the utility of HBMs to the understanding of pain or its treatment has not as yet been systematically undertaken. There would appear to be a number of promising avenues for exploration, but the specific value of these models in the pain field has not as yet been demonstrated empirically.

Types of cognitive processes in pain

In the pain field, consideration of cognitive processes has been derived mainly from systematic assessment of patients' presenting characteristics or from patients' responses to treatment. The major types of cognitive processes studied in the field of pain are shown in Box 2.11.

Box 2.11 The nature of cognitive processes

- Information processing: accuracy and discrimination
- Cognitive appraisal and distortion
- Social influences on the perception/report of pain
- Fear, catastrophising and depression

It is sometimes difficult to differentiate clearly amongst beliefs, appraisals and cognitive processes. Simply put, *appraisal* incorporates an element of judgement. Individuals differ not only in specific matters of appraisal, but also more generally in terms of their tendency to view events in a certain way.

Differences in the way information is processed

Experimental studies of various sensory modalities have shown differences in how different people process information in terms of accuracy and consistency of judgement. The 'demand characteristics' of the experimental setting can exert a profound influence on the responses elicited from a subject.

Studies of subjects faced with experimental pain stimuli have also shown consistent individual differences in how subjects respond to the same stimulus. Researchers have wondered whether such differences are consistent across other different pain stimuli (such as cold, heat and pressure) and whether it is possible to identify differences in the manner or style or response. Unfortunately with clinical pain it is not possible to examine the phenomenon with the same degree of precision since the 'pain stimulus' cannot be controlled with the same level of accuracy. Researchers, however, offered a number of ways of considering differences in how patients respond to pain.

Cognitive appraisal and distortion

Psychosomatic theorists interpreted coping with pain in terms of defences against physical threat. Subjects (or patients) thought to be underestimating the severity of pain (or perceived threat) were considered to be using 'denial' or 'repression'. This defensive style of coping was thought to be an automatic response to threat. Typically 'repressors' have low scores on self-report measures of anxiety, and high scores on measures of defensive avoidance or social disapproval. Such psychological mechanisms are considered to have their physiological and biochemical correlates. Simply put, the extent to which 'denial' or 'repression' is successful in reducing perceived threat or anxiety determines its success as a coping strategy.

Social influences on the perception of pain

The report of pain can be influenced by the social context not only through behavioural mechanisms (see above) but also by social desirability (or the desire to present oneself in a favourable light). Both Deshields et al (1995) and Haythornwaite, Sieber & Kerns (1991) found that patients with high scores on the Social Desirability Scale reported less depression, anxiety and disability than patients characterised as less susceptible to self-denial or impression management. The latter researchers accept this result as evidence that repressors (not described as such in either study) were a 'subgroup of chronic pain patients whose experience is less severe' than their counterparts. (Social, economic and occupational influences on pain and disability are addressed further in Chs 3 and 4.)

Fear, catastrophising and depression

One of the most common clinical features of chronic pain patients is catastrophising, which appears to be a type of cognitive distortion. According to Beck (1976), negative bias in information processing is maintained by general and systematic errors in logical appraisal. Catastrophising, which is characterised by profoundly negative ruminations about one's present and future ability to cope, though often included in measures of coping strategies, is probably best understood as a set of dysfunctional beliefs or appraisals (Jensen et al 1991). The tendency towards negative appraisal (or undue pessimism) has consistently been shown to be a better predictor of low pain tolerance, disability and depression than measures of disease activity or impairment, both at the time of testing and at long term follow-up (e.g. Keefe et al 1989). It may be based on mistaken beliefs about pain and outcome of treatment, but is most clearly associated with depression. The cognitive distortion is not, however, simply a facet of depression, for it has been shown to be a significant predictor of self-reported disability and work loss even when the influence of pain severity and depression had been taken into account (Burton et al 1995; Main & Waddell 1991).

Specific beliefs about pain and treatment

Investigation of cognitive factors in pain patients has been stimulated by research into depression and anxiety. Clinical investigation of distressed individuals commonly reveals patterns of predominantly negative thinking. This observation led Beck (1976) to identify patterns of thoughts in depressed and anxious individuals that he termed 'negative cognitive triads'.

The triad for depression is believed to consist of a negative view of the *self* (perceived as deficient, inadequate or unworthy), a negative view of the *world* (any and all interactions are perceived as frustrating, unrewarding and unsuccessful) and a negative view of the *future* (current difficulties or suffering will continue indefinitely). These thoughts exacerbate feelings of sadness, indecisiveness, apathy, avoidance, helplessness and hopelessness.

The negative triad of anxious patients relates to themes of personal danger. They view themselves as *vulnerable* people living in a world that is personally *threatening* (but not universally so), facing an *unpredictable future*. In addition to depressive symptomatology, anxiety is characterised by cognitive hypervigilance and heightened autonomic arousal.

A comparison can be made with pain patients who also demonstrate features of anxiety and depression. Similar pessimistic or negative beliefs are found regarding pain and outcome of treatment. Thus they believe that *hurt is synonymous with harm*, that *pain uniquely determines physical functioning* and that they face *inevitable structural and/or physiological decline* over the next few years. Such beliefs lead not only to demoralisation but also to debilitation. Patients avoid interactions or activities that are expected to elevate pain and/or suffering, and they become more socially isolated and physically deconditioned.

Box 2.12   Specific beliefs and appraisals about pain and treatment
• Nature of pain and controllability • Self-efficacy • Specific fears of hurting and harming

Research has tended to focus on a number of different types of belief or appraisal about the nature of pain and the development of new tests assessing different aspects of beliefs has become something of a 'growth industry' (DeGood & Schutty 1992). Although many of these tests seem to be of value, there is clearly much conceptual overlap amongst them. (Individual tests are discussed further in Ch. 10.)

Beliefs about pain

The perception of pain is complex and varies from individual to individual. Research studies, however, have highlighted a number of key themes that are commonly found amongst pain patients. The three clinically most important constructs are shown in Box 2.12.

The nature of pain. Patients often express puzzlement about the nature of their pain. The fact that their pain has persisted may seem to be a mystery. Questions about the nature of pain may need to be addressed as part of the initial clinical evaluation, and of course the nature of pain and disability is an integral part of the educational component of all pain management programmes. Indeed one of the recently developed psychological tests, the Pain Beliefs and Perception Inventory or PBAPI (Williams & Thorn 1989), contains a specific scale to assess this (Ch. 10).

Beliefs about control. Beliefs about the extent to which pain can be controlled would appear to be one of the most powerful determinants of adjustment to pain and the development of incapacity. In the psychological literature there has long been interest in the extent to which individuals believe they can control, or gain control over, aspects of their lives. Researchers have assessed specific beliefs about health (Wallston,

Wallston & deVellis 1978). The same scale was then adapted for the study of pain by simple substitution of 'pain' for 'health' throughout the questionnaire (Crisson & Keefe 1988, Toomey et al 1991). Other 'pain locus of control' scales have been developed (Main & Waddell 1991) and used in both health and occupational settings.

The role of perceived self-control as a factor that mediates pain and depression was explored by Rudy, Kerns & Turk (1988) using structural modelling techniques. Although the *direct* association between pain and depression was minimal, depression developed principally when pain significantly interfered with family, work and social interactions, and/or existed in conjunction with pessimism about being able to control pain. The issue of 'controllability' may be even more important in relationship to adjustment to pain and incapacity. In one interesting study (Affleck et al 1987), judgements of illness predictability were associated with perceptions of greater personal control over daily symptoms and disease course. Perception of a high degree of influence over medical care and intervention was associated with positive mood and psychosocial adjustment. Conversely, the belief that providers had greater control over *daily symptoms* was related to negative mood. Those who had a more severe disease and who believed they had no personal control over *disease course* experienced mood disturbance and exhibited less positive psychosocial adjustment. Optimal adaptation to a chronic condition thus seems to depend upon patients' ability to come to terms with what they can and cannot control.

Self-efficacy beliefs. Closely linked with the concept of controllability is that of self-efficacy. Described initially by Bandura (1977), self-efficacy refers to individuals' belief that they have about their capability to execute a behaviour required to produce a particular outcome. This general idea has been investigated in terms of the relationship between such beliefs and resultant behaviour in relation to treatment outcome. The theoretical perspective is offered by Bandura (1977), which can be paraphrased as follows: once a situation has been perceived as involving harm, loss, threat or challenge and individuals have considered a range of coping strategies open to them, what they do will be dependent on what they believe they can achieve. The action taken is a consequence of:

1. their conviction that they have the skill/ability to execute the behaviour required in order to produce the desired outcome (self-efficacy expectation)
2. their estimation that a chosen behaviour will lead to the desired outcome (outcome expectancy).

Turk (1996) describes four sources of information from which individuals make efficacy judgements: past performance on the task ('I've done it once, I can do it again'), or a similar task, performance of others judged to be similar to oneself ('if they can do it, so can I'), verbal encouragement from others that one can complete a task and finally perception of state of physiological arousal.

Self-efficacy beliefs therefore, both predict present behaviour yet can be used as mechanisms of change. Efforts however are not always successful. Clinical and experimental investigations suggest that perceived coping *inefficacy* may lead to preoccupation with distressing thoughts and concomitant physiological arousal, thereby increasing pain, decreasing pain tolerance and leading to increased use of medication, lower levels of functioning, poorer exercise tolerance and increased invalidism.

Such beliefs in combination with negative emotional responses frequently can lead to the following state of affairs (DeGood & Shutty 1992, p. 221):

Pain patients who perceive themselves lacking the capacity to acquire self-management skills might be less persistent, more prone to frustration, and more apt to be non-compliant with treatment recommendations. Hence, some patients might demonstrate adequate understanding of particular treatment rationale, yet be non-compliant due to their perceived inability to produce the behaviour necessary to follow treatment recommendations.

Most research into self-efficacy has ignored the outcome expectancy component of Bandura's theory, but a notable exception is a study conducted by Lackner, Carosella & Feuerstein (1996). They explored the relative contribution of predictors of disability, such as pain and reinjury expectancy, and self-efficacy beliefs in a sample of patients with chronic low back pain (LBP). Their results demonstrated that self-efficacy accounted for the greatest proportion of variance in physical performance even after anticipated pain and reinjury had been excluded. Pain intensity was also a significant (albeit limited) predictor of performance on four of the five tasks. The researchers challenge the view that harm expectancies and pain catastrophising are primary causal determinants of function, and argue that they are components of one's confidence of successful task performance. (Treatment recommendations derived from this interpretation emphasise the importance of goal and quota setting, and monitoring of pain and task performance as components of pain management.)

Specific fears of hurting, harming and further injury. Perhaps the most powerful yet least acknowledged cognitive factors are mistaken beliefs about hurting and harming. It is crucial to recognise the role of fear and avoidance as obstacles to rehabilitation following injury. Behavioural theorists such as Fordyce (1976) explained the development of 'avoidance learning' where successful avoidance of pain established a behavioural pattern that was successful in reducing pain but with the cost of maintaining the 'disability'. Vlaeyen et al (1995) found that fear of movement and reinjury were more related to depressive symptoms and catastrophising than to pain itself. (The role of mistaken beliefs and fear in the development of disability are discussed further in Ch. 5.)

Finally in a study of 300 patients attending their family doctor with acute back pain, fear-avoidance beliefs predicted outcome at 2 and 12 months (Klenerman et al 1995). The importance of addressing such beliefs and associated psychological mechanisms within a reactivation framework would seem to be compelling and the correction of mistaken beliefs has become an integral part of new approaches to the prevention of chronic incapacity both in health-care settings (Ch. 18) and in occupational settings (Ch. 19).

(Instruments for the assessment of fear and avoidance such as the Fear-Avoidance Beliefs Questionnaire (FABQ) (Waddell et al 1993) and the Tampa Scale of Kinesiophobia (TSK) (Kori Miller & Todd 1990, Miller, Kori & Todd, unpublished report, 1991) are discussed more fully in Ch. 10.)

Coping styles and strategies

Since the publication of Turk, Meichenbaum & Genest's textbook in 1983, there has been considerably interest in the styles and strategies demonstrated by patients in coping with pain. Jensen et al (1991) and Lazarus (1993) provide excellent overviews of the coping literature.

A range of psychometric instruments focusing on different aspects have been developed (Ch. 10) and, as a consequence, a number of different constructs have entered general parlance. The principal conceptual 'landmarks' are illustrated in Box 2.13.

It is perhaps helpful to begin with a definition of 'coping'. It has been defined as: 'ongoing cognitive and behavioral efforts to manage specific external and/or internal demands that are appraised as taxing or exceeding the resources of the person' (Lazarus 1993, p. 237). This appears to be a useful starting point, but in practice, of course, patients employ a range of coping *styles* and types of *strategy* in order to limit the effects of pain.

Coping styles

Letham et al (1983) described patients as *confronters* or *avoiders*; it has been observed (Waddell et

al 1993) that fear and avoidance of pain can become more disabling than pain itself as, although avoidance at early stages may reduce nocioception, the avoidance behaviours may persist in anticipation of pain rather than simply as a response to it. Whether this stable disposition leads to psychological and physiological consequences for pain patients may be extrapolated from research using global measures of flexible–accommodative versus rigid, less adaptive coping style. (According to Weinberger 1990, 'true' low anxious individuals are flexible copers whereas repressors have compulsive tendencies.)

Brandtstadter (1992) distinguished two fundamentally different styles of coping with chronic pain: *assimilative coping* (tenacious goal pursuit), involving active attempts to alter circumstances in line with personal preferences, and *accommodative coping* (flexible goal adjustment), or 'downgrading' of goals or expectations when goals are seen to be unattainable through active coping efforts. Two scales, tenacious goal pursuit and flexible goal adjustment, have been developed to measure these aspects of coping (Brandstadter & Renner 1990). In a recent study of coping style and pain-associated distress, it was concluded (Schmitz, Saile & Nilges 1996, p. 41):

accommodative coping functions as a protective resource by preventing global losses in the psychological functioning of chronic pain patients and maintaining a positive life perspective. Most important, the ability to flexibly adjust personal goals attenuated the negative impact of the pain experience (pain intensity, pain-related disability) on psychological well-being (depression). Furthermore, pain-related coping strategies led to a reduction of disability only when accompanied by a high degree of flexible goal adjustment'.

Coping strategies

The overall efficacy of coping techniques appears to be moderated by levels of pain intensity and appraisals of perceived pain control abilities (Jensen & Karoly 1991). Their role in pain management needs to be understood in the context of the specific beliefs and expectations already discussed. Individuals' choice of strategies will depend on their beliefs about pain, their

---

Box 2.13 Coping styles and strategies

- Styles:
  - avoiders and copers (confronters)
  - assimilative and accommodative
- Strategies:
  - active versus passive
  - adaptive versus non-adaptive
  - emotion-focused versus problem focused
  - avoidant and attentional
- Efficacy of coping strategies

confidence in being able to influence events (i.e. self-efficacy) and of course on their repertoire of coping behaviours. Over the last 20 years a wide range of psychological instruments have attempted to identify different ways of coping with pain and incapacity. A number of the more commonly used instruments are described in Chapter 10. At this juncture an attempt will be made only to identify the more important clinically relevant dimensions. (It should be remembered that there is a considerable degree of overlap amongst a number of these dimensions and constructs and that the categories are not mutually exclusive in that individuals may use combinations of coping strategies.)

Brown & Nicassio (1987) distinguished between active (adaptive) and passive (non-adaptive) coping strategies, the distinction depending on the relationship that a strategy has to variables such as psychological adjustment. Active strategies (e.g. taking exercise) require the individual to take a degree of responsibility for pain management by attempting either to control pain or to function despite pain. Passive strategies (e.g. resting) involve either withdrawal or the passing on of responsibility for the control of pain to someone else. Brown, Nicassio & Wallston (1989) found that depression was more severe when patients used high levels of passive coping strategies at high levels of pain intensity. No relationship between active coping and depression was found and it would appear that the use of active coping strategies does not act to mitigate the relationship between pain and depression.

Keefe, Salley & Lefebvre (1992) have criticised the concept of active and passive coping strategies arguing that no strategy is truly passive in nature. As they point out strategies such as taking medication may actually require the patient to comply actively with a treatment regimen.

The Coping Strategies Questionnaire or CSQ (Rosenstiel & Keefe 1983), is the most frequently used measure of pain-coping strategies and provides measures of both cognitive and behavioural coping strategies (Appendix to Ch. 10, p. 220). One of the major clinical findings from use of this questionnaire is that in chronic low back pain higher use of ignoring pain, reinterpreting pain sensations, diverting attention, and praying and hoping are related to increased pain and disability levels. Seven of the original eight scales on the questionnaire are often conceptualised in terms of either positive (adaptive) or negative (maladaptive) coping strategies. The *positive scales* encompass a range of cognitive and behavioural coping strategies such as diverting attention, ignoring pain, use of coping self-statements (reassurance), and increasing activity levels (as a pain management technique). The *negative scales* are passive praying/hoping and catastrophising ('fearing the worst'). The catastrophising scale in particular has been found to be highly predictive of outcome of treatment of acute back pain (Burton et al 1995). As Turner (1991) has pointed out, however, specific coping strategies are not inherently adaptive or maladapative. A strategy useful at one point in time may be of little value at another and some strategies may be of benefit if used in moderation but not if used to the exclusion of others. Indeed, as Keefe, Salley & Lefebvre (1992) have observed, the assessment of behavioural coping strategies can be problematic in that the distinction between behavioural coping efforts and outcomes of coping can become difficult to distinguish.

Emotion-focused and problem-focused coping strategies. Lazarus & Folkman's (1984) theory of stress and coping makes a clear distinction between problem-focused and emotionally focused coping. Emotion-focused coping strategies aim to control stress, in contrast with problem-focused coping strategies, which are aimed at attempting to relieve or solve a problem. This distinction seems to have inherent appeal and is certainly fundamental to psychologically oriented pain management programmes. These features can be assessed by the Ways of Coping Checklist (Folkman & Lazarus 1980). This instrument, which is widely used in the general stress and coping literature, measures the use of two major categories of coping efforts: problem-focused coping and emotion-focused coping.

Coping strategies have also been described as being attentional (e.g. seeking information) and avoidant (e.g. distraction). There is evidence to suggest that the different types of strategy are differentially effective at different stages in pain, thus in acute pain use of avoidant strategies is associated with decreased distress whereas in chronic pain the converse is the case.

Effectiveness

The relationship between use of these strategies and psychological adjustment is complex (Jensen et al 1991) and it has been suggested by Jensen & Karoly (1991) that pain duration has a moderating influence in that, for those with longer duration of pain, there is no relationship between use of such strategies and psychological adjustment. The overall efficacy of pain-specific coping strategies in enhancing pain tolerance was evaluated by Fernandez & Turk (1989) using meta-analytic techniques. Six major classes of cognitive coping strategies were conceptualised: external focus of attention, neutral imaginings, pleasant imaginings, dramatised coping, rhythmic cognitive activity and pain acknowledgement. They concluded that each class of coping strategy significantly attenuated reports of pain, imagery being the most effective and strategies involving repetitive cognitions or sensory focus being the least effective.

At present little is known about changes in use of coping strategy over time, about individual differences in use of coping strategy or about how the effectiveness of the same coping strategy varies from person to person. For example some individuals may use a variety of techniques, others only one. One of the few studies to examine the relationship between the day-to-day use of coping strategies, their perceived efficacy, and the effects on pain intensity and affect was conducted by Keefe et al (1997) in a sample of rheumatoid arthritis patients over a period of 30 consecutive days. Between-subject analysis demonstrated that individual differences in daily judgements of coping efficacy failed to correspond with either pain intensity or type of strategy used; greater pain intensity was associated with the use of a wider variety of coping strategies than low pain states. Using the day instead of the person as the unit of analysis, the authors demonstrated that perceived coping efficacy for that day was associated with greater use of relaxation, redefining of pain, spiritual support seeking and a consequent reduction in pain and negative affect and enhancement of positive mood. Furthermore, individual judgement of coping effectiveness resulted in lower pain levels on the following day, and improvements in next-day mood were also attributed to use of relaxation strategies.

PSYCHOLOGICAL FACTORS, STRESS AND THE DEVELOPMENT OF DISABILITY

Stress in various degrees is a facet of the human condition. Pain and pain-associated incapacity are stressful. As aforementioned, appraisal of threat leads to activities designed to reduce levels of stress. In the context of pain, a range of coping strategies will be evoked. With the passage of time, coping resources become exhausted, a decreasing number of options remain and significant disaffection with healthcare professionals may have become established (Chs 5 and 12).

How individuals react to pain is a function not only of the severity of the pain and its perceived significance, but also of their social and cultural background. The cultural, social and occupational influences on treatment seeking and response to pain will be considered in the next chapter (Ch. 3). Development of disability, however, is not only a psychological phenomenon but needs to be considered from a multidimensional perspective. The interaction between beliefs, emotions, physiology and pain behaviour will be considered in Chapter 5, where a new model of disability incorporating these features will be offered for consideration.

CONCLUSION

Psychological issues are at the heart of interdisciplinary pain management. The shift from the narrow biomedical model to the biopsychosocial model now permeates clinical service delivery and social policy. It is important to recognise, however, that the investigation of such factors has to be every bit as rigorous and systematic as investigation of fundamental physiology, anatomy and biochemistry. In historical terms, the psychology of pain is still a relatively young field of enquiry. In this chapter the nature of psychological influences on pain has been considered from a number of distinct perspectives. The ground-breaking work of the behavioural perspective offered by Fordyce (1976), and the cognitive framework stimulated by Turk, Meichenbaum & Genest (1983), has established the foundations for the psychology of pain in the context of interdisciplinary pain management. The multidimensional framework offered by the biopsychosocial model has required the integration of psychological concepts with both biomedical and socioeconomic perspectives (Chs 3 and 4). Understanding of psychological factors as part of the *process* of chronicity offers a new challenge in secondary *prevention* (Chs 18 and 19). Much remains to be done.

KEY POINTS

- Psychological factors have a considerable influence on pain and disability.
- They have a stronger influence on outcome than do biomedical factors.
- The shift from medical to biopsychosocial models of illness highlights the major importance of psychological factors.
- The most important factors are distress, beliefs or attitudes, pain behaviour and pain-coping strategies.
- Further research is needed into the interaction amongst these factors at various stages of illness.
- Psychological factors in response to acute pain are predictive of chronic incapacity.

- There needs to be a redirection from investigations into the nature of pain towards obstacles to recovery.
- Distress at and confusion about previous treatment have a powerful influence on patients' reactions to pain and disability.
- There is an urgent strategic need to develop the integration of psychological perspectives into the clinical practice of other professions.
- Better management of psychological reactions at early stages of treatment has the potential for reducing iatrogenic distress and preventing unnecessary chronicity.

REFERENCES

Affleck G, Tennen H, Pfeiffer C, Fiefield J 1987 Appraisals of control and predictability in adapting to a chronic disease. Journal of Personality and Social Psychology. 53:273–279

Agnew C 1998 Modal versus individually-derived behavioral normative beliefs about condom use: comparing measurement alternatives of the cognitive underpinnings of the theories of reasoned action and planned behaviour. Psychology and Health 13:271–287

Bandura A 1977 Self-efficacy: towards a unifying theory of behaviour change. Psychological Review 84:191–215

Banks S M, Kerns R D 1996 Explaining high rates of depression in chronic pain: a diathesis-stress framework. Psychological Bulletin 119:95–110

Beck A 1976 Cognitive therapy and the emotional disorders. International University Press, New York

Brandstadter J 1992 Personal control over development: some developmental implications of self-efficacy. In: Schwarzer R (ed) self-efficacy: thought control of action. Hemisphere, Washington DC, pp 127–145

Brandstadter J, Renner G 1990 Tenacious goal pursuit and flexible goal adjustment: explication and age-related analysis of assimilative and accommodative strategies of coping. Psychology and Ageing 5:58–67

Brown G K, Nicassio P M 1987 The development of a questionnaire for the assessment of active and passive coping strategies. Pain 31:53–65

Brown G K, Nicassio P M, Wallston K A 1989 Pain coping strategies and depression in rheumatoid arthritis. Journal of Consulting and Clinical Psychology 57:652–657

Bryant R A 1993 Memory for pain and affect in chronic pain patients. Pain 54:347–351

Burns J W, Johnson B J, Mahoney N, Devine J, Pawl R 1996 Anger management style, hostility and spouse responses: gender differences in predictors of adjustment among chronic pain patients. Pain 64:445–453

Burton A K, Tillotson K M, Main C J, Hollis S 1995 Psychosocial predictors of outcome in acute and subchronic low back trouble. Spine 20:722–728

Butcher J N, Dahlstrom W G, Graham J R, Tellegen A, Kaemmer B 1989 Manual for the administration and scoring of the Minnesota Multiphasic Personality Inventory-2: MMPI-2. University of Minnesota Press, Minneapolis

Cioffi D 1991 Beyond attentional strategies: a cognitive–perceptual model of somatic interpretation. Psychological Bulletin 109:25–41

Conner M, Norman P 1998 Editorial: social cognition models in health psychology. Psychology and Health 13:179–185

Costa P T Jr, McCrae R R 1985 The N-E-O Personality Inventory Manual. Psychological Assessment Resources, Odessa F A,

Crisson J E, Keefe F J 1988 The relationship of locus of control to pain coping strategies and psychological distress in chronic pain patients. Pain 35:147–154

DeGood D E, Shutty M S Jr 1992 Assessment of pain beliefs, coping and self-efficacy. In: Turk D C, Melzack R (eds) Handbook of pain assessment. Guilford Press, New York, ch 13, pp 214–234

Derbyshire S W, Jones A K, Devani P et al 1994 Cerebral responses to pain in patients with atypical facial pain measured by positron emission tomography. Journal of Neurology, Neurosurgery and Psychiatry 57:1166–1172

Deshields T L, Tait R C, Gfeller J D, Chibnall J T 1995 Relationship between social desirability and self-report in chronic pain patients. Clinical Journal of Pain 11:189–193

DSM-IV 1994 Diagnostic and Statistical manual of mental disorders, 4th revision. American Psychiatric Association, Washington DC

Eccleston C 1995 The attentional control of pain: methodological and theoretical concerns. Pain 63:3–10

Engel G L 1959 Psychogenic pain and the pain-prone patient. American Journal of Medicine 26:899

Fernandez E, Milburn T W 1994 Sensory and affective predictors of overall pain and emotions associated with affective pain. Clinical Journal of Pain 10:3–9

Fernandez E, Turk D C 1989 The utility of cognitive coping strategies for altering perception of pain: a meta-analysis. Pain 38:123–135

Fernandez E, Turk D C 1995 The scope and significance of anger in the experience of chronic pain. Pain 61:165–175

Flor H, Turk D C 1989 Psychophysiology of chronic pain. Do chronic pain patients exhibit symptom-specific psychophysiological responses? Psychological Bulletin 105:215–259

Folkman S, Lazarus R 1980 An analysis of coping in a middle-aged community sample. Journal of Health and Social Behaviour 21:219–240

Fordyce W E 1976 Behavioral methods for chronic pain and illness. C V Mosby, St Louis, MS

Gatchel R J, Polatin P B, Kinney R K 1995 Predicting outcome of chronic back pain using clinical predictors of

psychopathology: a prospective analysis. Health Psychology 14:415–420

Hathaway S R, McKinley J C 1967 Minnesota Multiphasic Personality Inventory manual (revised edn). Psychological Corporation, New York

Haythornthwaite J A, Sieber W J, Kerns R D 1991 Depression and the chronic pain experience. Pain 46:177–184

Jensen M P, Karoly P 1991 Control beliefs, coping efforts and adjustment to chronic pain. Journal of Consulting and Clinical Psychology 59:431–438

Jensen M P, Turner J A, Romano J M, Karoly P 1991 Coping with chronic pain: a critical review of the literature. Pain 47:249–283

Keefe F J, Brown G K, Wallston K A, Caldwell D S 1989 Coping with rheumatoid arthritis pain: catastrophising as a maladaptive strategy. Pain 37:51–56

Keefe F J, Salley A N Jr, LeFebvre J C 1992 Coping with pain: conceptual concerns and future references. Pain 51:131–134

Keefe F J, Affleck G, Lefebvre J, Starr K, Caldwell D S, Tennen H 1997 Pain coping strategies and pain efficacy in rheumatoid arthritis: a daily process analysis. Pain 69:35–42

Keller L S, Butcher J N 1991 Assessment of chronic pain patients with the MMPI-2. University of Minnesota Press, Minneapolis

Kerns R D, Rosenberg R, Jamison R N, Caudill M A, Haythornthwaite J A 1997 Readiness to adopt a self-management approach to chronic pain: the Pain Stages of Change Questionnaire (PSOCQ). Pain 72:227–234

Klenerman L, Slade P D, Stanley I M et al 1995 The prediction of chronicity in patients with an acute attack of low back pain in a general practice setting. Spine 20:478–484

Kori S H, Miller R P, Todd D D 1990 Kinisophobia: a new view of chronic pain behaviour. Pain Management Jan/Feb:35–43

Lackner J M, Carosella A M, Feuerstein M 1996 Pain expectancies, pain and functional self-efficacy expectancies as determinants of disability in patients with chronic low back disorders. Journal of Consulting Clinical Psychology 64:212–220

Lazarus R S 1993 Coping theory and research: past, present and future. Psychosomatic Medicine 55:234–247

Lazarus R, Folkman S 1984 Stress appraisal and coping. Springer-Verlag, New York

Letham J, Slade P D, Troop J D G, Bentley G 1983 Outline of a fear-avoidance model of exaggerated pain perception. Behaviour Research and Therapy 21:401–408

Magni G, Moreschi C, Rigatti-Luchini S, Merskey H 1994 Prospective study on the relationship between depressive symptoms and chronic musculoskeletal pain. Pain 56:289–297

Main C J 1983 The Modified Somatic Perception Questionnaire. Journal of Psychosomatic Research 27:503–514

Main C J, Spanswick C C 1995 Personality assessment and the Minnesota Multiphasic Personality Inventory 50 years on: do we need our security blanket? Pain Forum 4:94–96

Main C J, Waddell G 1991 A comparison of cognitive measures in low back pain: statistical structure and clinical validity at initial assessment. Pain, 46:287–298

Melzack R, Wall P D 1965 Pain mechanisms, a new theory. Science 150:971–979

Petrie K J, Weinman J A (eds) 1998 Perceptions of health and illness: current research and applications. Harwood Academic, Amsterdam, pp 2–3

Prochaska J O, DiClemente C C 1982 Transtheoretical therapy; toward a more integrative model of change. Psychotherapy: Theory Research and Practice 19:276–288

Quine L, Rutter D R, Arnold L 1998 Predicting safety-helmet use among schoolboy cyclists: a comparison of the theory of planned behaviour and the health belief model. Psychology and Health 13:251–269

Regier D A, Boyd J H, Burke J D et al 1988 One month prevalence of mental disorders in the United States. Archives of General Psychiatry 45:977–986

Robinson M E, Riley J L III 1999 The role of emotion in pain. In: Gatchel R J, Turk D C (ed) Psychosocial factors in pain. Guilford Press, New York, Ch 5, pp 74–88

Rosenstiel A K, Keefe F J 1983 The use of coping strategies in chronic low back pain patients: relationship to patient characteristics and current adjustment. Pain 17:33–44

Rudy T E, Kerns R D, Turk D C 1988 Chronic pain and depression: a cognitive mediation model. Pain 35:129–140

Schmitz U, Saile H, Nilges P 1996 Coping with chronic pain: flexible goal adjustment as an interactive buffer against pain-related distress. Pain 67:41–51

Skevington S 1995 Psychology of pain. John Wiley, Chichester

Sullivan M, Katon W 1993 Focus article: somatization: the path between distress and somatic symptoms. APS Journal 2:141–149

Toomey T C, Mann J D, Abashian S, Thompson-Pope S 1991 Relationship between perceived self-control of pain, pain description and functioning. Pain 45:129–133

Turk D C 1996 Biopsychosocial perspective on chronic pain. In: Gatchel R J, Turk D C (eds) Psychological approaches to pain management: a practitioner's handbook. Guilford Press, New York, ch 1, pp 3–32

Turk D C, Fernandez E 1995 Personality assessment and the Minnesota Multiphasic Personality Inventory in chronic pain. Underdeveloped and overexposed. Pain Forum 4:104–107

Turk D C, Meichenbaum D H, Genest M 1983 Pain and behavioral medicine: a cognitive–behavioral perspective. Guilford Press, New York

Turner J A 1991 Coping and chronic pain. In: Bond M R, Charlton J E, Woolf C (eds) Proceedings of the VIth world congress on pain. Elsevier, New York, pp 219–227

Vlaeyen J, Kole-Snijders A M J, Boeren R G B, van Eek H 1995 Fear of movement/(re)injury in chronic low back pain and its relation to behavioral performance. Pain 62:363–372

Wade J B, Doherty L M, Hart R P, Cook D D 1992 Patterns of normal personality structure among chronic pain patients. Pain 48:37–43

Waddell G, Somerville D, Henderson I, Newton M, Main C J 1993 A fear avoidance beliefs questionnaire (FABQ) and the role of fear avoidance beliefs in chronic low back pain and disability. Pain 52:157–168

Wallston K A, Wallston B S, deVellis R 1978 Development of the Multidimensional Health Locus of Control (MHLC) scales. Health Education Monographs 6:160–170

Weinberger D A 1990 The construct validity of the repressive coping style. In: Singer J L (eds) Repression and dissociation. University of Chicago Press, Chicago, pp 337–386

Williams D A, Thorn B E 1989 An empirical assessment of pain beliefs. Pain 36: 351–358

Wilson L, Dworkin S, Whitney C, LeResche L 1994 Somatization and pain dispersion in chronic temporomandibular disorder pain. Pain 57:55–61

Zimmerman M 1994 Diagnosing personality disorders: a review of issues and research methods. Archives of General Psychiatry 51:225–245

3

Social and cultural influences on pain and disability

Chris J. Main   Helen Parker

INTRODUCTION

In Chapter 2, the influence of beliefs and emotions on the perception of pain was reviewed. The response to pain in terms of pain-associated incapacity (or functional disability) has also been investigated and it appears that *adjustment* to pain is also subject to a wide variety of influences. The psychological factors affecting pain and disability have already been identified within a biopsychosocial framework, but before attempting a more comprehensive analysis of disability in the context of pain management (Ch. 5) it is important to appraise the nature of the 'social' component of the biopsychosocial model. The nature of social and cultural influences on pain and disability will be addressed in this chapter and an attempt will be made to appraise their influence on the perception of pain, the reporting of symptoms, health-care seeking and response to treatment. (Specific discussion of economic and occupational influences will be deferred until the next chapter.)

The evidence suggests that social factors have an influence on pain ranging from earliest experiences as a neonate to adjustment to chronic pain and incapacity in adulthood and old age. Prior to consideration of their specific spheres of influence it is important to consider briefly some of the underlying cultural, subcultural and social mechanisms that may shape our perceptions.

CULTURAL INFLUENCES

Culture can be defined in terms of individuals' sense of ethnicity, religion, historical roots and general value systems. Culture, as reflected in similarities amongst individuals within a society, forms the basis for the development of stereotypes, which essentially maximise the similarity within groups and focus on the differences between the groups. Cross-cultural differences are evident in many aspects of human behaviour, and certainly in prevalence of illness and in health-care usage. Volinn (1997) reports on the differing prevalence of back pain in different countries, but, as Waddell (1998) points out, the review tells us only about how different groups *report* back pain and not its physical or physiological basis. None the less, it would appear that report of back pain is associated with degree of urbanisation or availability of health care.

Cross-cultural differences in response to pain

There has been no research specifically into cultural differences in the *perception* of pain (which would require an experimental model), but a number of studies on back pain have addressed cultural differences in response to pain.

It is generally accepted that back pain is common in populations throughout the world, but the interpretation of the experience and the associated pain behaviours seem to differ significantly, depending on cultural norms. Sanders et al (1992) found differences in Sickness Impact Profile (SIP) scores of patients seeking help for back pain at pain clinics in different countries (USA, Japan, Mexico, Columbia, Italy and New Zealand). They found levels of psychosocial and vocational impact to be greatest in the Americans, then New Zealanders and Italians. (Unfortunately the study did not examine possible explanations for these differences, such as differences in work ethic, social support, economic factors, sickness entitlement and psychological factors such as beliefs or coping strategies.)

In a study in rural Nepal, for example, Anderson (1984) reported that, although back symptoms were very common, virtually no one sought help for the symptoms when medical services were made available. It appeared that back pain problems were not perceived as a medical problem, but rather as a normal part of life associated in part with the ageing process. In a study of back pain in an Australian aboriginal community, Honeyman & Jacobs (1996) reported that, when privately questioned, nearly one-third of men and half of women reported some long term problems with low back pain. However, they did not perceive back pain as a health issue and consequently did not report such symptoms openly, display pain-related behaviours or seek medical care. The provision of specialised services may in fact change the perception of musculoskeletal symptoms and the significance attributed to them. Waddell (1998) reported that before the introduction of modern medicine in Oman, although back pain was common, extended disability for back pain problems was virtually non-existent and there was no evidence that individuals became permanently disabled from non-specific back pain.

Cultural and subcultural context as a framework for socialisation mechanisms

As aforementioned, little is known in fact about differences in perception of pain. The stereotype of the stoical northern European and the more emotionally expressive southern European can be seen in the television coverage of reaction to disasters of various sorts. Although it may be helpful for some purposes to focus on features in common across cultures, ignoring differences can lead to overgeneralisation and caricature. In understanding how individuals react, subcultural factors may be more illuminating. Cultural factors can be best understood perhaps in terms of socialisation mechanisms, and how these may affect both the *perception* of pain and the *response* to pain (including both treatment seeking and response to treatment).

Box 3.1   Socialisation mechanisms

- Long term social influences on pain experience, beliefs, appraisals, pain behaviours and pain-coping strategies
- Role of direct instruction, reinforcement and punishment and observational learning
- Influence of emotional stress factors in the family context of pain experience and illness behaviour
- Specific influences of attachment, martial stress, family disturbances and family violence including physical and sexual abuse
- Role of sex differences in the socialisation of individual differences in pain and illness behaviour
- Influence of marital status, ethnicity and other socio-demographic characteristics on styles of socialisation
- Cross-cultural differences in the influence of health systems

---

SOCIALISATION MECHANISMS

A number of the key aspects of social aspects of pain have recently been identified (IASP 1997). They are summarised in Box 3.1.

A considerable body of research has been undertaken into many of these mechanisms (reviewed by Skevington 1997). Even though it may be extremely important to understand such factors from a societal perspective, and therefore from the viewpoint of education and social policy, individuals are seldom able to give a clear understanding of such mechanisms in their particular case. They will tend to recall significant events, and may be quite unaware of some of the social forces that have shaped their perception. In clinical decision making, clinicians have to rely primarily on the information immediately available to them in terms of medical documentation, and in terms of the clinical history and symptoms as presented by the patient. Some events of course may have considerable clinical significance (such as a history of sexual or physical abuse), but patients' clinical recall will tend to be focused on the supposed genesis of the current pain problem and the attempts to treat it. They will tend to be more accurate in their recall of aspects of history that are relatively recent and may be unable to clarify the origins of their beliefs about their pain. Such information frequently emerges during pain management as

patients refine objectives for treatment and become aware of obstacles to recovery. It is important therefore to consider some of these social mechanisms.

Social learning

Arguably one of the most important influences on the development of modern pain management has been the recognition that chronic illness needs to be understood in a social context. Pain behaviour can also be viewed from a social-learning perspective. A key feature in the early behavioural explanations was the recognition that pain behaviour was a consequence not just of nociception but of its social context. As such it needs to be understood not only as a response to nociception but also as a social event that may be subject to a wide variety of influences.

Most developmental psychologists would agree that a major feature of 'learning', as normally understood, is the conscious assimilation of information. The term 'social learning', as understood in the context of the development of chronic pain behaviour, needs to be understood somewhat differently, as a process by which pain behaviour, and even the experience of pain, may be shaped by the context in which it occurs. Furthermore, it is not always appreciated that social learning is an ongoing process and needs to be understood not only from the perspective of the young child, but also as a powerful force in the development of pain behaviour in adulthood. In the context of clinical pain management the power of social influences can often be identified particularly in the contexts of family interactions, and as an important aspect of the health-care consultation process. Patients may be mostly unaware of the power of such influences, and indeed may resist the suggestion that their incapacity is more than a direct result of nociception.

Spheres of influence of social factors

The major spheres of influence of social factors are shown in Box 3.2.

> **Box 3.2** Major spheres of influence of social factors
>
> - Understanding the meaning of pain
> - Communication about pain
> - Treatment seeking
> - Response to treatment
> - Development of pain-coping strategies

Understanding the meaning of pain

Although we are biologically programmed to respond immediately to sudden unexpected pain in terms of escape or withdrawal, our response to pain frequently also has to be understood in a social context. We arrive in the world with a set of instinctive responses which are then 'shaped' by social processes. As we mature from neonates into infants and then young children we learn about the meaning and significance of sensations, including pain. We observe how others react to situations and in turn develop behaviour repertoires of our own, initially by observation, then by imitation. Our first clumsy attempts are met with a variety of responses, but gradually through social learning processes we become more skilled and effective in our interactions with others, such that our needs are met.

These learning processes have been specifically investigated in children with pain. Craig, Prkatchin & Grunau (1992) have developed a sophisticated videotape rating system called the Neonatal Facial Coding System or NFCS (Grunau & Craig 1990), which has enabled research into the expression of pain in neonates. They report striking similarities between newborn and adult facial responses to events that are painful to adults. Parents are 'programmed' into responding to expressions of distress in their children. As non-verbal characteristics are integrated with verbal utterances, more sophisticated communication patterns are established between parent and child. Young children learn to attribute significance to various sensations and thus develop a set of responses, which become established behaviour patterns. 'Meaning' is thus learned and children learn to react to various levels of pain intensity. The

dual processes of observation and receiving various sorts of responses from others lead the child to develop not only a set of behavioural responses, but also a set of beliefs about pain and expectations about how others will respond. (A more detailed analysis of socialisation mechanisms is presented below.) As they grow older, children may experience new and different pain problems, and experience a different set of responses from others in their presentation of pain.

Communication about pain

As children mature into adults, they develop a wide range of communication skills. How they communicate about pain will depend on their experience of it. It is commonly observed among very young children who hurt themselves that their immediate response is to look at their parent. The response of the parent not only influences the child's response to that particular incident but also begins to establish a set of expectations and behaviour patterns in the child. By the time the child has reached adulthood they may have encountered other patterns shown by people with pain, and their understanding of pain may have been further developed.

Treatment seeking

Pain is a common fact of life, yet not everyone consults a professional about it. Whether individuals seek treatment seems to be determined not only by the severity of the pain but also by a further set of considerations, such as the significance given to the pain, the treatment options available and access to health care. Treatment seeking can also be understood from a social perspective (Mechanic 1977, 1986) and the term 'illness behaviour' was originally a social construct. These ideas have had a powerful influence on more recent terms such as chronic illness behaviour, 'invalidism', or the more specific 'pain behaviour' and 'chronic pain syndrome' (as viewed from a behavioural perspective).

Response to treatment

Prediction of individuals' response to treatment for pain is difficult, and their response seems to be determined by many factors. There is no doubt, however, that beliefs exert a powerful influence on response to treatment and may represent significant obstacles to treatment or recovery. Recent research (Burton et al 1995) has shown that psychosocial factors may be more important than medical factors in predicting future levels of disability. The most important feature of the psychological profile was found to be individuals' beliefs about the likely future course of their symptoms.

Beliefs have many origins, ranging from specific information conveyed to patients by health-care staff, to the views of family members or acquaintances, to articles in popular magazines and to television programmes. A key aspect in assessment of suitability for interdisciplinary pain management is the appraisal of such beliefs. Social factors may have a powerful influence on the degree of conviction with which patients adhere to a particular belief. Trust or confidence in influential friends or family may underpin development of a near unshakeable conviction in a belief that has been expressed by them about the nature of pain or treatment. If such an opinion is unhelpful or misguided, it may constitute an obstacle to recovery that is difficult to overcome.

Many patients who develop chronic pain problems express distress about opinions given to them by doctors. Unfortunately, information received by patients can be sketchy, inconsistent and sometimes wrong. Furthermore, information received from health-care professionals can also be contradictory or misleading. (As discussed in Ch. 5, with chronic pain patients such iatrogenically produced misunderstandings can lead to confusion and distress.) Understanding and managing the *social* aspects of the communication are therefore essential not only in the delivery of effective pain management, but also in the prevention of unnecessary incapacity. These are discussed in more detail later in this chapter.

Development of pain-coping strategies

Individuals present with a wide-range of coping strategies, which they have learnt, sometimes through trial and error, but frequently from their social and family environment. As discussed earlier in Chapter 2, there is a wide range of coping styles and strategies, which may be considered as appropriate or inappropriate depending on the specific context. A wide range of social influences may have had a bearing on the development of the particular repertoire of coping strategies evident at initial assessment. A detailed clinical history may indicate strong family influences. Locating management advice within an *appropriate* educational framework has been the guiding principle behind recent evidence-based guidelines for the management of back pain in primary care (CSAG 1994, Waddell 1998). (These newer initiatives are discussed further in Chapter 18.)

Conclusion

A proper understanding therefore of the social context in which the response to pain has been developed will often assist clinical decision making.

THE INFLUENCE OF AGE

Most clinical series of patients suggest that the peak incidence of back pain and sciatica is at about 40 years of age, and epidemiological studies (Consumer's Association 1985, Croft et al 1994) suggest that lifetime prevalence increases from the late teens up until the 45–55 years age group. According to Waddell (1998, p. 87): 'these studies all suggest that the peak prevalence of back pain is somewhere between 40 and 60 years. There is probably a slight fall later in life'. However, all forms of disability increase with age particularly among the elderly, and the proportion of individuals reporting *restricted activity* rises linearly until retirement age.

Physical changes in the musculoskeletal system are recognised as part of the ageing process. In the evaluation of the effects of accidents in cases of personal injury (such as road traffic accidents), there is frequently dispute among the medical assessors about the extent to which degenerative changes identified on X-rays can be attributed to the effects of injury received in the accident. Concepts such as 'acceleration' of pre-existing degeneration are based upon assumptions about normal changes in physical features with increasing age. To the extent that limitation in function is related to such changes, it is important therefore to evaluate an individual's disability in comparison with a reference group of the same gender and of a comparable age (Waddell & Main 1984).

Of more interest in the context of pain management, however, are the psychological and social changes that accompany increasing age. Unsurprisingly, work interference as such becomes statistically less problematic, as older people move to part-time work or cease work, but there is more to life than work. It is known that adjustment to pain is affected by the extent to which it interferes with valued activity (Rudy, Kerns & Turk 1988). Increasing age may bring increasing leisure opportunities, but also increasing dependence and the need for practical and social support. As far as pain management is concerned it is important therefore to consider age not necessarily as a barrier to treatment but as a factor that may influence the understanding of the individual's adjustment to pain-associated incapacity. It is important also to identify treatment goals that are appropriate for the individual's age and circumstances. Finally, it should be remembered that older patients are sometimes reluctant to disclose the extent of their difficulties to health-care professionals and may even hold the inappropriate view that they are 'troubling the doctor' in consulting for treatment.

THE INFLUENCE OF SEX AND GENDER

According to Unruh (1996), in most epidemiological research women are more likely than men to report a variety of temporary and persistent pains (in addition of course to sex-specific problems of menstrual pain, pregnancy and childbirth). Furthermore, women tend to report more severe pain, more frequent pain and pain of longer duration than men. The reason for these differences is not immediately apparent but seems unlikely to be explained simply by biological factors. The complexity of the situation is illustrated by the issues considered to be important by Unruh. In her judgement the key issues to be understood in trying to explain these differences are

- the way in which women and men perceive and respond to pain
- the biological, social and developmental factors that may affect gender variations in the pain experience and
- the response of the health-care system to the pain presented by men and women.

(Unruh 1996, p. 124)

Biological differences between the sexes

Some of the major biological differences between the sexes in response to pain are shown in Box 3.3.

Box 3.3 Biological differences between the sexes

- Pain specific to the sexes
- Pain associated with sex-specific disease conditions
- Sex-specific surgical procedures
- Central mechanisms
- Sex differences in perception of pain and in pain relief

Pain specific to the sexes

The experience of pain from adolescence through adulthood differs between men and women. Women are more likely to have had experience of recurrent pain as a result of menstruation. It is known of course that not all women are significantly troubled by menstrual pains and cramps, but such pains can usually be understood as part of a normal biological process, and as such essentially non-threatening. The extent to which women should expect to tolerate such pain is the subject of another debate. There seem to be differences across cultures in expectations of the sort of pain that women are expected to tolerate. Pregnancy and childbirth are further biological events that are sex specific. A proportion of women suffer chronic pain as a consequence of gynaecological problems or the physical demands of childbirth. Women need to distinguish between manageable and excessive pain due to normal processes. There is a danger that opportunity for appropriate pain treatment may be overlooked because the pain is viewed as a 'normal' phenomenon rather than as a consequence of disease or injury. As Unruh (1996, p. 157) has observed: 'pain for women is a monitor for health as well as a potential symptom of injury, illness or disease ... men have recurrent pains of lesser intensity, frequency or duration than women; however men are more likely to experience pain from injury, and acute and chronic life-threatening diseases'.

Pain associated with sex-specific disease conditions and surgery

These are important in terms of general medical management but of less relevance specifically to issues of pain management unless they have led to a chronic pain problem. In the latter event, the factors maintaining the chronic pain and the associated obstacles to recovery may be of more relevance than the genesis of the pain.

Sex differences in perception of pain and in pain relief

Women have higher pain morbidity from acute and non-fatal chronic diseases, and are more likely than men to report a variety of temporary and persistent pains, they also report more severe pain, more frequent pain and pain of longer duration (Unruh 1996). There is some evidence for a higher rate of headache and facial pain in women, possibly in the specific location of back pain and in thoracic pain, although the differences are relatively small. There is clear evidence that women report more

musculoskeletal pain than do men, report more multiple pain sites and have a higher prevalence of osteoarthritis, rheumatoid arthritis and fibromyalgia.

Biological mechanisms

There has been little research as yet on specific sex differences in biological mechanisms, although there appear to be some differences in brain chemical metabolism and in the biological mechanisms of pain transmission (Polleri 1992). Experimental pain research in animals has found differences in analgesic response, raising the possibility or oestrogen-dependent pain mechanisms as a partial explanation for sex differences. There do appear to be sex differences in pain-regulatory systems although it remains to be determined *which* aspects of the pain response differ according to sex. Both central and peripheral mechanisms have been investigated.

Central mechanisms. Experimental researchers have investigated both central and peripheral mechanisms. They have postulated differences both in primary afferent input to the central nervous system (CNS) (i.e. both long term developmental and phasic menstrual cycle-dependent changes in primary afferent function and coding) and in central processing of sensory–discriminative and motivational–affective information at several levels of the nervous system.

Peripheral physiological responses to noxious stimuli. Although sex differences in cardivascular response to non-painful stressors have been documented, there appear to have been fewer studies on sex differences in physiological response to tissue damage.

According to Fillingim & Maixner (1995, p. 216): 'Collectively, these findings suggest aversive stimuli and stressful tasks are less likely to evoke sympathetic nervous system and pituitary–adrenal responses while evoking greater negative psychological responses in females compared with males'.

A number of more specific conclusions also emerge from their review:

- overall, females exhibit greater sensitivity to laboratory pain compared with males
- these sex differences do not appear to be site specific
- although sex differences are reported for all pain induction procedures, some forms of stimulation have produced more consistent findings than others (e.g. pressure versus thermal)
- sex-associated differences appear to occur most consistently with pain induction procedures that mimic pain sensations similar to those experienced clinically (e.g. headaches, cramps and muscle soreness).

However, the authors acknowledge that further research is needed into different types of experimental pain, since experimental and biological factors do not appear to explain adequately gender differences, and that: 'pain responses are characterised by great inter-individual variability and this variability likely contributes to the discrepancies across studies' (p. 210).

Implications for understanding clinical pain

The specific relevance of experimental pain findings for the understanding of clinical pain or its management has always been problematic, and this is particularly true in the investigation of sex differences. As an example, greater use of morphine postoperatively by men has also been found, but it is not clear whether the difference is in nociception or in pain tolerance. In contrast, human laboratory studies have shown that women may have somewhat lower pain thresholds and increased muscle tenderness. Indeed the incidence of fibromyalgia is much higher in women. Thus, although there may be a biological component explaining some of the differences in pain perception between men and women, the size of the effect is neither large nor consistent. Even if it is accepted that there may be differences in how women and men react to pain, this difference does not appear to be attributable simply to differences in pain threshold. Even if it were accepted that experimental pain tolerance was an appropriate methodological framework

within which to investigate sex differences, there is abundant evidence that *clinical* pain tolerance is influ-enced significantly by psychosocial factors. Investigation of differences in response to pain by men and women would seem to require a broader biopsychosocial framework including a focus on gender role rather than the narrower biological construct.

The influence of gender

Men and women appear to differ in the significance they attribute to painful events. The reason for this is not entirely clear, but it may be related to differences in the interpretation of pain as well as socially determined differences in how they respond to pain. Some of the more important factors are shown in Box 3.4.

Box 3.4   The influence of gender

- Interpretation of pain
- Need to consult
- Reasons for consulting
- Willingness to consult
- Response to treatment
- Recovery from injury

The interpretation of pain

It has been observed that gender differences in the prevalence of recurrent pain appear from adolescence onwards. Interpretation is shaped by experience. It is easy to understand how differences in familiarity with different sorts of pain may lead to differences in the attribution of significance (and therefore action as a result of it). A key facet of clinical assessment is an appraisal of individuals' specific understanding of their pain, and the significance they attach to it (see Ch. 2). In the context of pain management it is important first and foremost as a determinant of consultation and may determine whether or not a patient is likely to benefit from pain management (Ch. 12). There is clear evidence of gender-specific differences in the interpretation of pain as such, but there may be important differences in the reasons for consulting.

The need to consult

There has been much speculation about the explanation for differing consultation rates between men and women. As mentioned above, women have different needs to consult health-care professionals, not only with reference to their own gynaecological and obstetric needs, but also as a consequence of their role as primary carers within the family. They may attend to pain sooner to prevent disruption of their wider social obligations to their family. Men may be more likely to consult if pain is perceived as a threat to work. The complexity of modern social structures and the marked variation within gender in consultation rates, however, make such generalities not only hazardous, but unhelpful in the context of pain management. The reasons for consulting would seem to be much more relevant.

Reasons for consulting

Differences in consulting may be a consequence of gender differences in the emotional response to pain and in types of coping strategies. Thus, whereas women may be more worried and irritated about pain, men may be more embarrassed about it (Klonoff, Landrine & Brown 1993). Men and women may differ in their use of coping strategies, whether 'problem focused' or 'emotionally focused' (Folkman & Lazarus 1980, Lazarus & Folkman 1984), and in their adoption of shorter term or longer term strategies (because of the potentially disruptive effects of the pain). Stress and depression may be more closely associated with pain in women than men (Magni et al 1990), although not all studies have found this.

Willingness to consult

There may be an element of truth in the ascription of gender differences in consultation to differences in the 'threshold' of self-disclosure or in willingness to discuss emotional issues.

Difference in the manner of presentation of symptoms, and in particular the emotional component, may have a significant effect on the patient–doctor communication process and the treatment actually received (see below).

Response to treatment

There are no controlled studies specifically on the influence of gender on outcome. Ascription of differences in treatment response specifically to gender would require control for possible biases in assessment, selection for treatment, goals for treatment and extent of engagement in treatment. (Unpublished data on the outcome of the interdisciplinary pain management programme at the Manchester and Salford Pain Centre has, however, shown some differences between men and women in the value they place on different aspects of the teaching programme, when reviewed 6 months post-treatment. It seems that women particularly appreciate discussing their difficulties within a group context, whereas men often seem to find the reactivation part of the programme more helpful.)

Recovery from injury

Although there is no clear evidence of differing effects of pain on activities of daily living in men and women, according to Unruh (1996) there is some evidence that there is a difference between men and women in the factors influencing return to work. She reports the study of Crook (1993) who found that men made more efforts to return to work, and returned sooner, whereas women had significantly more psychological distress and functional handicap than men as the time postinjury increased. It was reported also that the total number of painful sites and the extent of the psychological distress influenced the likelihood of a woman's return to work.

SPECIFIC INFLUENCES OF THE FAMILY CONTEXT

A number of specific influences of the family context are shown in Box 3.5.

> **Box 3.5** Specific influences of the family context
>
> - Complex role of family and social network in understanding of pain
> - Types of interaction between pain sufferers and their care givers
> - Contributions of the family and significant others to the maintenance of disability
> - Physical and psychological effects on the principal care giver
> - Economic effects of treatment on the family
> - Potential of the family and its members as powerful intervention agents.

Complex role of family and social network in understanding of pain

By the time many patients are considered for pain management, their pain behaviour is usually well established and it is often difficult to obtain a clinical history of sufficient accuracy to determine the precise mechanisms involved. It is important to appreciate that the report of pain intensity may be coloured by patients' suffering, the pain-associated disability influenced by responses of various family members and the ability to work affected by economic consequences of sickness not only on patients but on their family. Thus a pain problem that began with impact only on patients themselves may have become a problem of major significance to the entire family.

Types of interaction between pain sufferers and their care givers

Interpersonal communication comprises a complex set of signals, both verbal and non-verbal. Misunderstandings and miscommunications characterise dysfunctional families. When a pain problem arises amongst individuals who do not normally communicate adequately, major distress and disruption can arise. Families vary in sensitivity to self-report and non-verbal pain behaviour. It may be essential to identify and rectify such misunderstandings at the time of initial assessment before a pain management programme can be instigated. Indeed specific training in communication skills, such as

appropriate assertiveness, forms a key part of the psychological component of many pain management programmes.

Contributions of the family and significant others to the maintenance of disability

The most common interpersonal problems characteristic of chronic pain patients are anger (or hostility) and oversolicitousness.

Anger

Chronic pain and pain-associated incapacity are frequently very stressful (and indeed if there are no indications of distress then the patient may be insufficiently motivated to make a success of pain management). More specifically, chronic pain can create a profound sense of helplessness, resulting in feelings of frustration manifest as irritability, and sometimes anger, directed at other members of the family. Relationships may deteriorate. Patients may become even more demoralised and stressed. The diminished self-confidence may lead to avoidance of activities anticipated to be painful and they may feel unable to contemplate participation in active rehabilitation.

Oversolicitousness

Oversolicitousness on the part of family members is frequently easy to identify, but more difficult to address. Neither patients nor family members may be aware of the powerful influences their behaviour can exert on each other. It is important to consider oversolicitousness from two perspectives: first in the context of fear/avoidance and secondly in the context of enhanced well-being. If patients are confronted with an activity that is anticipated to be painful then, since pain is unpleasant at best, they will have some reluctance to undertake the activity. If their partner offers to assist them, they no longer have to face the situation. They feel relieved.

Unfortunately, this pattern of interpersonal behaviours can become generalised to more and more situations, until the patient becomes progressively more disabled. Unless patients are distressed about their level of disability and increasing dependence on their partner, it is perhaps unwise for the therapist to intervene. Many patients, however, become increasingly frustrated over their lack of independence. It can be difficult for both parties to accept that the oversolicitousness has contributed to the problem. The partner may have to be shown a more appropriate way of helping.

If the patient feels much happier with the increased attention then, provided the partner is willing to continue to provide it, it is perhaps necessary to view the oversolicitousness as an interactive pattern which meets the emotional needs of the parties concerned. As such the oversolicitousness may constitute a sufficiently serious obstacle to rehabilitation to permit acceptance for pain management. It may be, of course, that although it is possible to agree rehabilitation objectives that are achievable despite the oversolicitousness, they are not likely to be achieved. Certainly, where there is evidence of a clear mismatch between the needs of patients and their partners, some therapeutic attention may have to be directed at their relationships prior to the pain management programme. Only if the situation is successfully resolved will it be possible to proceed further with pain management.

Physical and psychological effects on the principal care giver

It is not always appreciated that members of the family can become significantly disaffected with chronic pain in their relative. They also may become tired, exhausted, demoralised and depressed. It is frequently found amongst chronic pain patients assessed for treatment that the needs of the partner have never been identified or even considered. As stated above, however, chronic pain can become a family problem. In some cases, the partner is the driving force behind treatment seeking. It is important therefore wherever possible to assess the needs of partners as well as patients in considering pain management. Sometimes partners will be demoralised to the extent of requiring treatment in their own right.

Economic effects of treatment on the family

For families in a difficult situation, the economic implications of continued incapacity may be considerable. Such difficulties are frequently found in the context of litigation. In considering pain management, it is important to attempt an appraisal in the context of the family unit and decide whether the perceived risk of improved function in terms of possible loss of benefits constitute an obstacle to acceptance for treatment. (The issue is discussed further in Chs 4 and 11.)

Potential of the family and its members as powerful intervention agents

The previous parts of this chapter have addressed possible mutually adverse influences of pain within families. Family members, however, can often be powerful influences on the *success* of rehabilitation. As aforementioned, it is important to include their contribution to the nature of the patient's difficulties. If they are given an appropriate understanding of the principles of pain management, with its core emphasis on the re-establishment of self-control, partners can help encourage and motivate patients, especially at times when their confidence wavers. They can be facilitators of change in family activity and equal beneficiaries of improvement in quality of life. Furthermore, after the pain management programme they may be able to provide the encouragement necessary to overcome 'flare-ups' and continue to improve function after completion of the programme, when patients are likely to miss the support and encouragement of their fellow patients (see Ch. 14 on maintenance of change).

PROFESSIONAL–PATIENT COMMUNICATION

In addressing aspects of professional–patient communication from a social perspective, it is important to appreciate the complexity of clinical assessment, as during a typical assessment there will be many and varied types of interaction. Strategies for maximising the effectiveness of interviewing will be addressed more specifically in Chapter 18, but in this chapter the focus specifically will be on the factors that influence the communication process.

A number of social aspects of the clinical assessment are shown in Box 3.6.

Box 3.6 Social aspects of clinical assessment

- Purposes of the clinical assessment
- Patient objectives for interview
- Factors affecting communication
- Potential biases affecting professional judgement
- Patient factors affecting self-disclosure
- Special features of different professional encounters
- Overview of the nature of communication

Purposes of the clinical assessment

Communication is at the heart of clinical assessment, yet the complexity of the communication process is seldom appreciated. It can be understood only with reference to the specific matter in hand. Simply put, even short interchanges on clearly focused topics contain a complex pattern of individual verbal and non-verbal communications that are then meshed so that responses from one person serve as cues not only as acknowledgements that the message has been received, but also as a cue for further discourse. In addressing the social aspects of clinical assessment, it may be helpful initially to consider the major purposes of clinical assessment. They are shown in Box 3.7.

Box 3.7 Purposes of the clinical assessment

- Eliciting information
- Clinical history
- Appraisal of presenting symptoms
- Seeking confirmatory physical signs
- Arriving at a clinical formulation
- Arriving at a clinical decision
- Communicating findings to patient
- Eliciting patient support for plan of action

By the time many pain patients come to see an interdisciplinary team, they are confused and distressed, and the assessment of suitability for pain management can represent another ordeal, particularly for patients who are apprehensive about doctors or have difficulty in communicating their fears and anxieties. It is most important not to contribute further to their confusion or distress by failing to communicate the clinical formulation and associated decision clearly and unambiguously. If further information is required prior to arriving at a clinical decision, the reasons for this should be clearly explained. If possible, the patient's partner or friend should be invited to attend the feedback session. Some clinics have a patient 'advocate' such as a nurse who will explain the outcome of the assessment in more detail to patients after the formal clinic interview. It is also good practice to summarise the clinical formulation and associated treatment decision to all interested parties in the form of a letter.

Patient objectives for interview

As has been already stated, almost all patients, if given a choice, would elect for a cure over and above all other possible outcomes. By the time chronic pain patients are referred to pain clinics, however, they may no longer believe that a cure is possible, and may present with a number of other, or additional, requirements. A summary of the most important patient objectives are shown in Box 3.8.

Box 3.8 Patient objectives for interview

- Obtaining cure or symptomatic relief
- Seeking diagnostic clarification
- Seeking reassurance
- Seeking 'legitimisation' of symptoms
- Expressing distress, frustration or anger

Obtaining cure or symptomatic relief

Pain is the single most common presenting complaint to hospitals. Direct referral from general practitioners, or re-referral to a pain clinic from other specialists, is often couched specifically in terms of pain relief or sometimes complete cure. This may have been 'promised' to patients, possibly in an attempt to get them to agree to the referral. In the majority of cases such an outcome is unattainable.

Seeking diagnostic clarification

Seeking diagnostic clarification is almost equally important. Any competent pain clinic should attempt to offer this. In pain management programmes in particular, clarification of the presenting characteristics in terms of the biological, psychological and socio-occupational dimensions is fundamental both in terms of specifying possible treatment targets (Ch. 13) as well as in identifying obstacles to recovery (Chs 8–11).

Seeking reassurance

Some patients are primarily seeking reassurance. They may have come to terms with the fact that there is no cure for their chronic pain. They may wish simply to confirm that there is no serious pathology (such as cancer) that has been missed, or that there has been no new treatment developed that would be of assistance to them. While it is often easy to reassure such patients, a thorough assessment should none the less be provided.

Seeking 'legitimisation' of symptoms

If patients have seen a large number of specialists, and been offered a wide range of different diagnoses, they may develop significant iatrogenic confusion and distress (Ch. 5). The intensity of such distress can be magnified by the medicolegal process, in which claimants may read reports expressing doubt about the validity of their symptoms or even describing themselves as malingerers. Alternatively, they may have heard doubts expressed by members of their family about the genuineness of their pain-associated symptoms. They may even have

begun to worry themselves that the persistence of their pain may be indicative of psychological disorder. In reassuring patients, it is important to identify the origin of the seeds of doubt. The powerful influence of the family has already been addressed earlier in this chapter. If the family are suspicious, it will be important to communicate also with them. Satisfactory 'legitimisation' of symptoms is a prerequisite for pain management.

Expressing distress, frustration or anger

By the time they are assessed in pain clinics, chronic pain patients may have developed significant distress and disaffection with health-care professionals. Referral to a tertiary centre specialising in interdisciplinary pain management may have necessitated a long wait before being seen. Whatever the reasons for the patient's distress, frustration or anger, it is important to give the patient time to express it. Preliminary questionnaires may have indicated a high level of emotion. Frequently emotionally charged issues are raised or become apparent only at the time of the initial interview. It is important to be empathic without becoming overtly supportive of an excessively negative view of previous treatment. It is important to remember of course that, in cases of medical negligence, patients have every right to redress. It should be made clear, however, that the purpose of the clinical assessment is to offer them appropriate advice or treatment, and not to offer an opinion whose prime purpose is to serve as part of a legal claim. If necessary, this should be made explicit (Chs 4, 11 and 12).

Factors affecting communication

Communication can be viewed from two distinct perspectives: either from a technical sociopsychological perspective, focusing primarily on the nature of the communication process, or from a psychotherapeutic perspective in which the emotional components of the doctor–patient relationship become the key ingredients of the therapeutic exchange. A number of the

---

Box 3.9 Factors affecting communication

- Verbal:
  - clarity
  - complexity
- Non-verbal:
  - general demeanour
  - eye contact
  - signalling continued attention
- Meshing of verbal and non-verbal signals
- Aspects of the therapeutic relationship:
  - practical considerations
  - familiarity
  - liking
  - trust
  - importance of the 'placebo response'

---

elements of communication (viewed from both perspectives) are shown in Box 3.9.

Communication characteristics

Analysis of communication has become almost a science in itself. It will be possible to consider only some of the major features in this chapter. Detailed analyses of communication using the NFCS (Grunau & Craig 1990) described earlier have illuminated understanding particularly of non-verbal communication of pain. As reported earlier, researchers have found striking similarities between newborn and adult facial responses to events that are painful to adults. An important finding of such research studies has been the importance of context. Development of florid pain behaviours can best be understood in a social context within which chronic pain behaviour patterns are displayed alongside a number that may be more 'context dependent' and 'triggered' by the consultation process itself. In clinical situations, during the course of a clinical assessment a vast quantity of social signals are emitted. The information has to be somehow integrated into a clinical opinion.

Verbal characteristics. A common language is a prerequisite for good communication. Special efforts need to be made to ensure adequate communication with patients who have a different first language. Interpreters may be needed. Where standardised questionnaires

comprise part of the assessment procedure, care should be taken to validate the questionnaires properly. Cultural differences in the meaning of pain are recognised (see above), but careful elucidation of their precise significance may necessitate a qualitative rather than a quantitative approach (Chew–Graham 1999).

In addition to consideration of the meaning of the words used, the complexity of the communication must also be addressed. Wherever possible, clear and simple sentences should be used. The time for interview is frequently constrained and patients may recall only the major points. Opinions should be stated clearly and the patient's understanding should be confirmed. It should be noted in passing that patients will tend to recall the points of most emotional significance, sometimes to the neglect of other important topics. (When one of our patients was told by a previous doctor that 'I am sure everything is all right, but I would like to ask Mr X., the consultant neurosurgeon, to have a look at you', she completely forgot the first part of the sentence and became convinced that she had been told she probably had a brain tumour.)

Non-verbal aspects of communication. There are many non-verbal aspects of communication and only some of the more important will be highlighted here. It should be recognised, however, that these can have a very powerful influence on the whole interaction. Many patients are apprehensive about consulting health-care professionals. Patients can be encouraged or discouraged in their presentation of symptoms simply by the professional's general demeanour. The power of 'social signalling' is perhaps most easily recognised amongst young people attempting to develop an intimate relationship. Establishment of eye contact and signalling interest by expression, orientation and reducing interpersonal distance are only some of the cues or signals learned in the socialisation process. Signals can of course be misunderstood.

In doctor–patient communication, the importance of establishing eye contact and signalling attention and willingness to listen are particularly important. Patients who are apprehensive about the encounter may become particularly aware of apparent 'mismatch' between cues (where for example the professional states interest, but communicates the opposite in terms of body language).

Meshing of verbal and non-verbal signals. Satisfactory meshing of verbal and non-verbal signals and keeping the discussion flowing (with appropriate reassurance or encouragement) are important in the facilitation of communication.

The therapeutic relationship. Communication can also be considered in terms of its emotional characteristics. Many encounters with primary care personnel are straightforward, focused and not particularly emotionally loaded. Chronic pain, however, is frequently accompanied by 'emotional baggage' and chronic disability is often best characterised as a 'psychologically mediated chronic pain syndrome'. The distress that accompanies chronic pain can be viewed from many aspects. Whatever its precise configuration, however, the level of distress can have a markedly inhibiting effect on self-disclosure, and thus compromise a clear assessment.

Practical considerations can have a powerful limiting effect on the quality of the therapeutic relationship. Making adequate time available for consultation and ensuring confidentiality (in terms of both records and privacy) are prerequisites of a good therapeutic context, although, as observed recently by Chew–Graham (1999), the typical 8–10 minute general practice interview is ill suited to a more than rudimentary exchange.

Many people find it difficult to disclose their feelings to others. In the assessment of chronic pain patients it is essential to facilitate this process. Although it may not be essential for patients actually to like their health-care professionals, it is important that they respect and trust them. Appropriate confirmation or clarification of the particular professional role may facilitate this process.

Studies of the 'placebo response' have demonstrated the importance of so-called 'non-specific effects' in treatment. Characteristics of the therapist seem to be amongst the more important of these (Richardson 1994). The same considerations should be borne in mind in establishing a satisfactory context for therapeutic exchange.

> **Box 3.10**   Potential influences on professional judgement
>
> - Technical skill:
>   — accuracy in identification of physical signs
>   — estimation of severity
>   — integration of elements
> - Prejudical biases:
>   — race, culture and gender
>   — nature of symptoms
>   — patient's clinical history
>   — ongoing litigation

Potential influences on professional judgement

Clinical decision making requires the integration of information of bewildering complexity. Studies on the interrater reliability of individual clinical signs have demonstrated that, even in the assessment of so-called objective physical signs, clinicians can vary considerably in their judgement (Waddell & Main 1984). There are two principal types of influence on clinical judgement: technical skill and prejudicial bias. Details of these are shown in Box 3.10.

Technical accuracy

Differences in the frequency with which certain features are identified by different raters indicate that raters differ in skill, in the way in which they are applying criteria and in prejudicial bias. There may be differences in the identification of specific clinical features, in estimation of their impact (or severity), or in their integration into a composite clinical grading or judgement. Many clinicians are unaware of their inaccuracies in assessment. Technical problems can be improved with training to criterion. (In clinical research trials for example it is customary to train interviewers or raters until they have reached an acceptable degree of consistency, see Ch 17)

Prejudicial biases

For the purpose of this chapter inconsistency in judgement will be examined from the standpoint of prejudicial bias, which can influence the judgement of the clinician irrespective of the symptoms the patient presents or of the manner in which they are presented.

Race, culture and gender. Deliberate discrimination on the ground of race, culture or gender is illegal. Unconscious or unwitting bias is harder to detect. Differences in diagnostic rates, in clinical features or in selection for different sorts of treatment may indicate such bias. It is important of course to examine referral patterns, as such a selected subgroup may have been referred. Comparisons within the team can, however, be made to determine whether clinicians indicate preferential bias of whatever sort.

Nature of symptoms. Clinicians may differ in the interpretation they place on different sorts of symptoms, or on the manner in which they are presented. Evidence of distress during clinical assessment may lead certain clinicians to pay insufficient attention to other aspects of symptom presentation and clinical history. Florid demonstration of pain behaviour may be viewed inherently with suspicion. This phenomenon is well illustrated in the medicolegal field in the interpretation of behavioural responses to examination (Main & Waddell 1998). Routine audit of decision making should indicate whether different clinicians place different weightings in arriving at an overall clinical judgement.

Patient's clinical history. It may become quickly apparent that a particular consultation is only the latest in a long 'patient career'. Expression of anger about previous healthcare encounters may make clinicians disinclined to be sufficiently objective in their assessment. If a treatment has not worked, it is easy to blame the patient. However, the patient may have been willing to undergo treatment and have been fully compliant with it. The treatment itself may have been ineffective, inappropriate or frankly contraindicated.

Ongoing litigation. In an increasing litigious society, because of the length of time until litigation is sometimes concluded, a significant number of pain patients may be still involved in litigation at the time of initial assessment. Determination of whether litigation should be considered a barrier to improvement can be difficult (Chs 11 and 12), but should not be taken as an excuse for an inadequate assessment.

Patient factors affecting self-disclosure

Clinical judgement has to be based on the best possible quality of information. The richest source of information is the patient. Patients' perception of their symptomatology and the interpretation they place on it are the cornerstones of modern pain management. Elicitation of the impact of pain on self-confidence, on relationships with others, on physical intimacy and on quality of life requires sensitivity on the part of the assessor. It is important to be aware therefore of a number of factors that can inhibit self-disclosure. These are shown in Box 3.11.

Box 3.11 Patient factors affecting self-disclosure

- Expectations
- Misunderstandings
- Nature of previous consultations
- Distress
- Fear
- Anger

Patient expectations

It is important, first and foremost to clarify the patient's initial expectations from the assessment. If some information has not already been obtained from questionnaires filled in by the patient, doctors need to clarify the issue at the outset of the interview. They should not assume that a third party (such as a referring doctor) has fully determined this.

Misunderstandings

It is equally important to address misunderstandings that may have arisen concerning the purpose, timing or content of the assessment. Dealing competently and promptly with such misunderstandings is important in establishing trust.

Nature of previous consultations

If doctors have a clear referral letter, and have obtained all relevant previous medical records, they may believe that there is little need to discuss the nature of previous consultations with the patient. It is important, however, to confirm the accuracy of the information that has been made available, and identify any discordance between the patient's perception of these encounters and those of the professional involved. A specific appraisal of their clinical history may be important not only regarding matters of fact, but also in terms of the emotional impact.

Distress

Many patients show evidence of distress. The reasons are not always immediately apparent. It is important to encourage distressed patients to clarify their concerns. This may take tact and patience. All clinical staff participating in pain management programmes have to be able to facilitate self-disclosure in chronic pain patients (Ch. 13). Videotaped training is recommended.

Fear

Patients may appear to be fearful. They may worry that they have significant structural damage or pathology that has been missed, that they are becoming mentally unstable or that they will become a permanent invalid. It is essential to establish a relationship with patients such that they feel able to disclose such fears. (Assessment directed specifically at fear of further injury is discussed in Chs 10 and 18.)

Anger

As indicated in Chapter 2, many chronic pain patients present with a mixture of emotions. Establishing a therapeutic climate with angry or hostile patients can be particularly difficult. As with the assessment of distress and fear, it is important to try to find out particularly what patients are angry about. They will usually tell the doctor. If it is a matter over which the doctor might have been expected to have some control, an appropriate apology should be made. If the matter lies outside the doctor's control, empathy should be shown as appropriate. Usually the doctor will be unable to right the wrongs of the past. The task, in the context of a clinical assessment, is rather to try to help patients to 'move forward'. Some patients can be 'defused' successfully at the time of the initial assessment. Others need the support of a therapeutic group. Doctors will have to decide whether the intensity or focus of anger can be dealt with therapeutically or whether it constitutes a major obstacle to rehabilitation.

Special features of different professional encounters

Finally, it is important to recognise that there are some differences in the social psychology of assessment in different sorts of assessment and therapeutic clinics. Encounters will differ not only in the specific objectives of the encounter, but also in patients' expectations of it. In general, however, the same principles regarding communication still apply. Whatever the purpose of the assessment, the trust of patients must be established, the purpose of the assessment agreed and a therapeutic style and context designed to maximise self-disclosure must be employed. A number of practical recommendations likely to lead to more successful interviews, particularly for single-handed practitioners, are offered in Chapter 18.

Overview of the nature of communication

It is hard to overemphasis the importance of focused, sensitive and skilled communication in the assessment of chronic pain patients. In most professions, such skills are not taught to a satisfactory level. New staff joining pain management teams frequently appear bemused about the nature of the interactions in which they find themselves. In the context of psychologically mediated chronic pain syndromes, attention to the communication process itself is as fundamental, as is the use of nuclear magnetic resonance (NMR) in the determination of structural damage. Individual communication skills are essential in careful assessment. Competent interdisciplinary clinical decision making requires furthermore adequate communication among members of the interdisciplinary pain management team. Finally, feedback to the patient at the conclusion of the clinical assessment often represents a critical moment in the patient career. Turning the patient from passive 'doctor shopping' towards active self-directed pain management sometimes requires finely tuned communication skills.

CONCLUSION

Experience of pain and response to it can be understood only within the individual's social and cultural framework. Beliefs about the nature of pain have a powerful influence on adjustment to pain and the development of incapacity. In addressing the impact of chronic pain within the context of pain management, it is important to consider not only the *content* of communication but also the *process* of communication. Consideration of the social factors may illuminate clinical history and help understand the patient's response to assessment. Furthermore, establishment of an appropriate 'atmosphere' or social climate is a prerequisite in gaining the confidence of the patient and in facilitating self-disclosure. Finally, social factors can also have a powerful influence on response to treatment, not

KEY POINTS

- Cultural and subcultural differences in the perception of pain and response to it need to be understood in terms of the underlying socialisation mechanisms and how they affect the individual.
- Social learning influences the meaning and significance ascribed to pain, communication about it, response to treatment and the development of pain coping.
- Evaluation of pain and disability and consideration for pain management need to include the influence of age.
- Differences in pain perception and response to treatment may be considered in terms of both biologically based sex differences as well as socially developed gender differences. In matters of general pain management, the latter appear to be of more importance.
- There may be a complex and significant role of the patient's family and social

network in understanding of pain and perpetuation of disability.
- Anger and oversolicitousness among members of patients' families may represent powerful obstacles to recovery if not addressed therapeutically.
- The sociopsychological factors involved in professional–patient communication need to be identified, understood and managed appropriately.
- Communication needs to be considered in terms of both the technical aspects of communication as well as the therapeutic perspective.
- Potential influences on professional judgement need to be recognised.
- Patient factors affecting self-disclosure also need to be addressed.
- Special features of different types of professional encounters may need to be recognised.

only in the context of group interventions, but also in the influence of staff and significant others, whether in the maintenance or enhancement of treatment gains or as contributory factors to lack of progress or relapse. (The influences on

treatment and outcome will be considered more fully in later chapters of the book.)

A number of key points and recommendations have emerged from this review of cultural and social factors. They are summarised opposite.

REFERENCES

Anderson R T 1984 An orthopaedic ethnography in rural Nepal. Medical Anthropology 8:46–59

Burton A K, Tillotson K M, Main C J, Hollis S 1995 Psychosocial predictors of outcome in acute and subchronic low back trouble. Spine 20:722–728

Chew-Graham C A 1999 Chronic low back pain: the interface between explanatory models of illness and medical communications. M D Thesis, University of Manchester, Manchester

Consumer's Association 1985 Back pain survey Consumer's Association, London

Craig K D, Prkatchin K M, Grunau R V E 1992 The facial expression of pain. In: Turk D C, Melzack R (eds) Handbook of pain assessment. Guilford, New York, pp 257–276

Croft P, Joseph S, Cosgrove S et al 1994 Low back pain in the community and in hospitals. A report to the Clinical Standards Advisory Group of the Department of Health. Arthritis and Rheumatism Council Epidemiology Research Unit, University of Manchester

Crook J 1993 Comparative experiences of men and women who have sustained a work-related musculoskeletal injury (abstract). Proceedings of the 7th world congress on pain. P293–294. IASP Press, Seattle WA

CSAG (Clinical Standards Advisory Group) 1994 Report on Back Pain. HMSO, London

Fillingim R B, Maixner W 1995 Gender differences in the responses to noxious stimuli. Pain Forum 4:209–221

Folkman S, Lazarus R 1980 An analysis of coping in a middle-aged community sample. Journal of Health and Social Behaviour 21:219–240

Grunau R V E, Craig K D 1990 Facial activity as a measure of neonatal pain expression. In: Tyler D C, Krane E J (eds) Advances in pain research and therapy. Raven, New York, vol 15, pp 147–155

Honeyman P T, Jacobs E A 1996 Effects of culture on back pain in Australian aboriginals. Spine 21:841–843

IASP 1997 The curriculum on pain for students in psychology. IASP, Seattle

Klonoff E A, Landrine H. Brown M A 1993 Appraisal and response to pain may be a function of its bodily function. Journal of Psychosomatic Research 37:661–670

Lazarus R, Folkman S 1984 Stress appraisal and coping. Springer-Verlag, New York

Magni G, Caldieron C, Rigatti-Luchini S, Merskey H 1990 Chronic musculoskeletal pain and depressive symptoms in the general population. An analysis of the 1st National Health and Nutrition Examination Survey data. Pain 43:299–307

Main C J, Waddell G 1998 Behavioural responses to examination: a re-appraisal of the interpretation of 'non-organic signs'. Spine 23:2367–2371

Mechanic D 1977 Illness behaviour, social adaptation and the management of illness. Journal of Nervous and Mental Diseases 165:79–87

Mechanic D 1986 The concept of illness behaviour: culture, situation and personal predisposition. Psychological Medicine 16:1–7

Polleri A 1992 Pain and sex steroids. In: Sicuteri F (ed) Advances in pain research and therapy. Raven New York, vol 20, pp 253–259

Richardson P H 1994 Placebo effects in pain management. Pain Reviews 1:15–32

Rudy T, Kerns R D, Turk D C 1988 Chronic pain and depression: a cognitive-mediation model. Pain 35:129–140

Sanders S, Brena S F, Spier C J, Beltrutti D, McConnell H, Quintero O 1992 Chronic low back pain patients around the world; cross cultural similarities and differences. Clinical Journal of Pain 8:317–323

Skevington S 1997 Psychology of pain. John Wiley, Chichester

Unruh A 1996 Review article: gender variations in clinical pain experience. Pain 65:123–167

Volinn E 1997 The epidemiology of low back pain in the rest of the world, a review of surveys in low and middle income countries. Spine 22:1747–1754

Waddell G. 1998 The back pain revolution. Churchill Livingstone, New York

Waddell G, Main C J 1984 Assessment of severity in low back disorders. Spine 9:204–208

4

Economic and occupational influences on pain and disability

Chris J. Main   A. K. Burton

INTRODUCTION

In the last chapter social influences on perception of pain, response to pain and the treatment process were considered. The social element of the biopsychosocial model (Ch. 5) and of the yellow flags initiative (Ch. 18), however, includes work. In this chapter, following a brief overview of economic influences on pain and response to treatment, the influences of occupational factors will be considered specifically. The primary focus will be on low back pain, for which the clearest picture is available (although clearer data recently have begun to emerge on upper limb disorders).

THE ECONOMIC IMPACT OF PAIN AND DISABILITY

Prior to the 1980s, clinical studies had highlighted the costs of chronic pain and disability to both the individual and society. Most such studies, however, were based in tertiary care facilities on chronic pain patients with significant levels of pain-associated functional incapacity. Indeed many of the early North American clinics were funded with the specific intention of returning individuals to productive work (Ch. 6). It was not, however, till the advent of population-based reports such as the Nuprin pain report (Taylor & Curran 1985) in the USA and the Consumer's Association report (Consumer's Association 1985) in the UK that a clearer picture began to emerge of the incidence and prevalence of pain

---

Box 4.1 Applications of epidemiology

- Health service planning
- Working of the health service
- Identification of syndromes
- Natural history of painful syndromes
- Prevention of disease

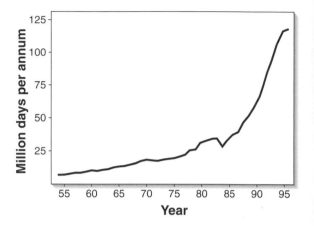

Figure 4.1 Trends in UK sickness and invalidity benefits for back pain. From Waddell The Back Pain Revolution 1998, Fig. 5.9 p. 83, based on statistics from the DSS, reproduced with permission.

in the community. The use of epidemiological methods such as surveys, cohort studies and case-control studies have since increased the accuracy of the information. Crombie (1999) has identified five distinct applications of epidemiology in the field of pain. These are shown in Box 4.1.

Of particular relevance at this juncture are the third and fourth of these (identification of syndromes and natural history of painful symptoms) since clarification of the nature of the disorders in the context of natural history allows a more accurate evaluation of specific economic and occupational impacts. In terms of economic impact specifically, most attention has been directed at low back pain (Linton 1998, Spitzer, Leblanc & Dupuis 1987) and, slightly more recently, at soft tissue injuries of the neck such as whiplash injuries and other upper limb disorders such as repetitive strain injury.

In the USA, for example, the cost of treating low back pain in 1991 was estimated at several billion dollars and, according to Deyo et al (1991), expenditure for low back pain was six times higher than for AIDS-related ill health. Van Tulder, Koes & Boulter (1995) estimated that the cost of back pain alone in the Netherlands was equivalent to about 1.7% of the gross national product (GNP). Even more striking was their finding that, of the costs incurred, only 7% of the expenditure was spend on actual health care, but 93% of the total was spent on the indirect costs of absenteeism and disability. Nachemson & Jonsson (2000) reported a similar ratio of direct/indirect costs in Sweden.

Differences in ways of estimating prevalence and cost make it difficult to obtain a precise estimate of the true costs of pain-associated impairment in performance and actual work loss, but the

economic burden is considerable A detailed analysis of economic impact is found in Waddell (1998, Ch. 5). Of particular concern has been the increasing trend in costs over the last 40 years. The UK sickness and invalidity benefits for back pain are shown in Figure 4.1. It should be acknowledged, however, that the overall trends in social security costs have not been clearly established.

The overall economic impact of musculoskeletal pain is considerable because, in addition to the costs of health-care provision, there are the costs of wage replacement, compensation and lost productivity. The position was summarised by Linton (1994, p. 164) thus: 'It is extraordinarily expensive to compensate sufferers for work loss because of pain and there is a tremendous disproportion of expenditures where the vast majority is spent on compensation'. The burden of the apparent epidemic is now widely recognised and there have been a range of different policy initiatives designed to prevent back pain becoming chronic, both in health-care and in occupational settings. (Chs 18 and 19). However, in considering the impact on the individual alone, the true economic impact may not always be appreciated. Goosens et al (1996), in a study of costs of fibromyalgia using a patient cost diary, found that only 51% of the total health-care expenditure was accounted for by direct health-care costs such as consultations and prescribed treatment, whereas the personal costs and out-of-pocket expenses accounted for 49%. In pain management, in the context of clinical decision making, it is essential to appreciate the influence of economic factors on the individual presenting for treatment and the possible effect on patients' participation in and response to treatment.

THE NATURE OF ECONOMIC FACTORS

As highlighted above, economic costs of pain can be considered at an individual as well as at a societal level. For a particular individual, the economic effects of pain and pain-associated incapacities can vary from the inconsequential to the catastrophic. The most powerful economic influences can be seen when individuals are compromised in their ability to work, but the economic impact on a particular individual will depend on a number of factors such as those shown in Box 4.2.

In a sense, for a particular individual, the overall economic impact can be most simply understood in terms of the *net costs of sickness*. The real costs may not be perceived by individuals until they actually find themselves in the situation. They may have made inadequate financial provision, or even no provision at all for such an eventuality. In the event of significant injury, pessimism about being able to obtain further employment may be considerable. It is not uncommon to find distress bordering on panic and despair amongst individuals who perceive their job to be at risk because of their sickness record. Response to painful injury is affected not only by the perception of pain and expectation of outcome of treatment, but also by attitudes

towards work and perceived entitlements in the event of work-related incapacity (whether temporary or permanent). Cross-culturally, there are major differences in social policy affecting injured workers.

THE RELATIONSHIP BETWEEN PAIN, INCAPACITY AND BENEFITS

Back pain as a biopsychosocial phenomenon can be considered from a variety of perspectives:

- from a *health-care* perspective, back pain is not a disease but a common bodily symptom, and chronic low back disability depends more on psychosocial factors than on physical pathology
- from an *epidemiological* perspective, back pain is not a discrete health problem, but is often associated with other pains, stresses and social problems
- from a *social* perspective, incapacity for work and pain-associated benefits have to be understood in the context of a country's economy and employment opportunities.

Over the last 30 years, however, as mentioned above, there has been a steady increase in the number of people on disability or incapacity benefits, and in the length of time people stay on benefits, *in the absence of any evidence of a corresponding increase in physical disease or impairment.* Furthermore, there has been a huge increase in the number of people being awarded retirement on health grounds, particularly non-specific low back pain. Improved clinical management has had no apparent beneficial impact on these social security trends. Significant alleviation of the increasing economic burden of back pain may require fundamental changes in levels of employment, in social policy and in cultural attitudes and behaviour about sickness. In does appear that sickness and incapacity benefit cannot be considered in isolation. In terms of clinical practical management the power of economic influences has to be recognised and an assessment of the significance of such factors has to form part of clinical decision making (Chs 11 and 12).

Box 4.2   Factors affecting the economic impact of inability to work

- Current financial commitments
- Length of work loss
- Entitlement to various benefits
- Insurance in the event of sickness
- Alternative sources of income

The psychological impact of economic factors will be addressed in the next section.

INFLUENCE OF ECONOMIC FACTORS ON THE INDIVIDUAL WITH PAIN

Economic hardship resulting from unemployment is well recognised, but an individual's economic situation can also directly influence treatment seeking and response to treatment. It also has to be taken into account as part of the assessment of the patient (Ch. 11) and in clinical decision making about whether or when to offer pain management (Ch. 12). The major spheres of influence are summarised in Box 4.3.

Box 4.3 Possible adverse effects of economic factors

- Increase in personal stress
- Increase in family hardship
- Strain on relationships
- Treatment seeking and legitimisation of symptoms
- Acceptance of treatment by the patient
- Acceptance or rejection for treatment by the health-care professional

---

Increase in personal stress

As highlighted in Chapter 2, pain itself can be considerably stressful, particularly if it is disturbing sleep and affecting activity. The unpleasantness of the pain and demoralising effects of its limiting effects can be enhanced still further if it has a significant financial impact, whether in terms of ability to work, or in terms of quality of life.

Increase in family hardship

The economic impact may be felt not only by individuals, but also by their family. This can further enhance feelings of despair, frustration and sometimes guilt. As aforementioned, the family may or may not have the arrangements or opportunities to mitigate the economic impact.

Strain on relationships

Families of chronic pain patients sometimes seem to have made remarkable adjustments to mitigate financial loss without apparent strain on relationships, but even the strongest of relationships can be strained by economic adversity. Even if it is possible to mitigate the hardship, this may be only at the cost of placing a significant strain on relationships. Frequently, partners of the major breadwinner will feel obliged to increase their hours of work or find a new or better paid job to compensate for the shortfall. This may result in increasing tiredness, impaired quality of life and resentment at having to make major changes to the pattern of family life. There may be effects also on relationships with the extended family, if help with childcare becomes necessary in order to obtain further paid work.

Treatment seeking and legitimisation of symptoms

First and foremost, consultation with doctors is motivated by a search for a diagnosis and cure. There are, however, other factors affecting treatment seeking. Sick certification by a medical practitioner may be necessary for entitlement to benefits of various sorts. In the UK, self-certification is permitted for up to 5 days, after which medical ratification is required for entitlement to benefit. Employers vary in the amount of self-certification they will tolerate in an individual period before formal appraisal of health status is initiated, but it is certainly the case that legitimisation of the complaint is a major factor in consultation with doctors. In families under strain, particularly with prolonged sickness absences, doubts may have been raised about the 'legitimacy' of the pain, and whether patients are genuinely as incapacitated as they claim. (As discussed below, such doubts may have been raised within medicolegal reports.)

Acceptance of treatment

Many chronic pain patients find themselves in a difficult situation. They may be dependent on the receipt of sickness benefits or some sort of compensation to avoid desperate financial hardship. Improvement as a result of treatment may put incapacity-related benefits at risk. While it could be argued that such a situation requires a 'social policy solution', it can none the less represent a real dilemma for pain patients whose medical history may decrease their chance of re-employment, irrespective of re-establishment of their physical capacity and perceived ability to work. Sometimes their pessimism is a function of their lack of confidence, but there may be significant economic anxieties about embarking on rehabilitation without satisfactory guarantees.

Acceptance for treatment and response to treatment

Consideration of economic obstacles to recovery is also important in the context of clinical decision making (Chs 11 and 12). It may be that the development of integrated clinical and occupational programmes, both for work retention and for rehabilitation into work, will overcome some of these obstacles to recovery. On a large scale, changes in social policy in terms of sickness benefit and phased return to work may also be required (Ch. 19). Such matters are beyond the influence of pain clinicians and the team may have to decide whether such influences constitute a relative or an absolute barrier to acceptance for treatment. In the former case, if change in economic circumstances is anticipated, it may be decided to defer treatment. Sometimes, however, the power of the economic obstacles to recovery may be considered to be a contraindication to pain management.

THE SPECIAL INFLUENCE OF COMPENSATION AND LITIGATION

Arguably, few issues in clinical medicine generate as much emotion as the nature of pain and pain-associated incapacity in the context of personal injury litigation. Indeed many of the early investigations into chronic pain and its psychological features were addressed from a forensic perspective from which apparent mismatch between symptoms and signs and persistence of pain beyond expected healing time

was viewed with innate suspicion. Many chronic pain patients today find themselves embroiled in litigation, at the heart of which is the acceptance or not of chronic pain as a valid clinical phenomenon and, sometimes, the legitimacy of psychologically mediated chronic pain syndromes. Involvement in personal injury litigation can not only be distressing, but may also adversely affect acceptance for treatment and response to it (Ch. 11). A brief appraisal of the influence of litigation on chronic pain and pain-associated incapacity will therefore be undertaken. The issue is discussed more fully in previous articles by the present authors (Main 1999, Main & Spanswick 1995, Main & Waddell 1998).

History of personal injury (PI) litigation

Although it is possible to find award of damages for emotional distress as early as the 14th century, a significant increase in PI legislation followed the construction of the railways in the second half of the 19th century. Mendelson (1988) offers a fascinating account of the polarisation that developed between those who considered 'railway spine' to be due to an *organic* cause and those who viewed the condition as a type of 'nervous shock'. In a legal context the phrase 'nervous shock' has been used to refer to identifiable psychiatric illness and not simply to emotional states such as anxiety, sadness or grief, which were not considered to be injuries, and were not therefore compensable.

In the evaluation of painful injuries, there are a small number of key questions. These are outlined in Box 4.4.

Box 4.4 Key questions in the evaluation of painful injury

- Has the individual been injured?
- What is the nature of the injuries?
- Has the individual suffered a 'psychological injury'?
  — psychiatric disorder
  — post-traumatic stress disorder (PTSD)
  — depression
- Is there any neuropsychological impairment?
- Is the patient suffering from a chronic pain syndrome?

As discussed in Chapters 2 and 10, there are established diagnostic procedures such as DSM-IV (1994) for the determination of psychiatric injury. The term 'chronic pain syndrome' or CPS is more problematic. A number of different terms have been used to address painful symptoms that are not considered fully explicable on the basis of physical findings. At the simplest level, CPS can be used to describe the symptoms and effects of chronic pain. In this usage, the term is defined essentially by a time parameter, time course and a range of effects (e.g. on function). There is no particular imputation regarding the nature of the symptoms themselves. Usually, however, in using the term CPS one infers that aspects of the symptoms are psychological in nature and either have a psychosomatic origin predating the injury in question or are indicative of a type of 'psychological injury' that is attributable to the accident. As has been suggested previously (Main & Spanswick 1995), the term 'functional overlay' is often used simply as a diagnosis of exclusion, since it is assumed *ipso facto* that if the symptom pattern is not considered fully explicable on the basis of the underlying physical characteristics then it must be psychologically mediated. Such an assumption is unsafe unless psychological factors have specifically been investigated. We recommend that where such influences have been identified, the term 'psychologically mediated pain syndrome' is preferred to CPS. Where no such influences can be identified, the persistence of the pain has not been explained, and the issue may amount to taking a view about the credibility of the pain complaint, about which a forensic rather than a clinical opinion may be required. The term 'chronic pain syndrome' is now increasingly referred to in medicolegal reports. It now seems that chronic pain in certain circumstances may be considered as compensable in its own right and not simply as a mental illness deemed to have resulted from the accident. Since it would now be accepted that psychological factors are an important component of chronic pain, it could be argued that psychological features not fulfilling classical psychiatric criteria are *de facto* being judged to be compensable as a feature of chronic

incapacity. This issue is of more than academic importance. Pain sufferers engaging in litigation may find themselves the recipient of vigorous attempts to challenge the legitimacy of their symptomatology in relation to the injury in question, or even more vigorous attempts to undermine their credibility or veracity.

The effects of compensation and litigation

Introductory note

The terms 'compensation' and 'litigation' can be somewhat confusing, since their precise meaning differs across different countries and in differing economic systems. In some contexts, 'compensation' is used in the literature as synonymous with 'financial influence' and in other contexts seems to refer to 'involvement in adversarial litigation'. The term 'litigation' itself will differ in interpretation depending on whether or not there is a 'no-fault' compensation system and on whether the system is essentially adversarial in nature.

The term 'secondary gain' is frequently found in medicolegal reports. The term is actually Freudian in origin. It referred originally to emotional benefits resulting from illness, which were being presented as distressing or unpleasant. In its original sense the term did not refer to a perceived benefit sought by the individual. In the medicolegal context, the term frequently has a pejorative or unsavoury connotation and is taken to refer to supposed advantages, whether realised or anticipated, as a consequence of being involved in litigation. Technically, the term is often used to imply that the claimant is at best exaggerating symptoms or incapacity for financial gain, and at worst that the individual is actually fraudulent. In such a context the term may be used in support of an allegation of deliberate exaggeration or even malingering.

In fact, all sorts of adversity may have their compensations. As mentioned in the previous chapter, pain-associated incapacity may lead to changes in family patterns. Sometimes adversity brings couples closer together. Most claimants pursue compensation or litigation with some expectation of outcome. The desired outcome is not always financial, although in high value claims, particularly in the context of current poverty, it may be the dominant feature. Some litigants want justice of a different sort, such as the righting of a perceived injustice, 'legitimisation' of their continued disability, or even retribution. Pursuit of litigation should not be viewed as inherently suspicious. It may offer the best or only way out of a major predicament.

In fact, impaired quality of life and inability to work often represent such an adverse set of circumstances that it is hard to imagine that such a 'career path' would have been chosen simply in pursuit of anticipated financial gain. Outcome of litigation is uncertain and pursuit of it is stressful (see below). Furthermore, statistics would suggest that litigants are seldom much better off even from the specific financial point of view.

According to Erens & Ghate (1993), half of benefit claimants receive less than 50% of their previous earnings, and only one in eight receives more than 80% of previous net earnings. According to Waddell (1998, p. 217, 218):

Looking at their whole social situation, the vast majority of people off work with back pain are much worse off in many ways. Workers' compensation or other sickness benefits are a very inadequate replacement … The average job tenure in the USA is now less than 3 years. This has inevitably changed attitudes to work, employers and unemployment.

These changed attitudes are probably much more important than the actual level of compensation.

In a review of 32 studies mainly involving pain clinic patients, Rohling et al (1995) found a consistent increase in reported pain severity of about 6%, and consistently poorer outcomes, for compensation patients in comparison with non-compensation patients, although the size of the difference seems to vary widely across studies and may reflect at least in part other clinical and psychological factors. Thus, differences in selection and referral pattern may explain the differences.

The effects of compensation on claims, surgical outcome and rehabilitation are shown in Box 4.5.

In conclusion therefore, it would appear that compensation claimants have a somewhat poorer prognosis in response to treatment, but the magnitude of the effect varies in different studies, and frequently research design does not permit determination of the specific effect of compensation over and above other factors.

Claim of benefits, whether state accredited, insurance based or worker's compensation, may be the only recourse open to many individuals following personal injury. In the process of legitimisation of their claim, they meet with frustration and sometimes disappointment. Their difficulties are heightened if they become

---

Box 4.5 Effects of compensation

Effect of compensation level on claims
- There is no evidence that it changes the actual injury rate
- 10% increase in compensation level produces 1–11% increase in claims rate
- 10% increase in compensation level produces 2–11% increase in duration of disability
- This affects 'verifiable' injuries such as fractures as much as more subjective soft tissue injuries

Effects of compensation on surgical outcome
- Compensation patients are less likely to have a good result of back surgery
- These findings have been criticised:
  — these people often have heavier physical jobs

- — they may get overaggressive surgical intervention
- Despite this, more than 75% return to their previous work

Effects of compensation on rehabilitation outcome
- Compensation patients respond less well to pain management and rehabilitation
- These findings have been criticised:
  — there are methodological flaws in many of these studies: often small samples of highly selected patients with poor diagnostic criteria. Follow-up is poor. There is a failure to allow for other factors such as job demands
  — differences are small
- Despite this, many compensation patients do benefit

From Waddell The Back Pain Revolution 1998, Box 13.5, p. 219, reproduced with permission.

involved in adversarial litigation in which their injury is contested and they are therefore obliged to win their case by demonstrating that they have received injuries as a result of a negligent act by the other party. The personal impact of such litigation will now be discussed.

The personal impact of ongoing litigation

The psychological impact of engagement in adversarial litigation can be considerable, and if sufficiently marked may constitute a psychological obstacle to recovery (Ch. 11). Some of the major influences of ongoing litigation are summarised in Box 4.6.

Need for additional assessments

In cases of personal injury, the litigation process almost always requires the claimant to undergo additional examinations specifically for medicolegal purposes. These often include a physical examination, which can be painful. The purpose of the assessment is not always made clear, and not infrequently claimants may believe they are being assessed with the primary purpose of offering treatment. Claimants who are fearful of pain or further injury find the prospects of such an examination extremely alarming. Patients with a history of distressing encounters with health-care professionals also may find the prospects of assessment distressing. A proportion of patients may have been emotionally traumatised by the accident and its sequelae. Even though only a minority of patients will

report symptomatology of a nature and severity sufficient to constitute an unequivocal post-traumatic stress disorder, many find it emotionally difficult to recall the details of the accident or injury. Finally, the adversarial nature of litigation does not encourage good doctor–patient rapport during assessments carried out on behalf of defendants.

Contrasting clinical opinions

Contrasting clinical opinions are frequently evident in reports prepared for medicolegal purposes. This can be confusing and distressing for pain patients, and may become part of significant iatrogenic distress (Ch. 5).

Protracted nature of litigation

Completion of the process of litigation may take years. Patients often are bewildered and distressed about this. They cannot understand why this should be so, particularly in cases such as motor vehicle accidents in which liability is frequently accepted and completion of the case hinges only on the extent of damages. Some claimants become extremely angry with their legal advisers, whom they blame for the delay. As time passes by, claimants' coping strategies may become exhausted and they may abandon the claim.

Adverse influence on decision to treat

It is perhaps not always fully acknowledged that clinical decisions are influenced by the fact of ongoing litigation. Although it may in certain circumstances be sensible to defer treatment until the conclusion of litigation (Ch. 11), some doctors are unwilling even to see patients with ongoing litigation, far less offer them treatment. Some doctors appear to view claimants with considerable suspicion and the doctor–patient relationship can be adversely affected on both sides. A minority of claimants find themselves in a virtually impossible situation in which their legal advisers recommend further treatment before they are willing to conclude the case whereas the

---

Box 4.6 The personal impact of personal injury litigation

- Need for additional assessments
- Contrasting clinical opinions
- Protracted nature of litigation
- Adverse influence on decision to treat
- Attributions of exaggeration, faking and malingering
- Videotaped surveillance
- Self-confidence and distress
- Need to convince

relevant clinicians are unwilling to undertake such treatment until the conclusion of litigation.

Attributions of exaggeration, faking and malingering

Possibly the most distressing aspect of litigation for chronic pain patients is that they may find themselves subject to attributions of exaggeration, faking or even malingering. Attribution of malingering as such is a matter for the court and not for a medical expert (Mendelson 1988) but medical experts are frequently asked by solicitors to give a view on whether they consider plaintiffs to be exaggerating their symptoms or even faking incapacity. Some clinicians none the less seem to consider that judgments do lie within their province as experts and appear to have considerable confidence in their ability to do so. According to Faust (1995), however: 'some malingerers practice deception for a living, and can easily outmatch the physician who lacks the same type of experience, mental set and willingness for exploitation that sometimes characterises the professional con artist'.

In addition to clinical interviews that seem to cast doubt on the their genuineness, patients may be subject to more formal assessment methods, such as those shown in Box 4.7.

These methods are described in a detailed critical evaluation elsewhere (Main 1999, Main & Waddell 1998). For the purpose of this chapter it is necessary only to recognise that any form of evaluation in which pain patients feel their credibility to be under question can be significantly upsetting.

Box 4.7 Formal assessment methods employed in the detection of faking

- Diagnostic assessment according to psychiatric criteria
- Self-report measures designed specifically to detect faking
- Symptom validity testing
- Elicitation of behavioural responses to examination
- Polygraphy

Videotaped surveillance

In potentially high value claims, it is not uncommon for defendants to engage surveillance operators to undertake covert surveillance of the claimant. Claimants are frequently distressed to see secret videos taken of themselves engaging in a variety of activities, particularly if it casts doubt on their credibility. (They may be even more distressed if they become aware of the surveillance at the time it is being carried out.) Experts are frequently asked to give a view on whether the behaviour displayed on the videotape is consistent with their own assessment of the claimant. Indeed videotape evidence, if it clearly discredits the claimant, can represent the turning point in a case. This is usually only the case if the video evidence clearly and unambiguously contradicts the claimant's self-report. The scientific basis of videotaped evidence has not so far been sufficiently developed to determine when a sample of behaviour obtained on a video can be said to constitute a fair and representative sample of the behaviour concerned. Visual evidence none the less appears to exert a powerful influence on judges, particularly when confronted with a claimant reporting pain (which the judge cannot see) in circumstances when the two sides offer markedly different medical opinions.

Self-confidence and distress

From the aforementioned it is easy to understand how claimants can become highly distressed about the litigation process. They may believe they established good rapport with the assessing clinician and feel that the latter was 'on their side', until they gain sight of the report that has been produced. Usually they will not know that they have been the subject of videotape surveillance. They may find sensitive aspects of their personal history revealed in reports. They may find significance that they do not accept given to aspects of their musculoskeletal history. Finally, they may find themselves the subject of what they perceive as a 'character assassination', with attributions of inconsistency, lack of motivation to get better and even lying. They may come to have doubts themselves about the reality or legitimacy of their pain or associated incapacities.

Need to convince

With genuine claimants such an emotional onslaught as described above can lead to the firm conviction that no one believes them, and they need to convince doctors of their bona fides. Ill-advisedly, they may exaggerate in an attempt to convince. They may not be entirely aware of this. Even when it is clear that a conscious element is present, a distinction should be made between 'exaggeration with the intention to convince' and 'exaggeration with the attempt to deceive'. This distinction, however, can be extremely difficult to establish, and may need a detailed history of the patient's symptom presentation to previous assessors (both clinical and medicolegal).

Conclusion

Economic factors can have a profound influence on treatment seeking and response to treatment. Financial difficulties as a result of inability to work and the need for benefits to ensure some sort of limited financial security are frequently the most powerful effects of painful injuries. The distress associated with such difficulties can be magnified considerably in the context of adversarial litigation, such that the litigation process itself can short-circuit recovery. Much of the helplessness is associated with fears about the future course of symptoms and lack of confidence in return to work. The specific influence of occupational factors will be addressed in the next section.

OCCUPATIONAL PERSPECTIVES ON THE WORKING ENVIRONMENT
Introduction

Spitzer, Leblanc & Dupuis (1987) have documented the return-to-work rates of those with sick certification amongst those with activity-

---

Box 4.8 Return-to-work rates (cumulative percentages)

- Within 4 weeks   74%
- By 7 weeks   83%
- By 3 months   87%
- By 6 months   92%
- At greater than 6 months 8%

---

related spinal disorders. The rates are shown in Box 4.8.

The last group accounted for 76% of the total compensation costs and 21% of the total compensation costs for all injuries within the Quebec compensation system. A high proportion of such injuries are classed as low back pain. Internationally, the economic costs of sickness absence due to pain are best documented for low back pain. It is one of the commonest medical reasons for work loss in the UK and most Western countries (CSAG 1994). Duration of work loss and rate of return to work following an acute attack of back pain have been documented in a number of studies in various countries. In Sweden for example the percentage of employees sicklisted for low back pain has risen from 1 to 8% between 1970 and 1987; the average number of days of sickness has increased by about 70% (from 20 to 34 days) resulting in a massive increase in the cost of lost production (Andersson 1999). Differences in employment legislation and in social security systems make accurate costings very difficult and cross-cultural differences problematic. Watson et al (1997), in a study of the working population of the States of Jersey, found that the incidence and prevalence of medically certified work loss for back pain were 5.6 and 6.3% respectively, and the cost of wages compensation was 10.5% of such benefits paid. They found furthermore that the cost of recurrent episodes (as measured by reference to the index year) was significantly higher than costs of the initial episode. Whatever the difficulties in attempting specific comparisons across different occupational and legislative systems, the overall picture is clear. Occupational difficulties associated with musculoskeletal pain problems appear to be considerable, whether considered from the perspectives of the individual

---

> **Box 4.9**   Fundamental questions concerning work incapacity
>
> ---
>
> • What is the nature of injury?
> • What is the relationship between injury and chronic incapacity?
> • What can be done to prevent chronic incapacity?

sufferer, the employer or indeed the society as a whole. Given the advances in medical technology, and the quantity of research into biomechanics and ergonomics, this failure to arrest the rise in back-associated disability would appear to be surprising.

Three fundamental questions need to be addressed. These are shown in Box 4.9.

The circumstances of the injury can frequently be identified, but there is only a relatively weak relationship between physical impairment, pain and disability (Ch. 5). Of more interest is the second question, which will be addressed later in this chapter, and the third question, which will be addressed primarily in Chapter 19. In order to consider further the nature of chronic incapacity, we should like to offer a review of psychological influences on work and an appraisal of the determinants of sickness absence.

Psychological perspectives on work

An historical perspective

In the next section of this chapter, we are indebted to Carayon & Lim (1999) for a helpful and interesting review of the nature of psychosocial work factors.

Early attempts in scientific management focused primarily on work efficiency and the division of labour. Essentially, work was simplified and standardised leading to the design of repetitive and monotonous jobs within which skill variety was minimal and workers had no control over the work processes. As the workforce became more educated, however, individuals aspired to better working conditions and job design theorists began to incorporate human performance factors, including individual needs. Herzberg (1974), in developing *job enrichment theory*, distinguished 'intrinsic' factors relating to

the work conditions (such as degree of control, relationships and skill development) from 'extrinsic' factors (such as financial rewards or benefits and the physical environment). Hackman & Oldham (1976) similarly, in their *job characteristics theory*, advocated the view that specific characteristics of the job (such as skill variety, task significance and autonomy) in combination with individual characteristics (such as growth need strength) would determine personal and work outcomes. Finally, Davis (1980), in his development of *sociotechnical systems theory*, recommended a 'flattened' management structure that would promote participation, interaction amongst and across groups of workers, enriched jobs, and, most important, the meeting of individual needs. According to Carayon & Lim (1999) this theory offers the foundation for current understandings of the relationship between social and technical factors. Thus, although certain 'objective' work characteristics can be distinguished from 'perceived' work characteristics, different work organisations will produce very different psychosocial work factors, and so these factors need to be understood within specific contexts.

Stress and work

The nature of work stress has been a major focus of research. It has been implicated as a cause of sickness absence, and by implication, as a potential obstacle to return to work, particularly important in the context of recovery from injury (whether considered in terms of work rehabilitation or work retention).

Smith & Carayon-Sainfort (1989), in the *balance theory of job design*, identified five elements of the work system, which interacted to produce a 'stress load'. These are shown in Box 4.10.

> **Box 4.10**   Elements of the work system producing 'stress load'
>
> ---
>
> • The individual
> • Tasks
> • Technology and tools
> • Environment
> • Organisational factors

Box 4.11 Selected psychosocial work factors and their facets

- Job demands:
  - quantitative work load
  - variance in work load
  - work pressure
  - cognitive demands
- Job content:
  - repetitiveness
  - challenge
  - utilisation and development of skills
- Job control:
  - task/instrumental control
  - decision/organisational control
  - control over the physical environment
  - resource control
  - control over workplace; machine pacing

- Social interactions:
  - social support from supervisor and colleagues
  - supervisor complaint, praise, monitoring
  - dealing with (difficult) clients/customers
- Role factors:
  - role ambiguity
  - role conflict
- Job future and career issues:
  - job future ambiguity
  - fear of job loss
- Technology issues:
  - computer-related problems
  - electronic performance monitoring
- Organisational and management issues:
  - participation
  - management style

From Carayon & Lim Psychosocial work factors, In The Occupational Ergonomics Handbook edited by Karwowski & Marras 1999, p. 278, reproduced with permission.

According to this theory, psychosocial factors are multiple and diverse. The principal psychosocial work factors and their facets suggested by Carayon & Lim (1999) are shown in Box 4.11. These authors stress that such factors need to be understood in the context of societal changes in the economic, social, technological, legal and physical environments.

Specific models of work stress (adapted from Cox 1993).

Cox (1993) identifies three different but overlapping approaches to the definition and study of stress. His three major models are shown in Box 4.12.

According to the *'engineering'* model, stress is conceptualised as an aversive or noxious characteristic of the work environment and is construed essentially as an environmental *cause* of ill health. The model has been criticised on the grounds of oversimplicity, since specific stimuli such as noise may be stressful or beneficial depending on a number of other factors.

In the *'physiological'* model, stress is defined in terms of the physiological *response* to a threatening or dangerous environment. This model has been criticised because differences in physiological responses to the same stressor, and difficulties in identifying unambiguously responses that are

---

Box 4.12 Major models of stress

- The 'engineering' model
- The 'physiological' model
- The 'psychological' model

---

specifically stress responses (rather than orienting responses, for example). Both models have been criticised for ignoring individual differences in the cognitive and perceptual processing of information, and ignoring the interactions between individuals and their environment and organisational *contexts* of work stress.

Finally in a third model, the *'psychological'* model, stress is conceptualised in terms of the *dynamic interaction* between people and their work environment. Lack of fit between these, whether defined objectively or subjectively (in terms of the individual's perceptions) has been recognised as a potential stress (French, Rogers & Cobb 1974). In such 'transactional' models, stress involves elements of both cognition (such as appraisal) and emotion. The appraisal process may be thought of in five stages, beginning with no more than a hazy recognition of the existence of a problem and leading to an ongoing process of interaction between coping strategies, reappraisal and redefinition of the problem.

According to Cox (1993, p. 17): 'The experience of stress is therefore defined, first, by the realisation that they are having difficulties in coping with demands and threats to their well being and, second, that coping is important and the difficulty in coping depresses or worries them'.

Coping with occupational stress

Stress affects people differently. Whether or not they become ill appears to depend to a considerable extent on what they think about the stressor and how they cope with it. Researchers have studied individual differences both in the way stressors are perceived and also in the extent to which these appraisals might moderate the relationship between stress and health (Payne 1994). A number of characteristics of the psychological processes mentioned in the literature are shown in Box 4.13. They are addressed in much more detail elsewhere (Griffiths 1998).

As can be seen, a wide range of work organisational characteristics have been associated with stress, ill health and musculoskeletal disorders, but they are confounded with physical work load (Bongers et al 1993, Davis & Heany 2000, Vingaard & Nachemson 2000); most studies to date have been unable to quantify either their individual importance or specific interactions. Nevertheless, the available evidence provides most support for influence of the factors shown

in Box 4.14 (Bongers et al 1993, Vingaard & Nachemson 2000), and it seems that workers' reactions to psychosocial aspects of work may be more important than the actual aspects themselves (Davis & Heany 2000), with stress acting as an intermediary (Bongers et al 1993).

Common sense would suggest that, with such a wide variety of working circumstances and individual differences in the perception of work, it would be inappropriate to try to develop a concept that encompassed all such factors within a single model. From a more general viewpoint, it would appear that negative appraisals associated with ineffective coping strategies appear to lead to frustration, even anger, and to significant work stress, deterioration in health and absence from work. In the context of musculoskeletal injury, however, there appears to have been no specific research into either the appraisal of stress at work or strategies specifically for coping with stress at work.

Box 4.14   Work organisational factors most clearly associated with occupational stress/musculoskeletal disorders

- High demand and low control
- Time pressure/monotonous work
- Lack of job satisfaction
- Unsupportive management style
- Low social support from colleagues
- High perceived work load

Box 4.13   Psychological features associated with poor health and well-being

- Working under time pressures
- Having too much or too little to do
- Monotonous tasks and too little variety
- Long working hours
- Poor communication systems
- Organisational change
- Lack of understanding of organisational structure or goals
- Lack of participation in decision making
- Lack of control (e.g. over work methods, pace or work environment)
- Inadequate and unsupportive supervision
- Poor relationship with coworkers

- Bullying, harassment and violence
- Isolated or solitary work
- Job insecurity
- Career stagnation
- Lack of recognition and feedback
- Unfair or unclear performance evaluation
- Being overskilled or underskilled for the job
- Unclear or conflicting roles
- Continuously dealing with other people's problems
- Conflicting demands of work and home

From Griffiths 1998, pp 217–218, reproduced with permission.

Conclusion: what lessons can be learned from the occupational stress literature?

The organisational stress literature has been important in the identification of adverse features of the working environment. Many different organisational characteristics have been associated with ill health, sickness absence or impaired productivity. Certain characteristics of the working environment appear to constitute risk factors in their own right, but it seems that *perceptual* factors may be even more important than objective characteristics. Most jobs have irritating, difficult or stressing features, which can be thought of as risk factors for sickness or ill health. Individuals, however, vary in their reaction to difficult circumstances or adversities and the extent to which a specific individual copes with such risk factors will influence job satisfaction, morale and psychological well-being. The principal lessons from the occupational stress literature are shown in Box 4.15.

In recovery from musculoskeletal injury, an adverse view of work may become an additional obstacle to return to work.

CURRENT CONCEPTS IN PREVENTION AND REHABILITATION

Identification of psychological features of work, and in particular the relationship between work

---

Box 4.15 Lessons from the occupational stress literature

- Aspects of work can have an adverse psychological impact in terms of stress
- Work stress can adversely affect health and lead to sickness absence
- A number of the key influences on health have been identified
- Coping styles and strategies may mediate or moderate the relationship between work stress, ill health and work absence
- Perception of work may be more important than actual working conditions or characteristics
- There has, however, been no systematic research into the relationship between occupational stress, musculoskeletal symptomatology and recovery from injury

---

stress and ill health, does not appear to have had a significant influence on the management of musculoskeletal symptoms or in the managment of injury. Currently, management appears to have been considered primarily from a biomechanical or ergonomic perspective.

Biomechanical and ergonomic perspectives

Burton (1997, p. 2575) has highlighted an apparent contradiction in the way in which occupational injury is viewed and managed: 'On the one hand, ergonomists and biomechanists strive to reduce physical stress in the work place with the intent of lowering the risk of musculoskeletal problems, while clinical scientists and psychologists are suggesting not only that psychological factors are important, but that rehabilitation of the back-injured worker should involve physical challenges to the musculoskeletal system.' This dilemma illustrates not only a management problem, as Burton asserts, but also illustrates a fundamental conflict in models of injury. At the heart of the debate lies the nature of mechanisms of chronicity.

The basic 'injury/damage' model is based on the commonly held view that physically demanding work is detrimental to the back in the sense that it can cause injury through sudden or cumulative trauma, and the injury in turn leads to pain and disability. Much clinical and nonclinical scientific research has been directed at the nature of injury and the possible underlying mechanisms. There have been many variants on the basic themes, but in the field of occupational injury the primary focus has been on biomechanical analysis of the physical stresses sustained during various movements or postures under various conditions of load. It might appear that there ought to be a direct relationship between the physical demands of work and the occurrence of injury, but in fact there are significant inconsistencies in the scientific literature (Burton & Main 2000a).

Certainly there is evidence of increased risk of work-related disorders affecting the back, neck and upper limbs with certain types of work, but not all workers become injured, and certainly not all become significantly disabled. Marras et al (1993) found that risk of musculoskeletal symptoms could be predicted from a combination of five trunk motion and workplace risk factors, but as not all jobs with high injury rates require the same physical abilities (Halpern 1992) the relationship between these risk factors and actual injury is not straightforward.

There is, however, evidence that many workers *perceive* their musculoskeletal symptoms to be work related. In a recent UK survey (Jones et al 1998) of individuals reporting musculoskeletal symptoms, nearly 80% identified a work task, or set of tasks, as leading to their complaint. The evidence seems to show that the back can certainly be injured in various ways (whether at work or leisure), but the 'injury model' is not able to explain the wide variation in resultant disability.

The primary focus of the biomechanical and ergonomic perspective has been on prevention. There have been energetic attempts to improve the working environment, with ergonomic redesign, to reduce the risk of injury. Most ergonomic interventions focus on strategies to reduce spinal loading, but the only intervention that has been formally evaluated has been worker training in manual handling techniques. Occupational guidelines for manual handling designed to constrain task performance to within safety limits of lifting and handling have been produced. It appears that, although lifting techniques can be improved, it has not been possible to demonstrate a corresponding reduction of injury rates (Smedley & Coggan 1994). The explanation for the lack of success in preventing injury is perhaps not all that surprising. According to Burton (1997), although epidemiological studies can link the occurrence of initial back pain with certain physical stressors (such as spinal loading and physical usage), there is little evidence that the symptoms are due to irreversible damage to spinal structures. Furthermore, there is increasing evidence that recurrence and disability are mediated by psychosocial phenomena such as the perception of comfort and the ability to cope (Hadler 1997).

In a recent review of the available evidence, Burton, Battie & Main (1998, p. 1134) concluded:

The possible role of ergonomics for reducing recurrence rates seems at best equivocal, but there is no convincing evidence that continuation of work is detrimental in respect of disability. It is likely that much back pain is only work-related in as much that people of working age get painful backs. It is becoming clear that reducing spinal loads or awkward postures is likely to have only a small impact on the overall pattern of back pain. Non-biomechanical approaches (organisational and social) seemingly are more effective in maintaining ability to work.

Risks of work-related illness and injury

Much of the emphasis on primary prevention of injury has relied on epidemiological studies that have addressed principally anthropomorphic and physical risk factors with a heavy biomechanical and ergonomic emphasis. This specific focus on primary prevention has perhaps hindered proper analysis of the mechanisms of recovery from injury, many of which seem to be psychosocial rather than biomechanical or ergonomic. Recognition, particularly in North America, of the increasing costs of longterm disability led to investigations into its predictors and a number of researchers examined a wide range of presenting characteristics in an effort to find predictors of chronicity. In a prescient review of risk factors in industrial low back pain, Bigos et al (1990) implicated four major types of risk factors; they are listed in Box 4.16. (In their view, however, methodological problems significantly compromised accurate evaluation of these factors.)

Box 4.16   Four major risk factors in industrial low back pain

- Individual factors (mainly demographic and anthropomorphic)
- Physical findings (mainly radiographic)
- Workplace factors (including various work characteristics)
- Psychological factors (determined from psychological tests or evidence of substance abuse)

Bigos and colleagues (1991) found that psychological distress, low job satisfaction and a history of back trouble were the strongest predictors of the report of back pain in the future. Cats-Baril & Frymoyer (1991), in a study of employees with between 2 and 6 weeks' incapacity, identified four main risk factors for long term disability. They are shown in Box 4.17.

Box 4.17 Four major risk factors for long term disability

- Job characteristics
- Aspects of job satisfaction
- Clinical history
- Educational level

Job characteristics considered important were: work status at time of the survey, past work history and type of occupation. The important elements of job satisfaction comprised preretirement policies and benefits, perception about whether the injury was compensable, who was at fault and whether a lawyer had been contacted. The utility of their predictive model, however, was criticised on methodological grounds specifically because of their failure to control for duration of disability, and because of the likely influence of psychological factors in terms of expectation. 'The population of patients who have already incurred two weeks of off-work time secondary to low back trouble probably are anticipating long-term disability, and, perhaps more importantly, so are their health-care providers, employers, and insurers. These expectations may trigger illness behaviours that help establish long-term disability' (Lehmann, Spratt & Lehmann 1993, p. 1110).

Specific psychosocial perspectives

Specific psychological features have been investigated in more detail in a number of more recent studies. Carosella, Lackner & Feuerstein (1994) found that patients with low return-to-work expectations, heightened perceived disability, pain and somatic focus had problems complying with an intensive work rehabilitation

programme. Haazen et al (1994) have shown that change in distorted pain cognitions, worker's compensation status and use of medication were the most important predictors in behavioural rehabilitation of low back pain. (They were, however, pessimistic about the overall level of prediction achieved.) The above studies, although tantalising, do not identify the putative psychological factors with a sufficient degree of accuracy to evaluate their specific importance.

Feuerstein et al (1994) categorised variables predicting return-to-work by 1 year into five categories: medical history, demographics, physical findings, pain and psychological indices. The specific psychological factors identified by them in different studies are shown in Box 4.18.

Box 4.18 Specific psychological factors predicting return to work

- Lower pain severity
- Pain-drawing scores
- Higher treatment satisfaction
- Higher cooperativeness during treatment
- Lower levels of hypochondriasis
- Distrust/stubbornness
- Depression
- Premorbid pessimism

In addition to these clinical psychological variables, Feuerstein & Huang (1998), grouped the factors associated with delayed recovery into medical, ergonomic and psychosocial, although they did not subclassify the latter specifically into clinical and occupational perceptions. Feuerstein & Zastowny (1999) did however recognise that in occupational rehabilitation the psychological problems specifically associated with job stress and work re-entry should be specific targets for psychological intervention (in addition to the usual clinical targets).

Finally, in two recent controlled studies, a large difference in prevalence of musculoskeletal disorders in Dutch and Belgian nurses was explained not by work load, or attribution of work as a cause, but by attitudes to work and depressive symptoms (Burton et al 1997). In another study, Burton et al (1996), in a comparison of musculoskeletal complaints among police in Northern Ireland and in Manchester (UK), found that the proportion of officers with persistent (chronic) back complaints did not depend on length of exposure to physical stressors, but rather to psychosocial factors such as distress and blaming work.

Conclusion

According to a relatively recent review (Bongers et al 1993, p. 297): 'Monotonous work, high perceived work load, and time pressure are related to musculoskeletal symptoms. The data also suggest that low control on the job and lack of support by colleagues are positively associated with muscuoskletal disease. Perceived stress may be an intermediary in the process.' It would seem that there is now overwhelming evidence that psychosocial factors influence musculoskeletal symptomatology and effect on work. Studies have been carried out in a wide range of settings, with varying degrees of precision and differences in measurement tools. The studies have offered evidence in the form of statistical associations between a range of psychosocial variables, work performance and illness characteristics. In an attempt to integrate some of these findings, consideration will now be given specifically to the psychological effects of work absence and on recovery from injury.

THE PSYCHOLOGICAL EFFECTS OF WORK ABSENCE

Stress, especially if prolonged, is likely to lead to ill health or sickness absence. Absence from work, however, is in itself a risk factor for further absence and delayed recovery. Extended absence from work can have a marked effect on the perception of the work environment. Interpersonal relationships at work for example may be an important determinant of successful return to work. Good relationships with colleagues, a sense of being valued and worry about letting one's colleagues down may act as important incentives to return to work after injury, whereas an unpleasant or difficult interpersonal environment may represent a significant

obstacle to return to work. The specific effect of these absences as a result of physical injury can have an even more marked effect since the individual may be anxious about coping not only with the stressful work environment but also with the physical demands of work. The combination of such factors, combined with a loss of self-confidence and anxiety about not being able to perform satisfactorily on return to work, may comprise a powerful set of obstacles.

A clinical perspective on chronic incapacity and recovery from injury

Recent clinical studies into the outcome of treatment for low backpain have, however, offered a more specific evaluation of the role of different sorts of psychological variables in the prediction of chronic incapacity (as determined by self-reported disability) than is currently available in most occupational studies. The findings of such studies for the understanding of the nature and development of chronic incapacity may have relevance also to secondary prevention in occupational settings. A number of these studies will now be reviewed.

In a study of attitudes, beliefs and absenteeism among workers in a biscuit manufacturing factory, Symonds et al (1996) showed that workers who had taken in excess of 1 week's absence due to low back trouble had significantly more negative attitudes and beliefs (when compared with workers who had taken shorter absences, or with those who reported no history of back trouble). Beliefs about the inevitability of back pain, fears of hurting or harming and perceived disability were significantly associated with absenteeism. In an associated study (Symonds et al 1995), introduction of a psychosocial pamphlet, designed to correct mistaken beliefs about back pain (e.g. confusing hurting with harming) and reduce avoidance behaviour, successfully reduced extended sickness absence resulting from low back trouble. It is clear from the aforementioned studies that there is a fair degree of consensus about the sort of factors that appear to affect recovery from incapacity in occupational settings, but there does not seem to be a conceptual framework within which to encompass the diverse and specific research findings.

Occupational factors and recovery from injury: a conceptual framework

Recognition of the sizeable costs of work-related incapacity has spurred considerable effort directed at the identification of risk factors associated with chronic incapacity. Although many of the studies have been able to quantify the relative risk of a range of factors in association with poor outcome, frequently they have had to rely upon the information which has been available and have not included standarised or validated assessment tools. Studies have frequently offered little more than a series of estimates of the specific importance of each of the variables with little attempt to examine their influence on each other or locate their findings within an overall theoretical framework. Although undoubtedly it is important to identify characteristics associated with chronic incapacity, not all such risk factors are targets for intervention and the risk ratios in many of the epidemiological studies are too low to inform clinical or management decision making in the individual case.

In the context of pain management, the focus needs to be on the identification more specifically of *obstacles to recovery*. Despite the acknowledged methodological weaknesses in many of the studies, the general picture is clear. Certain working conditions and adverse work characteristics place an individual at increased risk of ill health and associated absence from work. These occupational features, in the context of individual vulnerabilities or additional external stressors may lead to impaired performance and work absence. In the context of injury, they may delay recovery and return to work. It is within this framework that the importance of clinical and occupational features now will be considered. Initiatives in the field of non-specific low back pain will be used to illustrate this new perspective.

Red flags

Waddell et al (1992), as part of an assessment strategy for patients presenting with back pain,

recommends an initial diagnostic triage into simple back pain, nerve root pain or serious spinal pathology. The signs and symptoms considered indicative of possible spinal pathology or of the need for an urgent surgical evaluation became known as 'red flags'. These 'risk factors' for serious pathology or disease became incorporated into screening tools recommended for use in primary care by clinicians to identify those patients in whom an urgent specialist opinion was indicated (Ch. 18). Assessment of these risk factors were included within a new set of clinical guidelines for the management of acute low back pain (ACHPR 1994, CSAG 1994).

Yellow flags

The increasing costs of chronic incapacity, despite advances in technological medicine, stimulated the search for other solutions to the problem of low back disability. In New Zealand, increasing costs of chronic non-specific low back pain became an unmanageable burden. This fuelled a new initiative designed to complement a slightly modified set of acute back pain management guidelines with a psychosocial assessment system designed to address systematically the psychosocial risks factors that had been shown in the scientific literature to be predictive of chronicity (Kendall, Linton & Main 1997). This included a number of categories of the yellow flags, which are shown in Box 4.19. (A more detailed description is offered in Box 4.20.)

These flags are discussed more fully in Chapter 18 in the context of secondary prevention in health-care settings, but it is important to recognise here that they were developed not only

---

Box 4.19   Yellow flags

- Attitudes and beliefs about back pain
- Behaviours
- Compensation issues
- Diagnostic and treatment issues
- Emotions
- Family
- Work

Box 4.20   Clinical assessment of psychosocial yellow flags

Attitudes and beliefs about back pain
- Belief that pain is harmful or disabling resulting in fear-avoidance behaviour, e.g. the development of guarding and fear of movement
- Belief that all pain must be abolished before attempting to return to work or normal activity
- Expectation of increased pain with activity or work; lack of ability to predict capability
- Catastrophising; thinking the worst; misinterpreting bodily symptoms
- Belief that pain is uncontrollable
- Passive attitude to rehabilitation

Behaviours
- Use of extended rest, disproportionate 'downtime'
- Reduced activity level with significant withdrawal from activities of daily living
- Irregular participation or poor compliance with physical exercise; tendency for activities to be in a 'boom-bust' cycle
- Avoidance of normal activity and progressive substitution of lifestyle away from productive activity
- Report of extremely high intensity of pain, e.g. above 10 on a 0–10 visual analogue scale
- Excessive reliance on use of aids or appliances
- Sleep quality reduced since onset of back pain
- High intake of alcohol or other substances (possibly as self-medication), with an increase since onset of back pain
- Smoking

Compensation issues
- Lack of financial incentive to return to work
- Delay in accessing income support and treatment cost; disputes over eligibility
- History of claim(s) due to other injuries or pain problems
- History of extended time off work due to injury or other pain problem (e.g. more than 12 weeks)
- History of previous back pain, with a previous claim(s) and time off work
- Previous experience of ineffective case management (e.g. absence of interest, perception of being treated punitively)

Diagnosis and treatment
- Health professional sanctioning disability; not providing interventions that will improve function
- Experience of conflicting diagnoses or explanations for back pain, resulting in confusion
- Diagnostic language leading to catastrophising and fear (e.g. fear of ending up in a wheelchair)
- Dramatisation of back pain by health professional producing dependency on treatments, and continuation of passive treatment
- Number of times visited health professional in last year (excluding the present episode of back pain)
- Expectation of a 'techno-fix', e.g. requests to treat as if body were a machine
- Lack of satisfaction with previous treatment for back pain
- Advice to withdraw from job

Emotions
- Fear of increased pain with activity or work
- Depression (especially long term low mood), loss of sense of enjoyment
- More irritability than usual
- Anxiety about and heightened awareness of body sensations (includes sympathetic nervous system arousal)
- Feeling under stress and unable to maintain sense of control
- Presence of social anxiety or disinterested in social activity
- Feeling useless and not needed

Family
- Over protective partner/spouse, emphasising fear of harm or encouraging catastrophising (usually well intentioned)
- Solicitous behaviour from spouse (e.g. taking over tasks)
- Socially punitive responses from spouse (e.g. ignoring, expressing frustration)
- Extent to which family members support any attempt to return to work
- Lack of support person to talk to about problems

Work
- History of manual work, notably from the following occupational groups:
  — fishing, forestry and farming workers
  — construction, including carpenters and builders
  — nurses
  — truck drivers
  — labourers
- Work history, including patterns of frequent job changes, experiencing stress at work, job dissatisfaction, poor relationships with peers or supervisors, lack of vocational direction
- Belief that work is harmful; that it will do damage or be dangerous
- Unsupportive or unhappy current work environment
- Low educational background, low socioeconomic status
- Job involves significant biomechanical demands, such as lifting, manual handling of heavy items, extended sitting, extended standing, driving, vibration, maintenance of constrained or sustained postures, inflexible work schedule preventing appropriate breaks
- Job involves shift work or working 'unsociable hours'
- Minimal availability of selected duties and graduated return to work pathways, with unsatisfactory implementation of these
- Negative experience of workplace management of back pain (e.g. absence of a reporting system, discouragement to report, punitive response from supervisors and managers)
- Absence of interest from employer

Remember the key question to bear in mind while conducting these clinical assessments is '*What can be done to help this person experience less distress and disability?*'

From Waddell The Back Pain Revolution 1998, p. 327, after Kendall et al 1997, reproduced with permission.

from a clinical perspective but also from an occupational perspective and consisted of both psychological and socio-occupational risk factors. From these a number of specific guidelines for behavioural management were also produced, which are shown in Box 4.21.

Box 4.21 Behavioural management guidelines

- Provide a *positive* expectation that the individual will return to work
- Be directive in scheduling regular reviews of progress
- Keep the individual active and at work
- Acknowledge difficulties of daily living
- Help maintain positive cooperation
- Communicate that having more time off work reduces the likelihood of successful return
- Beware of expectations of 'total cure' or expectation of simple 'techno-fixes'
- Promote self-management and self-responsibility
- Be prepared to say 'I don't know'
- Avoid confusing the report of symptoms with the presence of emotional distress
- Discourage working at home
- Encourage people to recognise that pain can be controlled
- If barriers are too complex, arrange multidisciplinary referral

---

Further conceptual development

In tackling obstacles to recovery, whether from the perspective of actual clinical management or from that of occupational rehabilitation, it seems necessary to distinguish concerns that individuals have about their personal well-being from specific concerns about work. It was decided therefore to subdivide the yellow flags further into clinical yellow flags and occupationally focused 'blue flags' (Burton & Main 2000b, Main & Burton 1998).

The clinical flags include the sort of features that are recognised in the context of evaluation for pain management programmes or other clinically focused rehabilitation programmes. These include the range of cognitive, emotional and behavioural responses to pain and disability reviewed in Chapter 2. Such features can be thought of as risk factors for chronicity, which, after injury, may become obstacles to recovery. It will be argued in Chapter 18 that, particularly in

the context of individualised management, the clinical yellow flags can be separated into:

- general distress associated with adverse life events—found more in vulnerable individuals and in 'at risk' groups
- dysfunctional beliefs, negative emotions and inadequate coping responses to pain, injury and pain-associated disability.

Occupational factors as obstacles to recovery: the blue flags and black flags

The occupational component of the original New Zealand yellow flags focused on the perception of work, but in terms of obstacles to recovery it is necessary to make a distinction also between two types of occupational risk factors. They can be thought of as factors concerning the *perception* of work (blue flags) and *objective* work characteristics (black flags). The distinction is similar to the distinction between *intrinsic* and *extrinsic* factors by Herzberg (1974), but with a focus on obstacles to recovery—that is, potential targets for some sort of biopsychosocial intervention.

Blue flags

The blue flags have their origin in the stress literature reviewed above and some of them are illustrated in Box 4.11 on p. 74. They are perceived features of work which are generally associated with higher rates of symptoms, ill-health and work loss which in the context of injury may delay recovery, or constitute a major obstacle to it. They are characterised by features such as high demand/low control, unhelpful management style, poor social support from colleagues, perceived time pressure and lack of job satisfaction. Individual workers may differ in their perception of the same working environment.

According to Bigos et al (1990, p. 184), perception may be more important than the objective characteristics since: 'Once an individual is off work, perception about symptoms, about the *safety* of return to work, and about impact of return to work on one's personal life can affect recovery even in the most well-meaning worker'.

It should be emphasised that blue flags incorporate not only issues related to the perception of job characteristics such as job demand, but also perception of social interactions (whether with management or with fellow workers).

Black flags

'Black flags' are *not* a matter of perception, and affect all workers equally. They include both nationally established policy concerning conditions of employment and sickness policy and working conditions specific to a particular organisation. Some examples are shown in Box 4.22.

Box 4.22 Occupational black flags I: job context and working conditions

National
- Rates of pay
- Nationally negotiated entitlements:
  - sick certification
- Benefit system
- Wage reimbursement rate

Local
- Sickness policy:
  - entitlements to sick leave
  - role of occupational health in 'signing off' and 'signing on' requirement for full fitness
  - possibility of sheltered work
- restricted duties
- Management style
- Trades union support/involvement
- Organisational size and structure

It is not always possible to make an absolute distinction between black and blue flags, since there are also found content-specific aspects of work that characterise certain types of job and are associated with higher rates of illness, injury or work loss. They are shown in Box 4.23.

Box 4.23 Occupational black flags II: content-specific aspects of work

- Ergonomic:
  - job heaviness
  - lifting frequency
  - postures
  - sitting/standing postural requirements
- Temporal characteristics:
  - number of working hours
  - shift pattern

These features of work, following injury, may require a higher level of working capacity for successful work retention. After certain types of injury, such jobs may be specifically contraindicated and therefore constitute an absolute obstacle to return to work. It might be hoped that many such risk factors could be 'designed' out of the working environment, but such factors certainly need to be evaluated in the context of work retention or rehabilitation.

Is there any evidence for the need for a clinical–occupational interface?

In a recent predictive study, examining the transition from acute to chronic low back pain, Williams et al (1998) evaluated the influence of job satisfaction, pain, disability and psychological distress at baseline with outcome 6 months later. They found that job satisfaction may protect against the development of chronic pain and disability, and conversely that dissatisfaction may heighten the risk.

The need for an integrated approach to obstacles to recovery

There are in our view several major reasons that we have been so unsuccessful in work retention, and rehabilitation following musculoskeletal dysfunction. Some of the principal ones are outlined in Box 4.24.

Box 4.24 Possible reasons for failure of work retention programmes

- In general, we have failed to distinguish adequately between risks for chronicity and obstacles to recovery
- More specifically, we have failed to understand that sustained work retention or rehabilitation of the individual may require addressing both clinical and occupational obstacles to recovery
- Finally, even the most sharply focused intervention designed to remove the relevant yellow and blue flags may fail as a consequence of insuperable obstacles in the form of black flags

---

GENERAL RECOMMENDATIONS

The incorporation of the principles of pain management into work retention and work rehabilitation is discussed fully in Chapter 19, but it is important at this juncture to recognise the need for an integrated conceptual framework linking assessment and management. Our views are summarised in a recent article from which Box 4.25 is abstracted.

CONCLUSION

There is now considerable consensus that chronic pain and pain-associated incapacity need to be understood within a biopsychosocial perspective. This does not imply abandonment of biomedical factors but simply locates them in a wider framework. During the last two decades, the powerful influence of psychosocial factors has been demonstrated. Early studies into the psychological components have been followed by investigations into the influences of economic and occupational factors on the perception of pain and development of disability.

Disentangling of the complexity of psychological and social forces on the individual with incapacitating pain is frequently a daunting task, since the individuals themselves may not be fully aware of the influences that have shaped their beliefs, emotions and behaviour. In terms of pain management, however, economic and occupational obstacles must be addressed as possible obstacles to recovery (Ch. 11) in the context of clinical decision making (Ch. 12). It may be that, at the particular time of assessment, economic and occupational factors are considered to be insuperable barriers to recovery. It may be that consideration needs to be given to them prior to reconsideration for pain management. Individuals may need to make some difficult choices as far as their futures are concerned. It must be remembered above all, however, that failure to assess and understand the powerful influence of economic and occupational factors affecting symptom presentation and recovery will lead to ineffective or inappropriate treatment thus contributing to distress and chronic incapacity (Ch. 5), which pain management is designed to ameliorate.

Box 4.25 Recommendations for assessment and management of occupationally related musculoskeletal disorders

- Recognise that the workers' perception of their work is fundamental to understanding recovery from injury
- Understand the inherent risks in certain occupational environments for producing extended sickness absence and delayed recovery after injury
- Facilitate a system for early reporting of musculoskeletal symptoms to appropriately trained personnel
- Identify mistaken beliefs about the nature of pain, hurting/harming and unnecessary fears of prolonged injury, and recognise other psychological characteristics of the individual (yellow flags)

- Identify aspects of work perceived to be problematic by the injured worker (blue flags)
- Distinguish yellow flags and blue flags from lack of motivation to work
- Provide a psychosocial preventative approach to the individual, promoting self-help, establishing confidence and reducing unnecessary apprehension
- Facilitate return to work as soon as possible; restricted duties (if required) should be brief and time limited. Maintain management of the worker within the occupational environment so far as is possible

From Burton & Main 2000b, reproduced with permission.

KEY POINTS

- Economic and occupational factors can have an impact on the perception of pain, adjustment to it and response to treatment.

- With chronic pain patients, such factors need to be carefully evaluated before clinical decisions are made.

- It cannot be assumed that such factors influence all patients equally and patients should be assessed on an individual basis.

- Factors such as fear of further hurting or harming and lack of confidence may be important clinical obstacles to recovery in occupational as well as health-care settings.

- In chronic pain rehabilitation, the work environment should be considered not only in terms of its likely physical demands but also in those of work stress and work satisfaction.

- It should be recognised that *perception* of work may be more important than objective work characteristics.

- Successful rehabilitation may require attention both to clinical and to occupational characteristics, considered from the perspective of potential *obstacles to recovery.*.

REFERENCES

AHCPR 1994 Management guidelines for acute low back pain. Agency for Health Care Policy and Research, US Department of Health and Human Services, Rockville MD

Andersson G B J 1999 Epidemiology of back pain in industry. In: The Karwowski W, Marras W (eds) The occupational ergonomics handbook. CRC, Boca Raton, ch 51, pp 913–932.

Bigos S J, Battie M C, Nordin M, Spengler D M, Guy D P 1990 Industrial low back pain. In: Weinstein J, Wiesel S (eds) The lumbar spine. W B Saunders, Philaladelphia, pp 846–859.

Bigos S J, Battie M C, Spengler D M et al 1991 A prospective study of work perceptions and psychological factors affecting the report of back injury. Spine 11:252–255

Bongers P M, de Winter C R, Kompier M A J, Hildebrandt V H 1993 Psychosocial factors at work and musculoskeletal disease. Scandinavian Journal of Work and Environmental Health 19:297–312

Burton A K 1997 Back injury and work loss: biomechanical and psychosocial influences. Spine 22:2575–2580

Burton A K, Main C J 2000a Relevance of biomechanics in occupational musculoskeletal disorders. In: Mayer T G, Gatchel R J, Polatin P B (eds) Occupational musculoskeletal disorders. Lippincott Williams & Wilkins, Philadelphia, ch 10, pp 157–166

Burton A K, Main C J 2000b Obstacles to recovery from work-related musculoskeletal disorders. In: Karwowski W (ed) International encyclopaedia of ergonomics and human factors. Taylor & Francis, London, in Press

Burton A K, Tillotson K M, Symonds T L, Burke C E, Mathewson T 1996. Occupational risk factors for first onset of low back trouble: a study of serving police officers. Spine 21:2612–2620

Burton A K, Symonds T L, Zinzen E et al 1997 Is ergonomic intervention alone sufficient to limit musculoskeletal problems in nurses? Occupational Medicine 47:25–32

Burton A K, Battie M C, Main C J 1998 The relative importance of biomechanical and psychosocial factors in low back injuries. In: Karwowski W, Marras W S (eds) The occupational ergonomics handbook. CRC; Boca Raton, FA, chap 61, pp 1127–1138

Carayon P, Lim S-Y 1999 Psychosocial work factors. In: Karwowski W, Marras W (eds) The occupational ergonomics handbook. CRC, Boca Raton, ch 15, pp 275–283

Carosella A M, Lackner J M, Feuerstein M 1994 Factors associated with early discharge from a multidisciplinary work rehabilitation program for chronic low back pain. Pain 57:69–76

Cats-Baril W L, Frymoyer J W 1991 Identifying patients at risk of becoming disabled because of low-back pain: the Vermont Rehabilitation Engineering Center predictive model. Spine 16:605–607

Consumer's Association 1985 Back pain survey. Consumer's Association, London

Cox T 1993 Stress research and stress management: putting theory to work. HSE, Sudbury, Suffolk

Crombie I 1999 The potential of epidemiology. In: Crombie I (ed) Epidemiology of pain. IASP, Seattle, ch 1, pp 1–5

CSAG Clinical Standards Advisory Group 1994 Report on Back Pain. HMSO London

Davis K G, Heaney C A 2000 The relationship between psychosocial work characteristics and low back pain: underlying methodological issues. Clinical Biomechanics, in press

Davis L E 1980 Individuals and the organisation. California Management Review 22:5–14

Deyo R, Cherkin D, Conrad D, Volinn E 1991 Cost, controversy, crisis: low back pain and the health of the public. Annual Review of Public Health 12:141–156

DSM-IV 1994 Diagnostic and statistical manual of mental disorders, 4th edn. American Psychiatric Association, Washington DC

Erens B, Ghate D 1993 Invalidity benefit: a longitudinal study of new recipients. Department of Social Security Research Report no 20. HMSO, London

Faust D 1995 The detection of deception. In: Weintraub M I (ed) Neurologic clinics, malingering and conversion reactions W.B. Saunders, Philadelphia, pp 255–265

Feuerstein M, Huang G D 1998 Preventing disability in patients with occupational musculoskeletal disorders. American Pain Society Bulletin 8:9–11

Feuerstein M, Zastowny T R 1999 Occupational rehabilitation: multidisciplinary management of work-related musculoskeletal pain and disability. In: Gatchel R, Turk D C (eds) Psychological approaches to pain management: a practitioner's handbook. Gulford, New York, pp 458–485

Feuerstein M, Menz L, Zastowny T R, Barron B A 1994 Chronic back pain and work disability: vocational outcomes following multidisciplinary rehabilitation. Journal of Occupational Rehabilitation 4:229–251

French J P R, Rogers W, Cobb S 1974 A model of person-environment fit. In: Coehlo G W, Hamburg D A, Adams J E (eds) Coping and adaptation. Basic. New York

Goosens M E J B, Rutten-van Molken M P M H, Leidl R M et al 1996 Cognitive-educational treatment of fibromyalgia: a randomised clinical trial. II Economic evaluation. Journal of Rheumatology 23:1246–1254

Griffiths A 1998 The psychosocial work environment. In: McCaig R, Harrington M (eds) The changing nature of occupational health. HSE, Sudbury, Suffolk, ch 11, pp 213–232

Haazen I W C J, Vlaeyen J W S, Kole-Snidjers A M K, van Eek F D, van Es F D 1994 Behavioral rehabilitation of chronic low back pain: searching for the predictors of treatment outcome. Journal of Rehabilitation Science 7:34–43

Hackman J R, Oldham G R 1976 Motivation through the design of work: test of a theory. Organisational Behaviour and Human Performance 16:250–279

Hadler N M 1997 Back pain in the workplace. What you lift or how you lift matters far less than whether you lift or when. Spine 22:935–940

Halpern M 1992 Prevention of low back pain: basic ergonomics in the workplace and clinic. In: Nordin M, Vischer T L (eds) Common low back pain: prevention of chronicity. Baillière Tindall, London, pp 705–730

Herzberg E 1974 The wise old turk. Harvard Business Review. Sep/Oct:70–80

Jones J R, Hodgson J T, Clegg T et al 1998 Self-report of work-related illness in 1995. HSE, Sudbury, Suffolk

Kendall N A S, Linton S J, Main C J 1997 Guide to assessing psychosocial yellow flags in acute low back pain: risk factors for long term disability and work loss. Accident Rehabilitation and Compensation Insurance Corporation of New Zealand and the National Health Committee, Wellington N Z

Lehmann T R, Spratt K F, Lehmann K K 1993 Predicting long term disability in low back injured workers presenting to a spine consultant. Spine 18:1103–1112

Linton S J 1994 The challenge of preventing chronic musculoskeletal pain. In: Proceedings of the 7th world congress on pain: progress in research and pain management, vol 2. IASP, Seattle, pp 149–166

Linton S J 1998 (editorial) The socioeconomic impact of chronic back pain: is anyone benefitting? Pain 75:163–168

Main C J 1999 Medicolegal aspects of pain: the nature of psychological opinion in cases of personal injury. In: Gatchel R J, Turk D C (eds) Psychosocial aspects of pain. Guilford, New York, ch 9; pp 132–147

Main C J, Burton A K 1998 Pain mechanisms. In: McCaig R, Harrington M (eds) The changing nature of occupational health. HSE, Sudbury, Suffolk, ch 12, pp 233–254

Main C J, Spanswick C C 1995 'Functional overlay' and illness behaviour in chronic pain: distress or malingering? Conceptual difficulties in medico-legal assessment of personal injury claims. Journal of Psychosomatic Research 39:737–753

Main C J, Waddell G 1998 Behavioural responses to examination: a re-appraisal of the interpretation of 'non-organic signs'. Spine 23:2367–2371

Marras W S, Lavender S A, Leurgans S et al 1993 The role of dynamic three-dimensional trunk motion in occupationally related low back disorders: the effects of workplace factors, trunk position and trunk motion characteristics on injury. Spine 18:617–628

Mendelson G 1988 Psychiatric aspects of personal injury claims. Thomas, Springfield, II

Nachemson A, Jonsson E (eds) 2000 Swedish SBU report: Evidence-based treatment for neck and back pain. Swedish version: SBU, Stockholm; English version: Lippincott, Philadelphia, in press.

Payne R 1994 Individual differences in the study of occupational stress. In: Cooper C L, Payne R (eds) Causes, coping and consequences of stress at work. J Wiley, Chichester, pp 209–232

Rohling M L, Binder L M, Langhinrichsen-Rohling J et al 1995 Money matters: a meta-analytic review of the association between financial compensation and the experience and treatment of chronic pain. Health Psychology 14:537–547

Smedley J, Coggan D 1994 Will the manual handling regulations reduce the incidence of back disorders? Occupational Medicine 44:63–65

Smith M J, Carayon-Sainfort P 1989 A balance theory of job design for stress reduction. International Journal of Industrial Ergonomics 4:67–79

Spitzer W O, Leblanc F E, Dupuis M 1987 Scientific approach to the assessment and management of activity-related spinal disorders. A monograph for physicians. Report of the Quebec Task Force on Spinal Disorders. Spine 12(7):s1–s59

Symonds T L, Burton A K, Tillotson K M, Main C J 1995 Absence resulting from low back pain can be reduced by psychosocial intervention at the workplace. Spine 20:2738–2745

Symonds T L, Burton A K, Tillotson K M, Main C J 1996 Do attitudes and beliefs influence work loss due to low back trouble? Occupational Medicine 22:2612–2620

Taylor N, Curran N M 1985 The nuprin pain report. Louis Harris, New York

Van Tulder M W, Koes B W, Boulter L M 1995 A cost-of-illness study of back pain in the Netherlands. Pain 62:233–240

Vingaard E, Nachemson A 2000 Work related influences on neck and low back pain. In: Nachemson A, Jonsson E (eds) Swedish SBU report. Evidence based treatment for back pain. Swedish version: Swedish Council on Technology Assessment in Health Care (SBU) English translation: Stockholm; Lippincott, New York, in press

Waddell G 1998 The back pain revolution. Churchill Livingstone, New York

Waddell G, Somerville D, Henderson I, Newton M 1992 Objective clinical evaluation of physical impairment in chronic low back pain. Spine 17:617–628

Watson P J, Main C J, Gales T, Waddell G, Purcell-Jones G 1997 Medically certified work loss, benefit claims and costs of back pain: a one year epidemiological study of the Bailiwick of Jersey. British Journal of Rheumatology 37:82–96

Williams R A, Pruitt S D, Doctor J N et al 1998 The contribution of job satisfaction to the transition from acute to chronic low back pain. Archives of Physical Medicine and Rehabilitation 79:366–373

5

The nature of disability

*Chris J. Main   Chris C. Spanswick
Paul Watson*

INTRODUCTION

In a high proportion of patients who consult with pain, their reasons for consulting are the disabling effects of the pain. Non-specific low back pain is one of the most frequently presented pain problems in the NHS. A significant proportion of patients can establish reasonable control over their pain, but at a cost of restriction of activity. If the level of restriction is considered unacceptable, the patient will seek treatment. The relationship between pain, level of physical functioning and the ability to carry out activities of various sorts becomes critically important.

IMPAIRMENT, DISABILITY, HANDICAP AND FUNCTIONAL CAPACITY

There have been considerable efforts directed at trying to identify the precise relationships amongst impairment, disability and handicap. Unfortunately, the literature often confuses the terms. The World Health Organisation or WHO (1980) defined impairment as 'any loss or abnormality of psychologic, physiologic, or anatomic structure or function'. In the context of musculoskeletal problems, a sharper focus has been offered, and the relationship between *physical* impairment, pain and disability has been examined.

Physical impairment

Attempts to produce objective criteria for physical impairment in back pain were made by

Waddell & Main in the early 1980s. They defined physical impairment as: 'pathologic, anatomic or physiologic abnormality of structure or function leading to loss of normal bodily activity' (Waddell & Main 1984). They attempted initially to distinguish it from disability (as assessed on the basis of self-reported limitation in activities). Their early method of assessment formed the basis of the Glasgow Illness Model of disability (Waddell et al 1984b), which in turn led to the more fully developed biopsychosocial model of disability (Waddell 1987). Although useful as a starting point, the authors themselves recognised that not all the elements could properly be described as 'true structural impairments'. A further difficulty was that the elements could not be combined satisfactorily into a single dimension or scale. On the basis of further studies, they produced a revised impairment scale, comprising seven items (Waddell et al 1992). The assessment is considered in detail in Waddell (1998, pp. 124–131). Although specifically designed for the assessment of non-specific low back pain, the distinguishing of objective physical impairment from permanent structural impairment was an important stage in understanding the relationship between impairment and disability. Waddell (1998, p. 130) acknowledged, however:

We made every effort to separate our assessment of physical impairment from how patients respond to examination. Despite our efforts, we were only partly successful. All the tests in our scale still correlated to some extent with pain behaviour. Our final scale was still more closely related to the emotional than to the sensory scale of the McGill pain questionnaire (Melzack 1987). It correlated more with measures of illness behaviour than with pain itself. By their very nature, all of these tests may be open to exaggeration. It is never possible to separate clinical examination of pain wholly from such influences. Ultimately, this is a measure of physical performance.

In his recognition of the impossibility of *completely* separating 'objective findings' from effort in the assessment of non-specific low back pain, Waddell illustrates the necessity of moving beyond the Cartesian dualism that has constrained our understanding of pain and its effects. For many purposes, both clinical and medicolegal, however, it is necessary to evaluate the *relative* importance of physical and psychological factors. To clarify the picture, it is necessary to move back a step and clarify the WHO building blocks of 'disability' and 'handicap'.

Disability

The WHO (1980) offers the following definition: 'A disability is any restriction or lack (resulting from an impairment) of ability to perform an activity in the manner or within the range considered normal for a human being'. The definition attempts to distinguish performance from impairment (at least conceptually), and introduces the idea of disability being outside a 'range considered normal' but otherwise it is flawed, in that it assumes that it is possible to identify impairment that is absolutely distinguishable from disability, and a clear and unambiguous causal path between the two. As discussed immediately above, this endeavour may not only be impossible, but also misguided.

The assessment of disability is discussed in Chapter 9.

Handicap

The definition offered by the WHO (1980) for 'handicap' seems even less clearly focused than their definition of 'disability': 'A handicap is a disadvantage for a given individual, resulting from an impairment or a disability, that limits or prevents the fulfilment of a role that is normal (depending on age, sex, social and cultural factors) for that individual'.

The WHO model of an apparently simple causal relationship between impairment (e.g. fracture), disability (e.g. limitation in movement) and handicap (limitation in function) can be helpful in conceptualising someone's inability to work as a consequence of restricted movement resulting from an injury; in pain-mediated disability, however, the situation often appears much more complex than this (as illustrated in our staged theoretical model at the end of this chapter). Some of the specific conceptual and methodological problems are illustrated in Box 5.1.

Box 5.1 Conceptual and methodological difficulties

- It is possible to have a number of impairments and/or disabilities but no resulting handicap
- There is not a direct relationship between the severity of impairment or disability and handicap
- The same level of impairment may result in different levels of disability in different people and the same level of disability may result in different levels of handicap. Studies examining the relationship between impairment and disability have shown that there is not a one-to-one relationship between impairment and disability

---

A clinical example

The same mild degree of cervical spondylosis may result in the same moderate levels of pain and disability in two persons: a concert violinist and a bank clerk. However, the concert violinist is unable to play for long periods of time and is forced to give up work (i.e. suffers handicap in the areas of occupation and economic self-sufficiency) yet the bank clerk is able to continue with work after making only minor modifications to the working environment.

Functional capacity

Assessment of function, or functional capacity, is an integral part of assessment in pain management, but is also sometimes used as a measure of change or outcome (Ch. 17). The proponents of functional capacity evaluation, or FCE (Blankenship 1986) have developed a detailed system of evaluation that is claimed to be objective, thus removing the subjective component in the assessment of disability. FCE claims to measure whole body ability, cardiovascular capacity, lifting capacity and fitness for work. The system underpins the functional restoration programme (Mayer & Gatchel 1988), which is described further in Chapter 19. Simpler measures (Harding et al 1994) discussed in Chapter 9 are also available. Although clearly defined, reliable and clinically valid, they are essentially measures of *performance* and as such are influenced by *effort*, which is in turn influenced by a range of psychological factors including prior learning, fears, beliefs and expectations. Although physical capacity measures therefore can give a clear *description* of performance, their *interpretation* is a lot more complex and requires a biopsychosocial rather than a biomedical perspective.

A HISTORICAL PERSPECTIVE ON DISABILITY

Research into the multifactorial nature of pain has been paralleled by investigations into the nature of disability. One of the earliest attempts to examine the nature of disability scientifically was offered by Wilfling (unpublished work, 1973). Several previous studies had focused on work status as a sole index of disability, whereas others had attempted to understand disability simply on the basis of the patient's self-report. Wilfling followed Nashold & Hrubec (1971) in using multivariate statistical methods to identify types of disability. Having assessed 100 individuals after lumbar spinal fusion, Wifling identified 'eight independent basic dimensions of LBP disability'. From those he derived statistically 'four naturally occurring symptom complexes' from which he developed guidelines for management. Although statistically flawed, and perhaps conceptually somewhat muddled, his study was one of the first to attempt to disentangle physical and psychological factors and helped stimulate development of the original Glasgow Illness Model (Waddell et al 1984b).

MODELS OF DISABILITY

Many theoreticians and several different research groups have developed models of disability. Although some of the models are labelled as 'pain models', they are perhaps more appropriately understood as 'disability' or 'illness models'.

Emory Pain Estimate Model (EPEM)

The Emory Pain Estimate Model, or EPEM (Brena & Koch 1975), was one of the first to try to distinguish 'pathology' from 'behaviour'. The pathology dimension included the quantification of physical examination procedures, as well as diagnostic abnormalities for which a scoring system was devised. The behavioural dimension also consisted of a composite of scores from activity scales, reports of pain, drug use and MMPI scale elevations. Using median splits, patients were allocated to one of the four cells on a two-by-two grid. Although conceptually imaginative, the model is statistically flawed and has been superseded by classification systems such as the WHYMPI or MPI (see below), which are much more methodologically sound.

Glasgow Illness Model (GIM)

The original GIM (Waddell et al 1984a) resulted from an attempt to explain why some patients were more disabled than others with (apparently) the same amount of physical impairment. New measures of pain and disability (Waddell & Main 1984) were constructed and, using multiple regression models, the relationship between the two was examined. The additional influence of a number of other variables, particularly psychological variables, and also pain measures were then examined. The major findings of the set of research studies are shown in Box 5.2.

Box 5.2   Findings of the Glasgow illness studies

- The physical impairment variables explained about 40% of the variance in patients' disability scores
- There were slight gender differences
- Psychological factors explained about an additional 30% of variance in the disability scores
- Long-standing personality traits such as introversion or neuroticism, and hysteria or hypochondriasis, were relatively unimportant
- Current distress, in the form of heightened somatic awareness and depressive symptoms, and pain behaviour, in the form of behavioural signs and symptoms, were much more powerful influences on disability
- Even with statistical control for gender, and for differences on physical examination findings, distress and pain behaviour were significantly predictive of disability
- Development of pain behaviour was associated with the amount of previous failed treatment

---

These studies were important principally for three reasons. They demonstrated, first, that in patients with chronic non-specific low back pain the level of disability was only partly explicable by physical examination findings. Secondly the studies showed that the ways patients reacted to their pain was probably more important than had previously been understood. Finally, they suggested that explanation for high level of disability was more likely to do with the persistence of the pain and its effects, rather than some sort of pre-existing abnormality of personality.

The studies were, however, cross-sectional in design and so it was not possible to do more than suggest possible causal pathways. Little more than a rudimentary attempt was made to examine social and occupational variables, and the psychological measures available at that time did not include specific measures of beliefs about pain, fear or coping strategies.

The biopsychosocial perspective on disability

Turk & Rudy (1992) developed a classification system for chronic pain patients based on the empirical integration of biomedical, psychosocial and behavioural data that they labelled the Multiaxial Assessment of Pain, or MAP. The system was developed originally from a 64-item questionnaire called the West Haven–Yale Multidimensional Pain Inventory, or WHYMPI (Kerns, Turk & Rudy 1985). The first two sections of the questionnaire relate to patients' appraisal of pain and its effects on various aspects of life. The second part addresses patients' views of the reaction of others to their pain and its effects. The third part of the questionnaire assesses the frequency with which patients perform a range of activities. The authors claim wide empirical support for the validity of the questionnaire (Turk & Rudy 1992). The authors used cluster–analytic and multivariate classification methods to identify three different types of patient, which they have replicated across a wide range of pain patients with different pain diagnoses. The distinct patient profiles are shown in Box 5.3.

> **Box 5.3**   Turk and Rudy's MAP classification
>
> - *Dysfunctional*, characterised by patients who perceive the severity of their pain to be high, who report a high level of interference of pain in activities, indicate a high level of emotional distress and report a low level of activity
> - *Interpersonally distressed*, characterised by patients who view others as not very understanding or supportive of their problems
> - *Adaptive copers*, characterised by patients with high levels of social support, relatively low levels of pain, low perceived interference, low distress, higher activity and a higher level of perceived control

The MAP classification has been important in demonstrating that similar types of patients present with different sorts of pain disorders. A similar attempt was offered by the P-A-I-N clustering of MMPI profiles by Robinson, Swimmer & Rallof (1989). The MAP classification, however, has better statistical and clinical validation. It would appear to have merit as a general screening system, but is insufficiently accurate in the assessment of some of its elements to be used as a basis for individual clinical decision making in pain management.

During the last decade, a number of researchers have focused more specifically on specific cognitive factors. As discussed in Chapter 2, there has been increasing interest in specific beliefs about pain (such as its nature and controllability, the influence of fears of hurting or harming, expectations of outcome of treatment) and pain-coping strategies.

THE TRANSITION FROM ACUTE TO CHRONIC INCAPACITY

Gatchel (1991) put forward a three-stage model of the development of chronic low back pain disability, which differentiated pain into acute (stage 1), subacute (stage 2) and chronic (stage 3). (Frank et al (1996) later used the classification in the context of work loss.)

Obviously all chronic pain experiences start off with the experience of acute pain. Gatchel argues that pain at stage 1 is associated with emotional distress in the form of fear, anxiety and worry about the pain. If the pain does not resolve then after a period of about 2 to 4 months the patient then enters stage 2, the subacute stage. It is at this stage, Gatchel argues, that the patient may develop a range of psychological and behavioural disorders such as depression and anger. He hypothesises that the type of problems developed are related to both premorbid characteristics of the patient and to current socioeconomic and environmental factors. If the pain does not resolve, then the patient will develop chronic pain (stage 3).

In a later development of the model (Gatchel 1996) added a further dimension of physical deconditioning, described by Mayer & Gatchel (1988) in terms of losses of muscle strength, flexibility and physical endurance (see Ch. 9) As yet there is little empirical evidence to support this model, but the model has been very important in establishing the importance of factors at early stages of illness. Previously patients tended to be described simply in terms of acute pain (for which pre- or postoperative pain was frequently used as the model) and chronic pain (often studied on cohorts of patients having pain for a year or more). Unfortunately since the 'cut-off' for chronicity has varied between 3 and 12 months in different studies, it is difficult to integrate the findings.

The *development* of chronicity has been studied only relatively recently. Although acknowledging the important conceptual advance offered by Gatchel, there is a danger none the less of failing to recognise that there is much variation in clinical presentation by patients within each of the stages. Although comparison of cohorts of patients at different stages of chronicity has been illuminating, the framework is insufficiently powerful to examine the processes of change for which consideration of possible mechanisms is required. As a first step, it seems relevant to consider predictors of chronicity.

PREDICTING CHRONIC PAIN AND PAIN-ASSOCIATED DISABILITY

Of all pain syndromes, low back pain has been the most widely researched, and since it

> **Box 5.4**   Types of research into back pain and chronicity
>
> • Risk factors associated with the development of back pain
> • Clinical studies into the development of chronic back pain disability
> • Occupational studies into the recovery from injury, and return to work

comprises the most common diagnosis in most pain clinics it seems appropriate to review the relationship between back pain and disability. There have been a large number of studies attempting to identify risks of back pain, whether acute or chronic. These studies can be differentiated into three main lines of research, as shown in Box 5.4.

Risk factors associated with the development of back pain

Given the prevalence of chronic pain, particularly chronic low back pain, it is clearly important to find out whether it is preventable, and how it can be managed in terms of social policy. A large number of epidemiological studies have studied the characteristics of individuals with pain. Population studies of the incidence of back pain in various subgroups of the population may provide clues about the development of pain, and therefore its prevention. Waddell (1998, p. 99) has recently reviewed risk factors for low back pain, and summarised the finding as follows:

• Most people get back pain. Heredity, gender and body build make little difference.

• It is good general health advice to stop smoking, avoid excess weight and get physically fit. This may help to reduce the likelihood of developing new episodes of back pain, but such advice is more relevant to dealing with back pain after it occurs.

• Social class is probably the strongest personal predictor of back trouble. This is partly related to manual work, especially in men, and partly to social disadvantage, in men and women.

• Heavy manual work leads to slightly more short-term back pain, but this effect is soon swamped by stronger psychosocial influences on the reporting of symptoms, claims, workloss and the development of chronic pain and disability.

Clinical studies into the development of chronic back pain disability

Several studies have compared the importance of physical and psychological factors to the prediction of outcome of treatment. Most treatment and intervention are based on concepts of tissue damage and amelioration of biomechanical dysfunction following injury. Many studies have tried to identify the importance of all sorts of anthropomorphic, clinical and biomechanical factors in terms of risk of injury, or risk of continued incapacity. (Halpern 1992). Multivariable analyses of such data suggest that the relative contribution of the different classes of variable to prediction of chronicity is particularly complex (Burton & Tillotson 1991).

In chronic back pain patients the levels of distress at time of initial assessment were found to be as important as known risk factors (such as previous lumbar surgery) in outcome from conservative treatment 2–4 years later (Main et al 1992). The strong relationship between level of distress outcome was replicated in a study of chronic pain patients undergoing a rehabilitation programme based on McKenzie physiotherapy (Williams, Grant & Main 1995). Weiser & Cedraschi (1992) reviewed 16 predictive studies involving a range of healthy, acute and recurrent populations and concluded that psychological factors such as distress, symptom preoccupation, depression, anxiety, beliefs about pain and pain-coping strategies were associated with outcome of treatment. Similar findings were found in the recent study by Gatchel (1996) who found that depression, low activity–high pain behaviour and negative beliefs about pain and activity were predictive of chronic disability.

Specific beliefs and pain-coping strategies have also been addressed. Burton et al (1995) found that, for patients with acute back pain (a history of 3 weeks or less), the most significant predictor of disability levels at 1 year follow-up was the use of inappropriate coping strategies (catastrophising and praying/hoping) rather than measures of physical impairment. Disability levels at 1 year were also dependent on whether the person had a previous history of low back pain. (Interestingly, by far the most powerful predictors of outcome were found in the subgroup of patients with acute back pain, in which it was possible to explain 47% of variance in outcome from negative cognitive coping strategies alone.) In another recent review, Turk & Okifuji (1997) concluded that psychosocial factors were better predictors of chronicity than either clinical or physical factors.

It would therefore seem that levels of distress or dysfunctional thoughts may be important factors in the *development* of chronicity and thus represent psychological obstacles to recovery that need to be addressed as part of the rehabilitative process. Implications for prevention strategies are discussed further in Chapter 18.

Occupational studies into the recovery from injury and return to work

Burton and colleagues recently reviewed studies in occupational settings, mainly focused on work retention in employees with musculoskeletal difficulties. They concluded that (clinical) historical and psychosocial information rather than the socio-occupational or biomechanical variables that were associated with lack of recovery (Burton, Battie & Main 1998).

Conclusion

There appears to be considerable evidence that a wide range of psychological factors appear to be implicated in the development of disability (whether considered from a clinical or an occupational perspective). Overall, they appear to exert a more powerful influence on the development of disability than the traditional biomedical and ergonomic variables upon which most preventative and intervention strategies are based. It has been suggested in Chapter 4 that,

rather than focus on risks of chronicity as such, it may be advantageous to reconceptualise these psychological features in terms of obstacles to recovery. In order to understand the nature and development of disability, however, it is necessary now to consider how such factors in the context of pain and injury might interact with physiological factors to produce the sort of pain behaviour and chronic dysfunction so characteristic of patients attending pain management programmes.

PAIN, STRESS AND THE DEVELOPMENT OF DISABILITY

The psychological concomitants of chronic pain are now clearly recognised (Ch. 2), and it is increasingly accepted that chronic disability cannot always be explained simply on the basis of anatomical findings. The term 'chronic pain syndrome' can of course refer to almost any constellation of symptoms or incapacities associated with the persistence of pain, but it is becoming increasingly common, both in clinical and in medicolegal circles, to recognise disability as a *psychologically mediated* chronic pain syndrome. The specific mechanisms involved are a matter of much debate. Specific attention has been directed particularly at beliefs, mood and pain behaviour in Chapter 2. The significance of stress from a physiological and biochemical perspective will now be addressed.

The anatomical and physiological substrate

Clinical experience, and common sense, would tell us that pain is stressing, and of course it is common to report increased pain at times of stress (e.g. tension headache). Relatively little attention, however, has been paid specifically to the role of stress and to the possible anatomical and physiological substrates that might be involved. Since the 1960s, researchers in the fields of stress and pain have tended to work relatively independently. Recently, however, Melzack (1999) has offered a new perspective on the relationship between pain and stress that would appear to be of relevance to the understanding of disability.

Melzack's neuromatrix theory

Melzack offers a detailed exposition of the latest development of his theory elsewhere (Melzack 1999). The theory has a number of key features, which are summarised in Box 5.5.

The theory would seem to offer an explanation in terms of homeostasis for the development of chronic pain and disability. The emotional impact of chronic pain can be understood in terms of the stress of pain and other stressors (including specific pain-associated incapacities). The development of chronic disability can be understood within a homeostatic framework in terms of attempt to restore 'equilibrium' by engaging in attempts to minimise pain, if not escape from it, or to avoid pain altogether.

The development of the 'disuse syndrome', fear-mediated responses and guarded movements (frequently observed characteristics of patients attending pain management programmes) can also be understood within this general psychobiological framework as an example of a way of coping with persistent pain.

EXPERIMENTAL STUDIES INTO GUARDED MOVEMENTS, FEAR AND DISUSE

The relationship between emotion and physiological activity in pain has in fact been investigated in the laboratory. In one study of patients with back pain, heightened levels of muscle activity in the back muscles were found when the subjects were asked to imagine pain (Flor, Turk & Birbaumer 1985). Although the changes in the electrical activity in the muscles were relatively small, the effect was found only in response to painful or other stressful stimuli and was not therefore just a matter of attention. These psychophysiological responses can be considered as conditioned emotional reactions, or, (less technically) as residual effects of painful injuries.

Box 5.5 Melzack's neuromatrix theory

- Pain is a multidimensional experience … produced by characteristic 'neurosignatures' or patterns of nerve impulses generated by a widely distributed neural network: the 'body–self–neuromatrix'
- Neurosignature patterns may be triggered by sensory inputs but also independently
- The neuromatrix is genetically determined and modified by sensory experience
- Injury disrupts the body's homeostatic regulation systems thereby producing stress and initiating complex programmes to restore homeostasis
- Stressors activate programmes of neural, hormonal and behavioural activity aimed at restoring homeostasis
- If stress responses continue, they lead to immune system suppression and activation of the limbic system (which has a role in emotion, motivation and cognitive processes)
- Stress and pain perception possess overlapping mechanisms
- Neuromatrices' output determines whether pain will be experienced or suppressed
- Pain suppression must be determined not only by the release of endorphins and other opioids, but

also by sensory, discriminative and evaluative processes
- Prolonged activation of the stress regulation systems will lead to tissue breakdown and 'set the stage' for the development of fibromyalgia, osteoporosis and other chronic pain conditions
- The limbic system, being the neural substrate of the affective–motivational dimension of pain, is so interdependent that it should be considered to be part of a single system
- A number of chronic pain syndromes, as well as depression, may be linked to the stress regulation system
- All psychological stressors may contribute to the neuroendocrine processes that give rise to pain syndromes
- Individual variation in the enhancement of a given stress is a function of: other concurrent stresses, cumulative effect of prior stresses, kinds of concurrent or prior stresses and the severity and duration of stresses
- Even when pain is experienced, it may be a stressor if it implies danger and threat to the survival of the self, physically or psychologically

Adapted from Melzack R Pain and Stress. In Psychosocial Factors in Pain edited by Gatchel R J & Tusk D C 1999. Reprinted with permission from The Guildford Press, New York, USA.

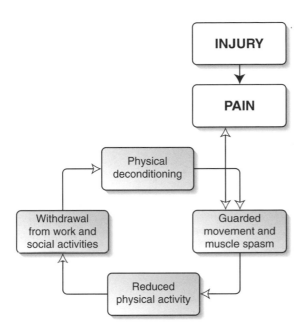

Figure 5.1   Model I: development of deconditiong and disuse.

Such findings are in accord with the common clinical observation that following injury many patients appear to show evidence of guarded movements.

Guarded movements have been investigated using surface electromyography (SEMG) on the lumbar muscles (Main & Watson 1996). Recently, a specific measure of the guarded movement during forward bending, the flexion relaxation ratio (FRR), has been developed and validated for use with low back pain patients (Watson et al 1997).

In a treatment study of chronic back patients undergoing a 3-week pain management rehabilitation programme (Watson, Booker & Main 1997), a significant correlation was found prior to treatment between fear-avoidance beliefs and abnormalities of muscle action. Following the pain management programme there were significant correlations between improvement in the muscular abnormalities, reduction in fear-avoidance beliefs and increases in self-efficacy beliefs (i.e. self-confidence).

These investigations into the development of chronicity suggest that psychological factors may be important mechanisms influencing recovery from injury. The above studies suggest that a number of specific pain-relevant psychological factors merit investigation. These are: the emotional impact of pain, the development of pain behaviour, beliefs about pain, treatment or outcome, and coping strategies.

A NEW MODEL OF DISABILITY

Stage 1. The development of deconditioning and disuse

A model illustrating the development of deconditioning and disuse is shown in Figure 5.1.

One of the major problems of avoidance of activity is that this can lead to physical deconditioning. The effects of physical deconditioning are widespread. Poor cardiovascular function, restricted joint range of motion, reduced muscle strength, reduced soft tissue extensibility, reduced soft tissue strength, poor physical endurance, poor sleep and alteration of mood (depression). These factors can serve not only to increase the perception of pain, poor sleep and depressed mood but they can make rehabilitation particularly difficult. Muscle weakness and

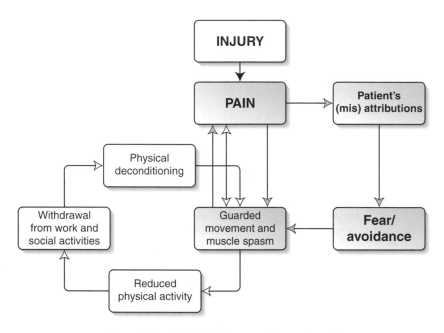

Figure 5.2   Model II: influence of fear and avoidance.

restricted range of joint motion can lead to an increase in pain on resumption of activity. If patients attempt to return to more normal physical activities they may experience an increase in pain owing to deconditioning. Poor physical endurance will result in excessive fatigue on resumption of activities. However, patients will most probably be unaware of the nature of this pain and fatigue and attribute it to the underlying condition that they believe they have. The fact that their pain has increased is seen as a reason for further avoidance, leading to further deconditioning, and a vicious circle develops leading to patients becoming more and more inactive and increasingly disabled.

Stage 2. The influence of fear and avoidance

Although it might be presumed that the initial reaction to acute pain is fairly 'instinctive', as the pain persists the role of fear and avoidance become important. The next stage of the model is shown in Figure 5.2.

Mistaken beliefs about hurting and harming, with fears about pain and future incapacity, are well-recognised features of patients attending pain management programmes. There is evidence that patients overestimate the amount of pain that they believe certain activities will cause and that they may have developed unfounded beliefs about the relationship of physical activity to pain. Indeed, by the time that patients are seen in tertiary treatment facilities, these beliefs, fears and behavioural patterns have often become clearly established and represent significant psychological obstacles to recovery.

As Philips (1987) has pointed out patients may come to view avoidance as the best way of managing their pain and that this avoidance may extend to avoidance of stimulation, movement, activity, social interactions and leisure pursuits. Although such avoidance behaviour may well be adaptive in certain acute disorders (for example if you have just broken your arm it would be adaptive not to use it prior to visiting hospital to have the arm set in plaster) and allow for natural healing to take place, in chronic pain conditions avoidance behaviour is maladaptive. There is little evidence that, in chronic pain, avoidance serves to decrease pain but patients may believe that by avoidance they have

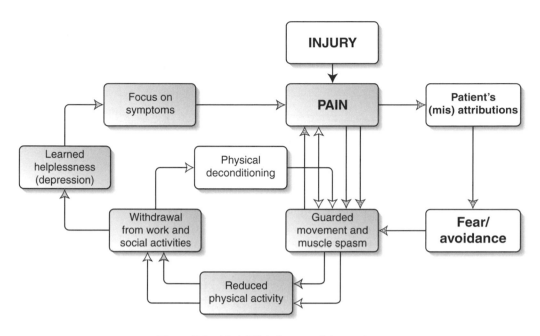

Figure 5.3   Model III: influence of depression.

prevented an anticipated increase in their pain severity. Philips (1987) discussing a study of patients with chronic headache reports that avoidance increases with time even though pain severity does not alter.

Waddell et al (1993) developed the Fear-Avoidance Beliefs Questionnaire (FABQ) to measure the degree to which patients held such fear-avoidance beliefs. Research using this questionnaire showed a strong correlation existed between fear-avoidance beliefs, disability levels and work loss. However, fear-avoidance beliefs were not related to the severity of patients' pain nor did they increase with increasing physical pathology. It seems that cognitive factors such as self-efficacy beliefs and memory for past pain have an important role to play in the development and maintenance of avoidance behaviour in chronic pain.

Stage 3. The influence of depression

As has been discussed above, perception of pain and mood is strongly related. The next stage of the model is shown in Figure 5.3.

Depression, anxiety and anger were the three emotions highlighted in Chapter 2. In the context of disability, depression is frequently the most common of these emotions. Depression influences both the perception of pain and the response to it, but can be best understood perhaps as a mediator between pain and disability. Simply put, pain is normally perceived as unpleasant. It can often be avoided, but only at a cost. If the cost of avoidance is too great, the person will attempt to engage in the painful activity. Judgement about this 'cost–benefit' ratio will be affected by a number of factors, but one of the most powerful is depression. Depression brings cognitive distortion and catastrophising (Ch. 2). This affects assessment of the 'cost–benefit' ratio. Patients may conclude that it is not worth making the effort to overcome their pain, that the perceived 'cost' is too high; that the likely 'benefit' is too low. As they become more avoidant, they may become socially withdrawn and isolated, and never hear an alternative more optimistic analysis of their situation. They become more aware of their pain and focused upon it. In the context of chronic disability, this

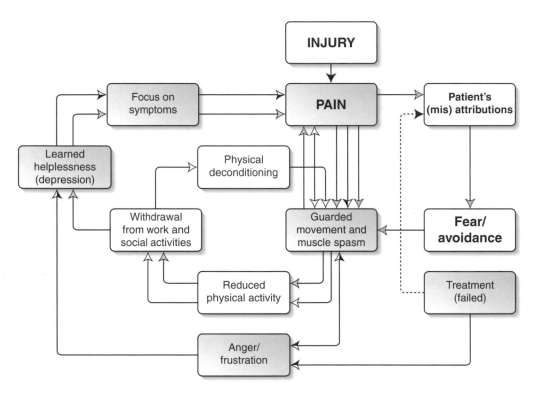

Figure 5.4 Model IV: influence of anger and frustration.

phenomenon can be understood as a sort of 'learned helplessness'.

Stage 4. The influence of anger and frustration

Anger and frustration also are frequent concomitants of chronic pain. Their influence on disability is illustrated in Figure 5.4.

Patients may have become angry for a host of reasons, and in consideration of their suitability for pain management it is important to assess whether or not the focus (or intensity) of their anger represents a significant obstacle to recovery (Chs 10 and 12). In consideration of disability, anger is important both for its physiological effects and for its psychological effects. Physiologically, elevated levels of tension may increase perceived pain intensity, which may in turn fuel the level of frustration and anger. Anger may affect compliance with treatment and benefit received from pain management. Not only are

stress and pain related (see above), but more specifically so are frustration, feelings of helplessness and avoidance behaviour. A powerful example of this interdependence can be seen in the effects of failed treatment (or iatrogenics).

Stage 5. The influence of iatrogenics

Treatment is not always effective and sometimes it is in fact detrimental (Loeser & Sullivan 1995). Adverse response to treatment is sometimes termed 'iatrogenic', which is defined as: 'a complication, injury, unfavourable result or other problem which can be directly attributed to medical care' (Churchill's illustrated medical dictionary 1989). Waddell et al (1984a) found that in a large sample of patients with chronic low back pain the amount of treatment received (e.g. bed rest, injections, physiotherapy) was related more to patients' level of distress and illness behaviour than to the presence of physical indications for such treatment. Patients attending pain

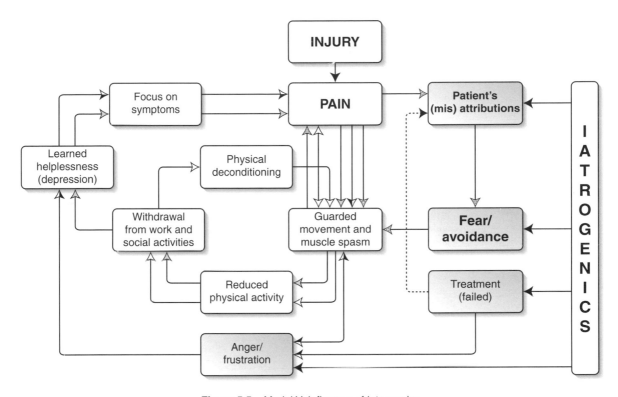

Figure 5.5   Model V: influence of iatrogenics.

management programmes frequently have had a lot of previous treatment, but, of all the sources of anger and frustration evident in patients attending pain management programmes, the influence of failed treatment among chronic pain patients is perhaps the most powerful. Specific iatrogenic influences are illustrated in the next stage of the model, shown as Figure 5.5.

Many patients are fearful of their pain and what it indicates (Ch. 2). They commonly have substantial misunderstandings about pain, the nature of tissue injury and healing. If such beliefs go unchallenged patients may continue to respond to their pain in an unhelpful way. On some occasions doctors and others actively reinforce such beliefs (more pain means more damage and therefore more pain) by telling patients to 'rest up' or 'let pain be their guide'. This will inevitably lead to the patient limiting their activity according to their pain. It will reinforce avoidance of any activity that is painful, thus leading to fear-avoidance

behaviour. Repeated failed treatment with unrealistic expectations of outcome may reinforce the patient's belief that there is something seriously wrong. Failure to improve may also contribute to the patient's sense of frustration. Patients may also perceive that the doctor doesn't really believe they have as much pain as they say or that it is all 'in the head'. This judgement may have been made on the basis of failure to respond to treatment. It serves only to make patients more angry and contributes to their sense of helplessness. They may focus more on the pain and seek further opinions.

Stage 6. The influence of the family

The role of the family has been discussed extensively in previous chapters, but it is important to consider its influence specifically on disability and response to treatment. The most powerful influence is usually from the patient's partner

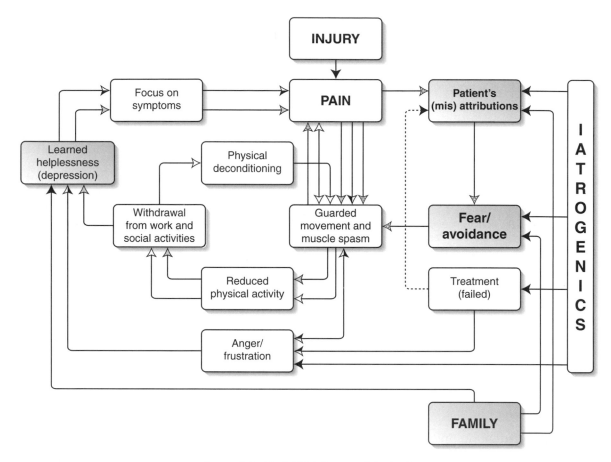

Figure 5.6 Model VI: influence of the family.

(Turk, Flor & Rudy 1987). The influence of the family is shown in Figure 5.6.

The family will have their own beliefs about the patient's pain, its cause and how it should be treated.

Persuading patients to undergo treatment

The partner may be the main instigator of the initial consultation. Many patients are anxious about consulting doctors, and partners can be helpful in encouraging patients to overcome such fears. They may insist that there *must* be something seriously wrong or there *must* be something that can be done. If, however, patients would rather remain incapacitated than undergo further treatment, they may feel resentful about being 'forced to undergo further consultations'.

Reinforcement of mistaken beliefs

The partner, like the patient, may mistake hurting for harming and believe, perhaps with even more conviction than the patient, that further treatment at best will be useless and at worse positively harmful. There is evidence that the response of partners can have a strong influence on rehabilitation outcome. Many clinics do not routinely incorporate partners into the management plan. In pain management programmes the inclusion of partners, both at the stage of assessment and also during the pain management programme, will diminish the likelihood of reinforcement of mistaken beliefs.

Undermining patient confidence

During pain management programmes, patients may need encouragement from time to time. A disinterested or dismissive attitude may undermine the patient's confidence. Some partners become overprotective and will not allow patients to do anything for fear of making their pain worse. Patients may then learn to become more and more reliant upon their family members for almost everything. This may lead to a decline in patients' sense of self-worth and they then become more depressed.

Undermining progress

Finally, family members may actually sabotage progress. This may not be deliberate. Partners may have emotional investment in the patient remaining incapacitated. A partner may have become the principal carer of the patient (and even given up paid employment to do so). The implication of such family dynamics must be addressed with both patients and their partners. The partner may be unaware that they are being overprotective. During group sessions in the pain management programme patients may have to be trained in assertiveness to overcome such difficulties and re-establish appropriate control over the management of their own pain-associated limitations. Conscious and deliberate attempts to sabotage progress are less common and constitute a barrier to inclusion in pain management.

Stage 7. The influence of socioeconomic and occupational factors

Socioeconomic and occupational influences on pain and response to treatment have been extensively discussed in the previous chapter, and they provide the final component in the model of disability, as shown in Figure 5.7.

Disability needs to be understood not only in terms of pain, suffering and pain-associated limitations, but also specifically in the context of economic and occupational compromise.

Financial effects

By the time patients attend a pain management programme they may have suffered a major decline in living standards and perhaps be faced with job loss and even loss of their property. As will be mentioned in Chapter 6, many pain management programmes are funded by occupational agencies or employers with the *specific* objective of return to work. Some patients may be faced with dire financial consequences if they cannot return to work. Some may fear loss of benefits if they improve their level of functioning as a consequence of treatment. Yet others may fear that improvement in functioning may compromise a medicolegal claim. Such factors can effect how patients present symptoms, and how they respond to treatment. Socioeconomic factors can serve both as powerful incentives for improved function and as powerful disincentives. Such factors must be viewed as possible obstacles to recovery (Ch. 4) and taken into account as part of clinical decision making (Chs 11 and 12). It is not possible, however, to make more than general observations as patients must be considered individually and a judgement made about the contribution of such factors to the overall level of disability in each case.

The interaction amongst these factors can be varied and complex, as is illustrated in Case study 5.1.

CONCLUSION

Disability needs to be understood as a biopsychosocial phenomenon that needs to be addressed from a range of perspectives and cannot be understood in terms of physical impairment alone. An attempt has been made in this chapter to examine discrete facets of the phenomenon, but, as was illustrated in the concluding case study, the challenge for the clinician is to understand how these various features interact in the individual patient. Only then can a competent decision be made regarding suitability for treatment and an appropriate 'patient path' identified.

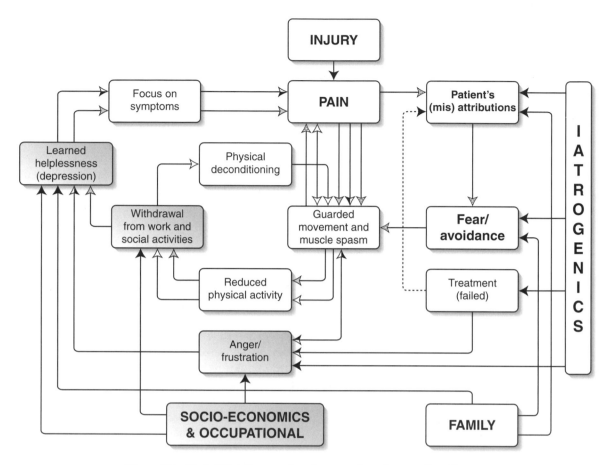

Figure 5.7 Model VII: influence of socioeconomic and occupational factors.

Case study 5.1 Model of disability

Stage 1
Mr S. was a very fit building labourer aged 30. He sustained a back injury at work when he fell off a plank, which had not been secured properly. He experienced immediate pain in his back. He had to leave work early and was taken home by a friend. By the next day he was in severe pain and was very stiff.

He was advised by his GP to rest up and was given analgesics and anti-inflammatory drugs. He was also given a sick note for 2 weeks. Mr S. did not notice any change in his pain. He felt unable to exercise (he was previously very active in sports).

Stage 2
By the end of the second week Mr S. was concerned that he had seriously injured his back. His pain was still severe and he had become progressively more and more stiff. Any attempt on his part to become more active produced excruciating pain and stiffness, which did not settle for several hours. Following further

advice from his GP he continued to rest and avoid activity. He was convinced that if he tried to do too much before his back 'healed' he would damage himself further.

Stage 3
As the weeks went by Mr S. became more demoralised. Not only was he not able to go to work, but he was unable to get out of the house. He could not go to the gym and he had lost contact with his workmates. Slowly his mood drifted down and he began to focus on his pain, which was preventing him from doing almost anything.

Stage 4
Mr S. tried on a number of occasions to 'get moving' as he was becoming very frustrated at his lack of fitness and reliance on others, including his wife, for trivial things. However, each time he tried to do something it simply caused a lot of pain and he would have to rest in

---

Case study 5.1   Cont'd

bed for days. His GP had sent him to physiotherapy. The physiotherapist tried some mobilisations but Mr S. had got very much worse afterwards. The physiotherapist was worried about Mr S.'s condition and had suggested a referral to a specialist. Mr S. was now convinced there was something seriously wrong. He avoided anything that would aggravate the pain until he saw the specialist.

Stage 5
Mr S. was eventually seen by a specialist. Some X-rays were taken and the specialist told Mr S. that he had arthritis of the spine. He suggested some injections and more physiotherapy. Unfortunately neither of these helped. In fact they seemed to make his pain worse. The specialist said there was no more he could do and that Mr S. would have to learn to live with it. If his pain got any worse he should come back. Mr S.'s worst fears had come true. He knew he had a progressive disease, 'arthritis'. He wondered how he would be when he was 60. He became very angry with his GP and his employer who he felt were not helpful. He was soon made redundant. He could not understand why more could not be done for him.

Stage 6
By now Mr S.'s wife had gone back to full-time work and had to do everything around the house. She left him meals ready each day so that he would not have to do too much. She would not let him do anything for fear of yet more pain. She went to her GP to insist on another specialist appointment. She felt there was perhaps something else wrong. She was worried her husband would end up in a wheelchair.

Stage 7
Mr S. had been called for a medical for his disability benefit. The examining doctor hurt him during the assessment. Mr S. later learned that the doctor felt there was nothing wrong with him and his benefits were withdrawn. Meanwhile Mr S.'s trade union was seeking compensation on his behalf. Mr S. therefore had to undergo a number of medical examinations from doctors instructed by his union's solicitors and those of his previous employers. Mr S. felt insulted when he read some of the reports, which seemed to imply he was putting it all on and malingering. He became very angry and depressed. His wife and family, meanwhile, had to adjust their lifestyle as the family's income had effectively halved.

KEY POINTS

- It is important to distinguish physical impairment, disability, handicap and functional capacity.
- Disability is multifactorial and changes with the passage of time.
- The relative contributions of biomedical and psychosocial components of disability have been quantified.

- Psychosocial factors are more powerful than biomedical factors in the prediction of disability.
- A new conceptual model of the influences of biomedical, physiological, psychological, socioeconomic and iatrogenic factors on disability is presented.

REFERENCES

Blankenship S K 1986 Functional capacity evaluation: the procedure manual. American Therapeutics, Macon, GA

Brena S F, Koch D L 1975 A 'pain-estimate' model for quantification and classification of chronic pain states. Anaesthesia Review 2:8–13.

Burton A K, Tillotson K M 1991 Prediction of the clinical course of low back trouble using multivariable models. Spine 16:7–14

Burton A K, Tillotson K M, Main C J, Hollis S 1995 Psychosocial predictors of outcome in acute and subchronic low back trouble. Spine 20:722–728

Burton A K, Battie M C, Main C J 1998 The relative importance of biomechanical and psychosocial factors in low back injuries. In: Karwowski W, Marras W S (eds) The occupational ergonomics handbook. CRC, Boca Raton, Ch 61, pp 1127–1138.

Churchill's illustrated medical dictionary 1989. Churchill Livingstone, New York

Flor H, Turk D C, Birbaumer N 1985 Assessment of stress-related psychophysiological stress reactions in chronic back pain patients. Journal of Consulting and Clinical Psychology 53:354–364

Frank J W, Kerr M S, Brooker A-S et al 1996 Disability resulting from occupational low back pain. Spine 21:2908–2929

Gatchel R J 1991 Early development of physical and mental deconditioning in painful spinal disorders. In: Mayer T G, Mooney V, Gatchell R J (eds) Contemporary conservative care for painful spinal disorders. Lea & Febiger, Philadelphia

Gatchel R J 1996 Psychological disorders and chronic pain. In: Gatchell R J, Turk D C (eds) Psychological approaches to pain management. Guilford, New York, pp 33–52

Halpern M (1992) Prevention of low back pain: basic ergonomics in the workplace and clinic. In: Nordin M, Fischer T L (eds) Common low back pain: prevention of chronicity. Baillière-Tindall, London, pp 705–730

Harding V R, Williams A C, Richardson P H et al 1994 The development of a battery of measures for assessing physical functioning of chronic pain patients. Pain 58(3):367–375

Kerns R D, Turk D C, Rudy T E 1985 The Westhaven-Yale Multidimensional Pain Inventory (WHYMPI). Pain 23:345–356

Loeser J D, Sullivan M 1995 Disability in the chronic low back pain patient may be iatrogenic. Pain Forum, 4:114–121

Main C J, Watson P J 1996 Guarded movements: development of chronicity. Journal of Musculoskeletal Pain 4:163–170

Main C J, Wood P L R, Hollis S, Spanswick C C, Waddell G 1992 The distress assessment method: a simple patient classification to identify distress and evaluate risk of poor outcome. Spine 17:42–50

Mayer T G, Gatchel R J 1988 Functional restoration for spinal disorders: the sports medicine approach. Lea & Febiger, Philadelphia

Melzack R 1987 The Short-Form McGill Pain Questionnaire. Pain 30:191–197

Melzack R 1999 Pain and stress: a new perspective. In: Gatchel R J, Turk D C (eds) Psychosocial factors in pain; critical perspectives. Guilford, New York, ch 6, pp 89–108

Nashold B S, Hrubec Z 1971 Lumbar disk disease: a 20 year follow-up study. CV Mosby, St Louis MO

Philips H C 1987 Avoidance behaviour and its role in sustaining chronic pain. Behavior Research and Therapy 25:273–279

Robinson M E, Swimmer G I, Rallof D 1989 The P-A-I-N MMPI classification system: a critical review. Pain 37:211–214

Turk D C, Okifuji A 1997 Multidisciplinary pain centers: boons or boondoggles? Journal of Worker's Compensation 6:9–26

Turk D C, Flor H, Rudy T E 1987 Pain and families. I. Etiology, maintenance and psychosocial impact. Pain 30:3–27

Turk D C, Rudy T 1992 Classification, logic and strategies in chronic pain. In: Turk D C, Melzack R (eds) Handbook of pain assessment. Guilford, New York, ch 23, pp 409–428

Waddell G 1987 A new clinical model for the treatment of low back pain. Spine 12:632–644

Waddell G 1998 The back pain revolution. Churchill Livingstone, New York

Waddell G, Main C 1984 Assessment of severity in low back disorders. Spine 9:204–208

Waddell G, Bircher M, Finlayson D, Main C J 1984a Symptoms and signs: physical disease or illness behaviour? British Medical Journal 289:739–741

Waddell G, Main C J, Morris E W, Di Paola M, Gray I C M 1984b Chronic low-back pain, psychologic distress and illness behavior. Spine 9:209–213

Waddell G, Somerville D, Henderson I, Newton M 1992 Objective clinical evaluation of physical impairment in chronic low back pain. Spine 17:617–628

Waddell G, Newton M, Henderson I, Somerville D, Main C 1993 A Fear-Avoidance Beliefs Questionnaire (FABQ) and the role of fear avoidance beliefs in chronic low back pain. Pain 52:157–168

Watson P J, Booker C K, Main C J 1997 Evidence for the role of psychological factors in abnormal paraspinal activity in patients with chronic low back pain. Journal of Musculoskeletal Pain 5(4):41–56

Watson P J, Booker C K, Main C J, Chen A C N 1997 Surface electromyography in the identification of chronic low back pain patients: the development of the flexion relaxation ratio. Clinical Biomechanics 12:165–171

WHO 1980 International classification of impairments, disabilities and handicaps. World Health Organisation, Geneva

Weiser S, Cedraschi C 1992 Psychosocial influences in the prevention of chronic low back pain—a literature review. Baillière's Clinical Rheumatology 6:657–684

Williams M M, Grant R N, Main C J 1995 The Distress Risk Assessment Method (DRAM) as a predictor of outcome in chronically disabled workers attending a physical rehabilitation programme. Abstracts International Society for the Study of the Lumbar Spine, Helsinki, Finland, p 46

6

The origins and development of modern pain management programmes

Chris J. Main   Chris C. Spanswick

INTRODUCTION

In his textbook of pain, Bonica (1990) outlines the origins and development of multidisciplinary and interdisciplinary pain programmes. Bonica (1990) reports that his experience as a military anaesthetist led him to appreciate the difficulty in managing some of the more complicated pain problems. He developed the view that such patients could be best managed by a multidisciplinary/interdisciplinary team, all member of which contribute their own specialised knowledge. Shortly after the Second World War, the first such clinic was established in Tacoma General Hospital in Washington State. Interestingly the initial group of specialists included an anaesthesiologist, a neurosurgeon, an orthopaedic surgeon, a psychiatrist, an internist and a radiation therapist. This group met approximately fortnightly to discuss complex cases. The clinic ran for 13 years. The problems encountered at that time seem strikingly familiar (Bonica 1990, p. 198):

They included (a) the resistance by many physicians to accept the team approach and their reluctance to refer patients to the group, especially if the physician was in the same speciality as one of the members of the group; (b) difficulty in co-ordinating the time of conferences so that all of the key persons and the referring physician could attend; (c) difficulty in discussing the problem frankly, especially failure(s) of the referring physician and other specialists to make a correct diagnosis or to carry out effective therapy; (d) the cost of the comprehensive evaluation which was then considered too high.

In the 1950s a number of other truly multidisciplinary clinics were those established at the VA hospital in McKinney, Texas by Alexander and at the University of Oregon in Portland by Livingston. According to Bonica, these three facilities were the true forerunners of the modern pain management programmes. Although this may be historically accurate, the programmes developed in the 1960s have had most influence. Pre-eminent is the University of Washington Pain Clinic established by Bonica himself from 1960. Around the same period, Crue together with Pinsky established the programme at the City of Hope Medical Center in Los Angeles and Seres together with Newman established the first private multidisciplinary programme in Portland, Oregon. There followed a rapid and widespread development of pain management programmes. No less than 327 pain clinics appeared in the first directory of pain clinics (Modell 1977). It was of course immediately apparent that the range and quality of services offered under the name of a 'pain clinic' were widely variable, ranging from single-handed anaesthetists delivering nerve blocks to comprehensive pain services such as those at the University of Washington.

The history of pain management has been bedevilled by matters of definition, but in 1979 a second survey was carried out and resulted in an important fourfold classification of pain centres/clinics (Carron 1979). The essential features are outlined below.

Modality-oriented pain centre. This offers appropriate therapy *as defined by the specialty of the centre.* These might include nerve-block clinics, transcutaneous electrical nerve stimulation (TENS) clinics, acupuncture clinics, biofeedback clinics and mental health centres.

Syndrome-oriented pain centre. In such facilities a range of treatments is offered for a particular syndrome. Examples include headache clinics, facial pain clinics and low backpain clinics.

Comprehensive pain centre. In such a facility, a large variety of pain syndromes are dealt with. Psychosocial as well as physical aspects of pain are managed. At least two-thirds of the criteria listed under 'major comprehensive pain centre' must be available.

Major comprehensive pain centre. This is the 'Rolls-Royce' of pain facilities, with adequate space and a wide range of personnel, committed to comprehensive assessment of all aspects of pain and capable of developing a multidisciplinary approach to pain management. The following prerequisites are necessary (Bonica 1990, p. 200):

space and beds assigned solely to the pain center; a professional staff representing five or more disciplines; full-time support staff (secretaries, nurses, therapists etc) organised evaluative process for screening and selecting of patients; review and maintenance of records; participation of consultants of various disciplines; routine psychologic assessment; ongoing research activities; organised training programs; availability of therapy appropriate for the physical and psychosocial problems found; and periodic evaluation of treatment results.

It is clear that if there is a move towards a 'hub-and-spoke' system of health-care delivery in the UK (Ch. 15) then some sort of classification will have to be adopted. The fourfold classification might serve as a useful starting point.

Brena (1985) reviewed the distribution of clinical models and medical specialties in pain control facilities. They are summarised in Table 6.1. It can be seen that at that time the majority of clinics were either modality oriented or syndrome oriented, and about two-thirds of the clinics were in the USA. The table also illustrated that the majority of clinics were anaesthetically led.

The rapid development in pain clinics led to concern for quality. The American Pain Society therefore developed a set of guidelines, which were adopted by the Commission for Accreditation of Rehabilitation Facilities (CARF), a non-profit organisation supported by a number of other organisations. The evolution and function of CARF are detailed elsewhere (Morse 1985).

SEATTLE MODEL

The University of Washington Pain Centre in Seattle, hereafter referred to as the 'Seattle model', has become world renowned. It has pioneered multidimensional treatment, research, education and interdisciplinary working. Its

Table 6.1 Distribution of models and specialties in pain control facilities

	Asia	Australia New Zealand	Canada	Europe	Latin America	USA
Major comprehensive pain centres	1	1	1	6	0	41
Comprehensive pain centres	10	7	9	17	1	78
Modality-oriented pain clinics	13	2	13	40	1	97
Syndrome oriented pain clinics	6	1	4	16	1	62
Department with primary responsibility						
Anaesthesiology	14	7	11	35	3	96
Neurosurgery	2	1	1	6	0	31
Orthopaedic surgery	0	0	0	1	0	8
Psychiatry	0	1	2	0	0	9
Psychology	1	0	2	0	0	7
Oral surgery	1	1	3	0	0	13
Rehabilitation medicine	2	0	2	3	0	35
Others	1	1	4	13	0	18

From Brena Pain Control Facilities 1985, reproduced with permission.

specific missions are declared as follows (Bonica 1990, p. 202):

1. To enhance the quality of care of patients with chronic pain referred to the University of Washington Medical Center and affiliated hospitals and to have the Clinical Service to serve as a model of a multidisciplinary/interdisciplinary facility for the diagnosis and therapy of complex pain problems.
2. To contribute to the education in algology of graduate students of medicine, dentistry, clinical psychology and other health professions.
3. To encourage the study of the basic mechanisms and the anatomic, physiologic, behavioral and psychosocial aspects of acute and chronic pain, through individual research projects, program projects and demonstration projects.
4. To encourage the development of research teams composed of critical masses of scientists and clinical algologists from the appropriate disciplines to study some of the more important clinical pain syndromes, to evaluate current therapeutic modalities, and to develop new and better procedures for diagnosis and treatment of such syndromes.
5. To enhance interaction and communication among all pain investigators at the University of Washington and to encourage cross-fertilisation of ideas on pain research and therapy.
6. To educate and train biomedical scientists who will pursue careers in pain research.
7. To enhance the transmission of new knowledge about the diagnosis and therapy of pain to all practitioners of the health profession.

Perhaps the most important aspect of this statement is the breadth of perspective illustrated. The conceptualisation of pain as consisting of nociception, suffering and pain behaviour represents a radical departure from the traditional medical model (Ch. 1). Their mission is not only an example of a practical implementation of a biopsychosocial model of pain (Ch. 5), but also an illustration of the mutual interdependence of clinical practice, teaching, training and research. In an almost immeasurable sense, the Seattle model has served as an inspiration to the rest of the world.

More specifically, in the early days, the Seattle group promoted a view of illness that incorporated both physical and behavioural aspects. Although the behavioural perspective has broadened from its original fairly narrow origins in behaviourism (both experimental and sociological), the importance of the introduction of this perspective as as alternative to a a narrow pathology-based medical view cannot be overemphasised. Although most pain management programmes now would define themselves as cognitive–behavioural in their orientation, the power and incisiveness of the behavioural component (Fordyce 1976) in the original Seattle model was critical to the development of modern interdisciplinary pain management.

COGNITIVE–BEHAVIOURAL MODEL

During the last 20 years, there has been increasing interest in cognitive aspects of pain. The arrival of a major textbook on cognitive–behavioural approaches to pain (Turk, Meichenbaum & Genest 1983) represented another significant phase of conceptual development. It had been observed that there were similarities between chronic pain patients and depressed patients both behaviourally and cognitively. Aspects of the treatment of cognitive distortion and learned helplessness in patients with depression were blended with training in cognitive coping strategies for pain derived essentially from the hypnosis literature. These cognitive approaches were combined with some of the behavioural methods outlined by Fordyce into a comprehensive approach to pain management known as cognitive–behavioural therapy, or CBT. This has become the framework from which most current pain management programmes are derived. Simply put, the behavioural model focuses primarily (and some would say exclusively) on what patients are *doing*. Cognitions, if deemed relevant at all, are seen as being of secondary importance. In contrast to the radical behavioural approach, CBT aims to change the way patients think, challenge their beliefs about their pain and therefore influence how they behave.

DEVELOPMENTS IN THE UK

The first out- or day-patient pain management programmes were developed at Walton Hospital in Liverpool and at Hope Hospital in Salford in 1983. Since then there has been a progressive development. A number of other hospitals offered group therapy for pain patients but would not meet the criteria for a pain management programme. There were programmes established in psychiatric wards in Gartnavel Hospital in Glasgow and at Manchester Royal Infirmary, but the first fully funded in-patient pain management programme was opened at St Thomas's Hospital in London in 1988. A number of smaller programmes were also established at Gloucester Royal Hospital and Whittington

Hospital. During the 1990s there has been a rapid development of treatments for pain by an increasing number of health-care professionals and many other pain management programmes have been established. They have varied in complexity, content, context and organisation, but in general they have focused on the care of the chronic pain patient. Unfortunately this development has been somewhat chaotic and frankly entreprenurial, which has been confusing both for patients and for purchasers of health care. The British and Irish Chapter of the International Association for the Study of Pain (IASP) therefore, inspired by the IASP report (IASP 1990) and by Sanders (1994), recently produced a set of 'desirable characteristics' for pain management programmes (Pain Society 1997). They are discussed in relationship to service development and competencies in later chapters of this book (Chs 15 and 16).

INGREDIENTS OF A PAIN MANAGEMENT PROGRAMME

Pain management programmes contain many ingredients. Loeser, Seres & Newman (1990) identify 23 different assessment and treatment modalities that include: medical assessment, psychological assessment, diagnostic procedures, medical treatment, physical therapy, occupational therapy, psychological treatment, vocational counselling, vocational aptitude testing, family therapy, nerve blocks, trigger point injections, acupuncture, biofeedback, relaxation therapy, autogenic training, education, assertiveness training, communication training, massage therapy, TENS, ablative neurosurgery and implanted stimulators. Recent interest in complementary medicine in the UK has seen the promulgation of a host of other treatments, which are sometimes incorporated into pain management programmes.

As early as 1980, the National Institute of Drug Abuse in the USA commissioned a conference at the National Institute of Health in Bethesda, Maryland charged with carrying out a review of multidisciplinary pain clinics and pain centres. The subsequent publication (Ng 1981)

Box 6.1   Elements of the pain management programme

Identified problem
- Nociception
- Lack of knowledge
- Stiffness/immobility
- Loss of strength/fitness
- Distress
- Depression
- Pain behaviour
- Cognitive dysfunction
- Maladaptive coping
- Ergonomic mismatch

Therapeutic solution
- Pain reduction
- Education
- Activation
- Functional restoration
- Counselling
- Pharmacotherapy or CBT
- Respondent and operant behaviour therapy
- Cognitive therapy
- CBT
- Work redesign

---

illustrated the considerable diversity even at that time in the philosophy, administration, funding, clinical focus and diagnostic conditions targeted by the pain management programmes then established. There are, however, a number of common themes and key elements and the development of the modern interdisciplinary pain management programme has to be seen against the backdrop of these earlier programmes. Every programme contains a number of discrete elements blended into a package of care. Each of these elements has its own pedigree as an approach to treatment, and each element has its origins in a particular perspective on the nature of pain.

A number of the elements in a pain management programme are highlighted in Box 6.1. The shift from the Cartesian to the biopsychosocial model of pain is clearly demonstrated.

Pain modality techniques

Specific pain reduction techniques such as nerve blocks or neuroablative techniques are offered by certain pain centres in order to assist rehabilitation. Since they are completely passive in nature, however, they may lead to patients ascribing change to the techniques concerned rather than their own self-directed effort. Pharmacological assistance in terms of analgesics, non-steroidal anti-inflammatory drugs (NSAIDS) or antidepressants may be offered, but in pain management programmes they should be used in order to facilitate recovery of function and not as the primary or sole treatment strategy (Ch. 8).

Back schools

The proliferation of back schools as a form of education was based on the assumption that the principal reason for the development of unnecessary disability was mistaken beliefs or lack of knowledge. They were introduced originally into occupational settings to try to prevent the development of chronic incapacity in workers who had been injured. Misinformation or lack of appropriate education, however, should be recognised as significant obstacles to change. Presentation of an appropriate 'pain and disability model' and delivery of the self-help message are critical to the success of the rehabilitative process. An appropriate educational component is a major ingredient of all pain management programmes but it seems that education, although necessary, may not be sufficient (Ch. 19). It seems that unless increased understanding leads to significant behaviour change it is of little value.

Individualised approaches to the treatment of stiffness and immobility

Treatment of stiffness and immobility are cornerstones of individualised approaches to manipulation and mobilisation, as offered by many physiotherapists, osteopaths and chiropractors. Recent systematic reviews have found some evidence of effectiveness in the very acute stages of incapacity, but there is no evidence for their effectiveness for chronic pain (Ch. 17). As passive techniques, they do not assist patients to help themselves. More appropriate self-directed physiotherapeutic approaches are discussed in Chapter 13.

The loss of fitness, loss of strength and the 'disuse syndrome'

Many chronic patients are characterised by the 'disuse' syndrome (the development of which is discussed in Ch. 5). Loss of strength and fitness are key features of many chronic pain patients. Sophisticated functional restoration programmes, or FRPs, (Mayer & Gatchel 1988) place considerable emphasis on restoration of muscle power and fitness as a way of achieving increased functional capacity. The 'sports medicine' approach has often been attempted by the time patients arrive on pain management programmes. In most such programmes there is insufficient time to achieved significant changes in strength or aerobic fitness by the end of the programme. A large proportion of therapeutic effort is directed at educational and psychological obstacles to change. It is not possible to schedule as rigorous a programme of activity as is found on most FRPs. It is expected none the less that some progress in restoration of strength and fitness will occur and this will serve as the basis from which further change will develop.

Treatment of distress and depression

The treatment of distress or depression on an individual basis will not often be necessary and indeed will often not be appropriate. To the extent that distress is based on loss of confidence and misunderstanding about the nature of the pain, being part of a group may alleviate the problem to a considerable extent. Most depression is reactive to (or secondary) to the pain-associated incapacity (Ch. 2). Restoration of function with associated increase in quality of life will 'treat' the depression.

Cognitive therapy or CBT is the treatment modality of choice for cognitive dysfunction or maladaptive coping strategies (Ch. 2). In pain management programmes such problems are tackled primarily within groups. The more recent focus on the role of fear and avoidance behaviour (Ch. 5) can be seen as a further development of this integrated perspective.

Modification of pain behaviour

Modification of pain behaviour may take many forms. In many of the early clinics, biofeedback was routinely used to try to reduce physiological arousal in general and muscle tension in particular. Stress reduction programmes are now part of every competent pain management programme although its specific effects are unclear. The psychological boost to re-establishing some control over patients' incapacity may be as important as specific counterconditioning of the pain response. Operantly maintained pain is hard to assess and even harder to 'treat' but the focus of attention may be the family, the work environment or the economic milieu (Chs 3 and 4). Although it may be extremely difficult to effect change in such parameters within the context of such a programme, clarification of their nature may enable patients to make more informed choices. Considerable change can be effected within pain management programmes, particularly on in-patient programmes, but unless changes are made also in a patient's own environment the programme will lead to only short term changes (Ch. 17). Assessment of such factors is extremely important in clinical decision making and they may best be viewed as potential obstacles to change rather than patient goals that are likely to be achievable (Ch. 12).

The development of occupationally oriented rehabilitation

Finally, sources of funding and specification of outcome in terms of occupational parameters have led to a number of programmes that are particularly occupationally focused (Chs 4 and 19). Some incorporate ergonomic assessment of the workplace and simulate specific work tasks. As such they resemble some of the FRPs. In some countries there are strong interfaces between health and education, which have allowed the development of shared initiatives including both

---

Box 6.2   Defining characteristics of the pain management programme

- Behavioural rather than a disease perspective
- Focus on pain management rather than cure
- Blend of ingredients
- Interdisciplinary skill-mix
- Incorporation of group therapy
- Emphasis on active rather than passive approaches to treatment
- Promulgation of self-help and patient responsibility

---

clinical management and ergonomic redesign. Pain management programmes differ in the extent to which such arrangements are possible, perhaps because specific competencies in biomechanics and ergonomics are necessary (Ch. 16). Increasing emphasis on reduction in sickness absence as an outcome criterion (Ch. 17), however, is likely to lead to the development of this aspect of pain management.

Defining characteristics of pain management programmes are listed in Box 6.2.

It is not possible to overstress the importance of the behavioural perspective as an alternative to the disease/pathology model in offering a new and alternative understanding of pain. It has led to the focus on pain management as an alternative to cure, which is not available for many pain conditions.

The widely varied content of pain management programmes has already been highlighted. The precise package offered by a particular centre may depend more on the opportunistic 'hijacking' of enthusiastic staff and 'carpet bagging' rather than an articulated and well-reasoned plan. The requirements of evidence-based medicine, with the focus of purchasers on much clearer outcome-related funding (Ch. 17), will make such chaotic service development much less common. There will be not only a requirement to justify the costs of the whole programme but, as is happening increasingly in North America, an examination of specific aspects of care from the perspective of managed care plans. The establishment of desirable characteristics of such programmes has begun (IASP 1990, Pain Society 1997,

Sanders 1994) and the setting of standards seems inevitable. Perhaps this development should be welcomed rather than resisted (Ch. 20).

Whatever the blend of therapeutic ingredients, an interdisciplinary skill mix is required and the group milieu is essential. Arguably, patients learn as much from each other as from staff. It should be remembered, however, that there is more to group therapy than sitting in a circle. Specific competence in the therapeutic use of groups is exceedingly important (Ch. 16).

Perhaps most important of all as a defining characteristic of pain management programmes is the promulgation of self-help and personal responsibility. This is evident particularly in the emphasis on active rather than passive approaches to treatment.

CONCLUSION

The specific focus on pain reduction for chronic pain patients was seen as a logical extension of skills developed by anaesthetists in the management of postoperative pain. Unfortunately, such pharmacological and modality treatments proved less successful in treatment of complex or long-standing pain problems than was hoped. Agencies such as the Workmen's Compensation Board (WCB) found themselves carrying increasing costs of chronic incapacity in injured workers unable to return to work. The shift in emphasis led to the identification of a wider set of objectives for treatment than pain reduction. Behavioural analyses of the circumstances in which pain occurred shifted focus to individuals' responses to their pain and the determinants of pain-associated incapacity. The broader perspective required a broader range of skills packaged into treatment programmes, which included a variety of components delivered by several health-care professionals. The modern interdisciplinary pain management programme for the chronic pain patient represents the latest development in a process that began 40 years ago with the recognition of the limitations of traditional 'nociceptive' models in the conceptualisation of chronic pain and pain-associated incapacity.

The powerful influence of iatrogenic distress and dysfunction as a consequence of excessive and inappropriate treatment has been recognised. The lessons learned in pain management programmes about the characteristics of chronic pain have highlighted therapeutic possibilities for early intervention. It seems likely that the first years of the this century will be characterised by a significant shift from primary prevention to secondary prevention and from chronic care to subchronic care.

KEY POINTS

- Pain management began as pain relief clinics, using a range of specific modalities designed to relieve pain.
- The first multidisciplinary pain management clinics were established in North America in the late 1950s and early 60s.
- During the 1970s there was a progressive growth in the number of pain management centres in North America (many funded by Workmen's Compensation Board schemes). Since the 1980s, pain management programmes increasingly have become established in other countries.
- Clinics ranged in sophistication from single-handed modality clinics to fully comprehensive multidisciplinary centres.
- Larger centres integrated service delivery with clinical research and teaching.
- The earliest programmes were primarily behavioural in orientation. Most now offer an approach to pain management that is both cognitive and behavioural.
- There is now clear scientific evidence of their efficacy.

REFERENCES

Bonica J J 1990 Multidisciplinary/interdisciplinary pain programs. In: Bonica J J (ed) The management of pain 2nd edn. Lea & Febiger, Philadelphia, ch 9, pp 197–208

Brena S 1985 Pain control facilities: patterns of operation and problems of organisation in the USA. Clinics in Anaesthesia 3:183

Carron H 1979 International directory of pain centers/clinics. American Society of Anaesthesiologists, Oak Ridge, Il

Fordyce W E 1976 Behavioural methods for chronic pain and illness. C V Mosby, St Louis, MS

IASP 1990 Desirable characteristics for pain treatment facilities. Report of Task Force on Guidelines for Desirable Characteristics for Pain Treatment Facilities. IASP, Seattle

Loeser J D, Seres J L, Newman R I 1990 Interdisciplinary, multimodal management of chronic pain. In: Bonica J J (ed) The management of pain, 2nd edn. Lea & Febiger, Philadelphia, ch 100, pp 2107–2120

Mayer T G, Gatchel R J 1988 Functional restoration for spinal disorders: the sports medicine approach. Lea & Febiger, Philadelphia

Modell J 1977 Directory of pain clinics. American Society of Anaesthesiologists, Oak Ridge, Il

Morse R H 1985 Accreditation of the USA chronic pain treatment facilities: current status. Clinics in Anaesthesia 3:197

Ng L K Y 1981 (ed) New approaches to treatment of chronic pain: a review of multidisciplinary pain clinics and pain centers. NIDA Research Monograph 36, Rockville, MD

Pain Society 1997 Desirable characteristics for pain management programmes: report of a working party of the Pain Society of Great Britain and Ireland (the British and Irish Chapter of the International Association for the Study of Pain). Pain Society, London

Sanders S H 1994 An image problem for pain centers: relevant factors and possible solutions. APS Bulletin 4:17–18

Turk D C, Meichenbaum D H, Genest M 1983 Pain and behavioural medicine. A cognitive–behavioural perspective. Guilford, New York

Assessment

Adequate assessment is a necessary precursor of successful pain management. After consideration of a number of general issues in Chapter 7, the ensuing Chapters 8, 9, 10 and 11 address respectively a number of discrete facets of assessment: medical assessment; assessment of pain, disability and physical function; psychosocial assessment and finally socioeconomic and occupational assessment. Each aspect of assessment is designed to yield information principally in terms of either targets for treatment or obstacles to recovery. The process of integrating individual clinical opinions into collective interdisciplinary decisions is addressed in Chapter 12. Clinical decisions need to be made in the knowledge of available patient pathways (or treatment options). During the feedback process to the patient, the various options should be outlined. In considering the process of 'negotiation' with the patient, the importance of recognising the interface between assessment and clinical intervention and of understanding the use of 'motivational interviewing' techniques becomes particularly apparent.

7

General issues of assessment

Chris C. Spanswick

INTRODUCTION

Assessment of patients and their pain is a standard and essential part of pain management, whatever type of treatment options may be available. Indeed treatment begins during the assessment process. This chapter discusses the important general issues of assessment irrespective of the type of pain problem that is being assessed or the profession of whoever is doing the assessment.

Essentially the assessment process is an exercise in information gathering to enable rational treatment planning. The information must be gathered in a consistent and accurate way. The information should be reliable and if, for example, it includes a measure of a particular parameter (e.g. depressive mood) the measurement of that parameter must have been shown to be valid. This is vital if decisions are to be made on the basis of this information.

There are a number of sources of information and different methods of gathering information about the patient (Box 7.1). The sources include: the referring letter, the GP, the hospital notes, the history elicited directly from the patient, observations of the patient in the clinic, specific responses to physical examination, information gathered directly from the patient's partner or 'significant other' and information gathered from questionnaires given to patients and/or their partners. All of these sources of information will help provide a broad picture of patients, their pain and other problems, and how the patients manage their pain and related problems.

117

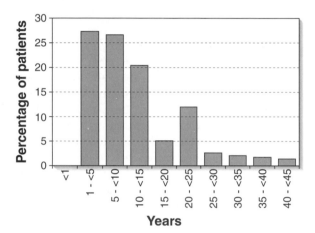

Figure 7.1 Length of history of pain at patient presentation.

Many patients presenting at pain centres have had their pain for some considerable time (Fig. 7.1). They often present with complex medical histories and there are frequently difficulties in diagnosis. Often there is no 'specific' diagnosis at all. For example White & Gordon (1982) indicate that for 85% of episodes of back pain the diagnosis is unclear. Great care must be taken to assess the problem with an open mind to exclude carefully any treatable pathology that may have been missed. It is important not to jump to conclusions or to make judgements but to concentrate all efforts on careful dispassionate data collection.

The pain will have had an impact on the patient, their family, their ability to work and their leisure activities (Chs 3 and 4). The family may inadvertently compound the problem by kindness and overprotection. Patients will have

adopted a number coping styles and strategies and hold a number of beliefs relating to their pain and its treatment. Many of these coping methods and beliefs may not be helpful and indeed may be counterproductive (Ch. 2).

It is essential that careful enquiry is made into all of these areas. The enquiry must be unbiased, non-judgmental and accurate (Box 7.2).

ACCURACY OF INFORMATION GATHERING

For information to be of any value it must be accurate and reproducible. In other words the same test or question must elicit the same response whoever is observing. If there is great variation in the response to that question or test then that information is of little value.

Many tests of differing variety may be used. These must have been shown to be valid and reproducible, particularly in the population in which they are being used. For example straight leg raising not only shows a considerable variation within patients but also between observers. In addition, although it may be a measure of 'severity', however poor, it is not an accurate measure of 'root irritation'. Therefore the results of this test should not be used as a reliable measure and specifically not as a measure of root irritation. Straight leg raising is not an accurate enough measure to allow any clinical decision to be based upon its result.

The importance of using assessments that have been validated for the clinical population in which they are to be used, is particularly highlighted when it comes to choosing measures of

---

Box 7.3   Principal uses of information

- Patient and population description (case mix)
- Clinical decision making (treatment allocation)
- Outcome measurement (audit)
- Specific research investigations

Box 7.4   Basic skills needed by team members

- Good communication skills (ability to put the patient at ease)
- Good working knowledge within own profession
- Good working knowledge of pain management
- Self-confidence
- Ability and willingness to work within a team

---

psychological distress. For example a depression rating scale designed for general practice may not be a good measure for the population of patients attending a pain centre. The spread of scores in the general population will be very different from the spread of scores in a pain clinic population. Therefore if depressive symptoms are to be measured a scale that has been designed and demonstrated to be accurate in the pain clinic population should be used.

It is easy to collect too much information, much of which may be redundant or simply not used. The purpose of the collection of any piece of information must be explicit. There is little point in collecting information unless it is to be used for a specific purpose. Information will be used for a limited number of purposes. These include population description, to aid clinical decision making (treatment allocation), for measurement of outcome or for a specific research (Box 7.3).

Use of information obtained for clinical decision making, for outcome measurement and for research are obvious reasons for collecting such material; however, the population description is also very important. This will provide the centre with information that will identify changes in case mix and other details, which will help greatly in negotiations for resources with administrators, purchasers and others. It will enable changes in allocation of staff and other resources, including the type of service provided to be made on the basis of data rather than clinical impression, which has a tendency to be biased and inaccurate (Ch. 8).

TECHNIQUES OF GATHERING INFORMATION

It is impossible for one single person to gather all of the relevant information about a given patient.

A team of professionals from a number of different disciplines is required. There is a set of common skills required by all professionals working in an interdisciplinary team in order to ensure accurate and consistent data collection (Box 7.4).

Communication skills

All members of the team must possess a number of basic skills in addition to those specifically related to their own profession. Good working communications are essential, both between members of the team and between the team members and the patient. Team members must have a clear understanding of their own areas of competence and their responsibility for information gathering. The team member requires a degree of maturity and should not be thrown off course, be disconcerted, or become defensive when faced with patients who become very distressed or angry. Frequently patients will display quite 'bizarre behaviour'. It is important that team members should be able to ignore this in their interactions with the patient and not allow it to colour their assessment or communications with the patients. This is vital as patients will not only pick up on judgemental statements but will also notice changes in the behaviour and attitude of the team member. This will have an immediate impact upon the willingness of patients to disclose information and may affect their responses to 'objective' examination. Team members must, therefore, take great care with not only what they say, but also how they speak and behave. They should have the ability to put patients at their ease. Patients will disclose more information only if they have confidence that clinicians are being honest and non-judgemental.

Patients will have been seen by a number of other specialists. Usually these consultations have been very short, often not with a consultant but a trainee, whose communication skills may not be well developed. It may have been implied that the pain is 'all in the head' or that patients are exaggerating their pain. The patient may have even been invited to see a psychiatrist. The team member, therefore, generally has a considerable amount of repair work to do in order to gain the patient's confidence and impress upon the patient that this consultation will be different. It is important that team members have a level of communication skills that will enable them to identify the problems with previous consultations and address these early on in the interaction with the patient. The team member needs to be able to put the patient at ease quickly and explain that the team will take the patient's pain seriously. Only then will the patient begin to 'open up' and disclose perhaps important and sensitive information, which may have a bearing on diagnosis and treatment.

Professional skills

This is not the place to discuss the specific requirements for individual professions involved in pain management (Ch. 16). However, all those involved in pain management must have several years' experience within their own profession. They must have an in-depth knowledge of their own subject. They should not only have the basic qualifications required for their profession but a further qualification within their field. They should be mature enough to know and understand their clinical limitations and be prepared to ask for advice from colleagues and peers when appropriate.

There are a number of reasons for having a minimum level of professional experience. The patient will pick up quickly on team members who are neither knowledgeable nor confident in their field. The patient will then lose confidence not only in that individual but, potentially, the whole team, thus putting the whole assessment

into jeopardy. In addition the team has to be able to rely on competent advice from each member. All members must, therefore, have an in-depth knowledge of their own professional skills.

Finally team members will on frequent occasions need to communicate with their contemporaries. It is therefore important to have good standing with contemporaries in order to be able to communicate with them as an equal. If team members need to refer the patient for other treatment and or assessment their contemporaries are likely to communicate their own feelings about the team member and the team to the patient either directly or by implication. If patients are to have any confidence in the pain team they must feel that it and its members are held in high regard by their contemporaries. Certainly if the patient feels that this is not the case all hope of helping the patient will be lost.

Core knowledge

Team members not only need a good background in their own field, but they must also have a good understanding of the 'core subjects' in the management of pain. This is outlined in the International Association for the Study of Pain's 'core curriculum', which is discussed in more detail in Chapter 16.

There are two major areas that each team member must understand. First, all team members must have a basic knowledge of the physiology and psychology of pain, the potential treatments available, common pathology, the treatments the patient may have been offered by others and the potential outcomes. Secondly they must have a high level of knowledge and skill in 'pain management', the specific skills required to help patients cope with and manage their pain more successfully. This is, of course, achieved by means of the team approach. All the members of the team must have the same objectives and use similar techniques for this to be successful.

Self-confidence

Self-confidence may be an innate characteristic (i.e. some people are generally more self-confident than others). Professional confidence usually comes with the development of professional skills. Staff require the right level of self-confidence. It is important that they should be neither over- nor underconfident; both can lead to problems when working in a team. They should know their own limitations professionally but be prepared to offer their professional opinion and defend it if necessary.

The self-confidence must not only enable constant peer review and competent team working, but more importantly it must enable confident handling of patients and their families. The ability to gain the confidence of patients and their families is of prime importance, not only in the gathering of information during assessment but also during the treatment process.

Ability and willingness to work in a team

There is no room for 'egos' in teamwork. The team is more important than is any individual member. Individual team members should not feel threatened by others in the team. The decision to treat is a team one and is reached by mutual consent. This means that the individual may be overridden by the team. All members must feel that they are part of the decision-making and treatment process. Each team member must be willing to support other members of the team. This is not to belittle individual skills but to be prepared to put them into the context of the common goal. After a team has been working together for a while the members should begin to work intuitively, often predicting what others will say before they do so. This allows team members to interject during the interview with the patient, without feeling constrained, if they feel that the patient has misunderstood or misinterpreted what another team member has said. This produces a very powerful effect during assessment and treatment. However, if the team does not 'gel' and some members remain separate philosophically then disasters may often follow.

This latter point is perhaps one of the most important. If the team works well together and all members feel their opinion is respected it works very well. In addition patients quickly pick up on any discord within a team and will take the advice less seriously. Conversely there is probably a profound non-specific effect upon patients when they are assessed and managed by a team who clearly agree and are focused on the patients' needs rather than their own agendas.

SELF-DISCLOSURE

For the team to arrive at an appropriate conclusion as to the problems that patients have and how they may be tackled, accurate information is required (Ch. 12). The patients must feel that they are able to disclose sensitive information safely. If patients do not feel comfortable in doing so they will neither disclose such information nor will they take an active part in the treatment process. Throughout the whole of the assessment patients must be put at ease to allow sensitive information to be revealed and to let patients effectively drop their guard. This is true not only of information that might be gained from interview, but also of that from physical examination.

Interviewing techniques should be non-threatening. It is important to be candid and honest with the patient, even to the extent that interviewers may say how they feel. For example if patients have totally unrealistic expectations and are fixed on a cure for their pain the doctor might say 'I don't like to have to say this but … your pain is not likely to go away'. Patients will appreciate honesty from the team members. Patients will often have been through previous assessments when their assessors may have been judgmental or dismissive. Often enquiries will not have been made about patients' opinions as to what is wrong with them and their worries and fears are not addressed. The patient may have been physically hurt during examination, as assessors may not have believed the level of pain and restriction of movement. Little time will have been spent in explaining the nature of the problem to the patient.

It is vital that patients are given an understanding that their pain and associated problems are taken seriously and that they will be given an unbiased hearing. Patients should be told that they will be assessed thoroughly and the results of that assessment will be discussed with them honestly, with no hidden agendas. This will take a positive effort on the part of the team, given the natural scepticism that patients may have as a result of their previous contact with the medical and other professions. Unless a positive approach is taken, the information revealed by the patient at assessment will not only be incomplete, but may also be totally inaccurate. This will inevitably lead to unhelpful and inappropriate treatments being offered, or the patient declining to take part in any treatment.

STRUCTURED ASSESSMENT

There is no perfect way of organising the assessment of patients in a pain centre. An example of a system is given in Table 7.1. It is structured and based on screening the information at various stages. It allows patients to be fast tracked if there are any indicators of important issues that need to be addressed urgently (e.g. cancer-related pain, or major suicidal risk).

Initially the pain management programme at Salford was run separately from the pain clinic. It was then necessary for patients who had already been assessed in the pain clinic to be assessed again before being offered a place on the pain management programme. The pain management programme also took direct referrals from other specialists and under certain circumstances from GPs. This led to considerable confusion for the referring agents. To whom should they refer patients with chronic low back pain? Patients were receiving subtly different assessments, being offered different treatments initially and then ultimately having to wait twice to be considered for the programme. A decision was made to combine both units and develop a single port of entry to treatment with a broad-based assessment that would allow the patient to be directed to the most appropriate treatment, whether that be physical intervention, pain management or a combination of treatments given either concurrently or sequentially.

The referral letter

The assessment process begins immediately following receipt of the referring letter. All referral

Table 7.1 A patient assessment system at a pain centre

Action	Issues considered	Types of information
Initial referral	Letters triaged by senior nurse. Urgent referrals (e.g. cancer) dealt with rapidly. Inappropriate referrals forwarded or returned	
Questionnaires sent to patient	Triaged by team. Allocated appropriate clinic appointment	Free text open questions. Measures of pain, physical/social function, beliefs, coping and distress
Clinic interviews by team (including partner if appropriate)	History of pain, impact of pain, previous treatments, investigations, etc.	Structured interviews with patient and partner
Clinic examination	Medical, physical and behavioural assessment	Structured medical assessment; physical and behavioural assessment
Case conference	Clinical opinions. Discussion of treatment options: Pain Management programme; Intermediate treatment/assessment; Alternative treatment; Discharge. Plan for feedback	Review of all information available including: X-rays, scans and other tests. Consider need for further information e.g. physical, functional and/or psychometric tests
Feedback to patient (and partner)	Negotiation with patient (and partner). Check patient's understanding. Further information given if necessary. Agreed plan of action	Further specific information re patient's understanding, beliefs and motivation
Clinical decision	Specific plan of treatment and/or further assessment. Need to opt into treatment	

letters are screened by the pain centre's senior nurse to identify patients with cancer-related pain and those in whom there appear to be problems that may need addressing urgently. Any borderline cases are discussed with members of the team at the regular team meetings. If further information is required urgently the referring agent is then contacted by phone so that the patient can be offered the most appropriate assessment.

The degree of urgency expressed in the letter may sometimes reflect the helplessness of the referring agent and that of the patient. The patient may well have pressurised the referring agent 'to get something done'. Such patients *cannot* be assessed in 5 minutes at the end of a clinic. The more distressed the patient is the more important it is to offer a full assessment rather than a quick assessment. Such patients are offered the opportunity to choose between a 90-minute assessment (the next available appointment) or literally 5 minutes at the end of a clinic. To date no patient has opted for the 5-minute appointment! When it is explained to patients, they usually understand that they will require some time to be made available for a proper assessment to be completed and all of the issues surrounding their pain to be addressed.

Inappropriate referrals (e.g. patients with a clear need for surgery) are either sent back to the referring agent or redirected to the most appropriate specialist immediately.

Questionnaires

Not all patients attending a pain clinic require a full assessment by a team of doctors, physiotherapists and clinical psychologists, although probably more require this form of assessment than one might initially think. Nevertheless, resources are finite and a decision has to be made to allocate patients to the most appropriate form of assessment for their given problem.

The information provided in the referral letter is extraordinarily variable and only represents the referring agent's view of the problem. It may therefore be inherently very biased and not include much useful clinical information. It is essential to gain more objective information, or at least the patient's perspective of their problem, before they are allocated to an assessment clinic. Questionnaires (see Appendix to this chapter, p. 131) are an essential part of the triage system at Salford (Table 7.2); these are sent to the patient's home with an invitation to return them

Table 7.2 Purpose of patient questionnaires

Information	Purpose
Gather further information about nature and site of pain problem	Identify complexity of the problem. Possible obvious straightforward organic problem. May not require full team assessment
Gather further information about previous investigations, treatments and outcome	Allows details of investigations etc. to be obtained prior to clinic attendance. Helps team tackle misunderstandings about the nature of pathology
Gather information about the patients' understanding of their problem	Enables team to address major misconceptions about causation early on in the assessment
Enquire about the patients' expectations of treatment and major concerns about their pain	Enables team to address issues the patient feels are important early on. Helps to gain the patient's confidence. Team can focus on the questions the patient wants answering
Enquire about any concurrent medical/surgical problems	If major other problems and therefore not suitable for a PMP, allows team to allocate shorter appointment and consider other options
Enquire about any other current treatment or anticipated other consultations	Avoid unnecessary appointments for patients awaiting or listed for other treatments
Assess level of psychological distress	Enables allocation of psychology resources according to need
Assess level of physical and social functioning	Helps identify potential physical goals for management
Assess other psychological factors including coping styles and strategies	Enables positive skills to be reinforced and challenging of unhelpful coping styles during interview
Enquire about socioeconomic impact of pain and associated disability	Helps identify potential barriers and incentives to progress

completed. There are potential problems of compliance and understanding, but the accompanying letter should explain the importance, provide a phone number for those who require help and be explicit that the questionnaires need to be completed to help allocate enough time for the clinic assessment. The questionnaires and the accompanying letter were developed in conjunction with the local community health council (see Appendix, p. 131). The letter is explicit in explaining that patients must either contact the clinic or return the questionnaires completed before they can be given an appointment. Approximately 40% of questionnaires do not get returned.

It is important not to overface the patient with questionnaires sent to their home. It may be more appropriate to gather some of the information (in particular any psychometric questionnaires) by administering these at the time of the first clinic appointment. This will enable checking of compliance and accuracy of completion (see Appendix, p. 131).

The questionnaires include items requesting details of the patients' pains, previous treatments and investigations. Patients' understandings of their problems are asked for, together with an enquiry into their goals and expectations and an opportunity to identify specific questions or worries they may have. An enquiry into the site and nature of the pain is made using standardised pain measures. These comprise, the Short-Form McGill Pain Questionnaire (Melzack 1987), the Pain Drawing (Ransford et al 1975) and the Pain Diary. These are illustrated on pages 133–134. Finally, standardised psychometric questionnaires designed to measure the patient's level of distress using the Distress Risk Assessment Method (Main et al 1992) shown on pages 142–143 and a measure of physical and social functioning using the SF36 (Ware & Sherbourne 1992) are included (Chs 9 & 11).

A patient who does not return the questionnaires is contacted by letter again after 4 weeks and a second set of questionnaires is sent with another explanatory letter. If the questionnaires are not returned or the clinic contacted within another 4 weeks the patient is removed from the waiting list and the referring agent, the GP (if different) and the patient are informed. Very few of those who do not return questionnaires first time do so following the second contact.

This may seem very severe. However, like most clinics the rate of referral surpasses the ability to deliver any service by a large amount. Resources are therefore allocated in a way that will produce the best outcome.

Triage of questionnaires and referral letter

The returned questionnaires and the information in the referring letters are then triaged by

Table 7.3 The triage decision process

The team must decide:	Examples:
• Should this patient have a full team assessment with a view to considering a place on a pain management programme?	• Long history of pain. All treatment finished. Very distressed. Wants to learn to cope better
• Should this patient be seen by a single professional with a view to other specific treatment?	• Elderly patient with specific localised pain • Straightforward sciatica with no obvious major distress
• Does this patient need to be seen by another department first?	• Very short history of acute sciatica with significant weakness
• What specific barriers are there to considering a Pain Management Programme and can they be dealt with at assessment?	• Long history. Patient convinced there must be something wrong in spite of a normal MRI scan
• Is there any important other data that must be obtained prior to the assessment?	• Substantial root pain. MRI scan performed at another hospital. Report unknown
• What degree of priority should be given to this patient?	• Off work for 6 months. Job on the line

members of the team (Table 7.3). The team must allocate specific time to perform the triage on a regular basis. This should be protected time as the triage process is the key to efficient running of the service. Explicit rules are used for allocating patients to the appropriate clinic. Each team member is responsible for some of the triage. If there is any doubt the case can be discussed with other team members and a collective decision made. If further information is required in order to allocate the patient to the appropriate clinic this is sought and the decision to allocate is deferred.

The team may request that other information must be available at the time of assessment. This may include hospital notes from elsewhere, scans and the results of other tests, etc. Primarily such information is not only to aid the team at assessment in diagnosis or assessing previous treatment, but also to help address some of the questions that the patient may ask.

Patients frequently have misconceptions about the nature of their problem, previous investigations, their interpretation and subsequent treatment. These issues must be addressed by the team at the assessment. Such information is therefore essential and a clear decision for treatment and management can often not be made until such issues have been specifically addressed.

The prime task of the triage is to allocate the patient to either a full assessment with a pain clinician, physiotherapist and clinical psychologist or to an assessment with just a clinician with or without other support. The full team assessment will take a minimum of 90 minutes of contact time and require the patient to attend with a partner (if applicable) for a whole morning or afternoon. The assessment with just the pain clinician allows only 30 minutes' contact time. Some patients will require a joint assessment with the physiotherapist as well. Individual patient needs will be identified at triage and the relevant patients will be allocated to the appropriate assessment clinic.

The triage system is simply a screening system. The administrative system must allow for patients who have been allocated to a short assessment to be seen quickly by the rest of the

team if the clinician identifies important issues that need addressing by the whole team.

The triage system should be audited regularly by the team to ensure that similar decisions are made at the triage meetings irrespective of the individual members involved. In addition the rules for triage will become more refined and explicit with time and experience, being continuously subject to review.

Information gathering in the assessment clinics

The specific issues of assessment are dealt with later in other chapters (Chs 8, 9 and 10), as are the detailed issues of clinical decision making (Ch. 12). The main 'general' issue in the assessment clinics is creating an environment in which patients feel comfortable and able to disclose information either in consultation with the various members of the team or during physical examination and assessment. Patients should be made to feel that their pain problem is taken seriously and they are being subjected to a thorough and complete assessment. Any fears that patients may think that the pain is all in the head must be specifically allayed.

The interview techniques should include non-threatening, non-judgemental style of questioning and open-ended statements to encourage patients to disclose information that they may feel to be sensitive. This will enable the team to gain an understanding of patients' beliefs about their pain and associated problems. Table 7.4 gives some examples of ways of allowing patients not only to disclose specific information but also to say what they feel about their problems. It invites the patients' thoughts rather than just yes/no answers. Much more information can be gained in this way. Not only will patients express their feelings, but also they are likely to be more open and honest with their answers. Table 7.4 is not meant to be complete but simply gives some examples.

The options for treatment and management should be discussed openly and honestly with patients and where relevant their partners. The risks—physical, emotional and financial—must

Table 7.4 Examples of open-ended statements and non-threatening questions as alternatives to direct questions

Team member	Patient's thoughts	Potential alternative statement or question
Do you get depressed?	They think it's all in the head	Many patients we see tell us that their pain has made them very irritable and feel depressed
Are you working at the moment?	They think I am just trying to get out of work	Most of the patients we see find that their pain stops them from doing a lot of things including work
What stops you from doing more?	Are they trying to trick me? It's the pain of course	A lot of patients tell us they are frightened of damaging themselves when they try to do more
What have you been told about the cause of your pain?	Nothing!	Some patients feel confused because they have been told different things by different doctors about their pain. Has this happened to you?
Do think you have something seriously wrong with you?	I am a hypochondriac?	Some patients we see have not been told in English what is wrong with them. Sometimes they feel their doctors have treated them rather dismissively
Are you suing any one at the moment?	This means they won't give me any treatment and probably think I am just after the money	About one in five of our patients are in the process of taking legal action for their pain. They tell us that it is stressful and feel as if they are not taken seriously. This makes them feel very angry sometimes

be explained openly, together with the potential benefits. The requirement of the active participation of the patient in not only the decision process but also the treatment should be stressed. Even if physical intervention is deemed necessary the patient's responsibility to make the most of the treatment should be made explicit. It may be necessary to make an explicit contract with the patient—for example: 'If I do this injection for you, I need you to work on the movement and regain as much function as you can. If you don't there will be little point in me doing the injection, as it will not last for long'.

Occasionally further advice from other specialists may be required either to address a diagnostic problem or to answer a specific question, which the team members do not have the knowledge to answer. In such cases a referral to a specific 'trusted' colleague is made. The colleague will be given specific instructions regarding the question(s) the team wishes to obtain answer about. The colleague is invited to answer directly to the patient as well as to the team. Sometimes it requires a specific specialist to correct the patient's misconceptions. For example it may require a spinal surgeon to say to the patient 'you do not need an operation'.

Joint clinics run with a trusted clinician from a different speciality can be of much value in addressing specific issues and may prevent inadvertently giving mixed messages to the patient. Both clinicians seeing the patient at the same time, rather than communicating by letter, is much more effective in ensuring that the same message is given and that no misunderstandings arise. For example, it is common for patients referred to pain management programmes to believe still that there is a surgical answer to their pain problem. If patients are simply referred to an orthopaedic surgeon they may become lost in the system and be seen by a trainee who is not aware of the issues and the importance of reassurance (if appropriate). The patient may then be unnecessarily reinvestigated or offered other treatment. Even if the patient is seen by the consultant, the consultant may not communicate in quite the same way as the team and may make slightly different emphases. This may simply confuse the patient further. In some centres joint clinics are held, allowing the referring team to 'present' or 'introduce' the patient to the specialist. This enables the important issues to be explained. It allows the referring team to know exactly what the specialist (e.g. spinal surgeon) said and if necessary the specialist and team member are able to agree a form of words to use in communicating with the patient. Thus all concerned—the team, the specialist and the patient—can be quite clear as to the outcome of the consultation.

At the end of assessment (case conference)

Having each conducted their own discipline specific assessment the team members meet together (without the patient) and discusses the findings of each (Ch. 12). All members of the team will present their own view of the patient and any relevant positive and negative findings. Each member will outline whether any further therapeutic interventions are indicated and whether any further tests or investigations are required to complete the assessment. Thus the possible barriers to the use of 'pain management techniques' are identified or excluded.

Providing there are no specific outstanding matters the team will then discuss the potential for 'pain management' and whether there are any other barriers to rehabilitation that need to be addressed (Table 7.5). These potential barriers to progress will be discussed amongst the team members to ascertain whether they represent an absolute exclusion from pain management or whether they are relative and further exploratory discussion with the patient is necessary.

The feedback

Once the team is agreed on the specific issues that need to be addressed they 'feed back' their thoughts to patients and their partners. The team should agree about who will lead and who will act in a supporting role in this interaction. It is important that information is imparted in a logical order, clearly and in terms that the patient will understand. The team should be explicit in allowing patients or their partners to stop the proceedings and ask questions. It must be said that both the patient and the partner may become overloaded with new information. The team must constantly appraise whether patients and their partners understand what has been said by checking this. It is occasionally worth asking them to go away, think the whole issue over and come back at another time to discuss any aspects they do not understand. At this stage some form of written material to focus thoughts is helpful. Neville Shone's (1995) book 'Coping successfully with pain' has been very useful in our practice (also see Parker & Main (1993), Sternbach (1988)). The written material should also give detail of the treatment package(s) on offer, so that patients can make a rational judgement based on a knowledge of what is being offered and what is expected of them.

Sometimes the patient may have appeared very resistant to using self-control techniques

Table 7.5 Examples of barriers to progress (Ch. 12)

Nature of problem	Example	Potential decision
Medical	Severe asthma, angina	Not physically fit enough for exercise part of programme. Consider other options
Physical function	Substantial loss of fitness. Cannot sit for more than 5 minutes. Spends 6 to 8 hours laying down each day	Set task (usually physical goal, e.g. walking distance or sitting tolerance) to confirm or refute motivation. Reassess after a set time. If goal achieved, list. If not, ask patient to contact the team when goal has been achieved
Psychological	Continuing grief reaction to recent bereavement	Individual psychological help to address grief issues. Relist for final assessment for programme after psychological treatment completed
Socioeconomic	Involved in legal case that will not be settled for some time	Asked to go away and consider risks and benefits of pain management programme. The patient to contact team again if willing to accept risks and be listed for programme

Table 7.6 Some examples of what can go wrong

What can go wrong	Potential reason(s)	Resolution
Patient ends up in the wrong type of clinic (e.g. a doctor-only clinic instead of full-team assessment)	Triage error. Either missed evidence of distress or not evident on questionnaires	Audit decision making at triage. Consider revision of questionnaires. May need to be less threatening
Patients very angry with team because they feel they will be treated dismissively	Experience of previous assessments. Misunderstanding of reason for questionnaires	Specific reassurance on following points: pain taken seriously by the team, understand previous experience, explain reasons for questionnaires
Patients not willing to consider pain management	Offered treatment elsewhere. Does not want management. Wants cure	Encourage having realistic expectations regarding other treatment offered and returning when willing to address management of pain rather than cure
Patients become very angry about previous treatments	Inadvertent criticism of previous treatment by team member	Explain reasons why many treatments do not provide long term help. Explain that other doctors try their best to help. Evaluate communication techniques
Patients suddenly change from resistant to compliant during feedback	Team misinterpreted patients' responses during interview and examination. Patients began to take on realistic expectations	Team must change tack during feedback and reinforce compliance rather than discharge patients
Patients refuse physical examination	Fear from previous experience	Explain the need for thorough assessment. Reassure that patients will not be hurt or harmed
Major drug misuse discovered when on programme	Patients felt too threatened during assessment	Consider changing interview technique
Patients on programme still not convinced hurt does not mean harm. Want a scan	Team failed to assess patients' beliefs. Patients not given time to consider implications of entering the programme	Evaluate assessment process. Allow patients time to consider and positively opt into treatment

and may unexpectedly change during feedback from being resistant to very accepting of the pain management model. The team must be able to adapt and change quickly without the need for another case conference. The team will have to run with this by intuition. The converse may also happen: patients may become more entrenched in their ideas and be totally unwilling to change.

COMMON THINGS THAT GO WRONG

Table 7.6 outlines a few of the problems that may arise either during the assessment process or afterwards on a pain management programme. In general most problems arise from communication errors either on the team's part or due to patients' misunderstanding. Whatever the cause the team members must constantly check the patient's understanding of the nature of the assessment

and the treatment offered. They should be given time if necessary to consider their options and should in any case opt positively into treatment. The assessment process must be audited continuously. This should lead to continual changes designed to improve assessment and ultimately the outcome of treatment.

CONCLUSION

The quality of interaction at assessment is vital. Patients and their partner must sense that their pain and associated problems are taken seriously by a team of professionals well versed in their own discipline. The quality of the communication is vital if patients are to feel comfortable with disclosing sensitive information and to consider an alternative view of their problem, which they will not have anticipated. The team must remember that their job has to be done

KEY POINTS

- Treatment starts with the assessment process.
- Information must be gathered in a consistent and accurate way; measures used should be both reliable and valid.
- Interview techniques must be non-threatening and encourage self-disclosure of sensitive information.
- A triage system is needed to ensure that patients receive the most appropriate assessment.

- Team members require both good communication and good professional skills.
- Patients must feel that their pain problem is being taken seriously by the team.
- The end process of assessment is the formulation of a plan of action and feeding this back to patients in a way that is understandable and acceptable to them.

frequently in the face of significant sensitisation of the patient against addressing certain issues, particularly those of a psychological nature.

Formulation of a plan of action and feeding this back to patients is the most important part of the assessment. It is ultimately at this point when the final clinical decisions are made. The decisions should only be made on objective, accurate and reproducible data. The reasoning behind the decisions should be made explicit not only amongst the members of the team, but also to patients and their partners.

REFERENCES

Main C J, Wood P L R, Hollis S, Spanswick C C, Waddell G 1992 The distress and risk assessment method. A simple patient classification to identify distress and evaluate the risk of poor outcome. Spine 17 (1)

Melzack R 1987 The short-form McGill pain questionnaire. Pain 30: 191-197

Parker H, Main C J 1993 Living with back pain. Manchester University Press, Manchester

Shone N 1995 Coping successfully with pain, revised edn. Sheldon Press, London

Ransford A O, Cairns O, Mooney V 1976 The pain drawing as an aid to the psychological evaluation of patients with low back pain

Sternbach R 1988 Mastering pain: a twelve-step program for coping with chronic pain. Ballantine, New York

Ware J E, Sherbourne C D 1992 The MOS 36 item short-form health survey (SF - 36) I. Conceptual framework and item selection. Medical Care 30(6): 473-483

White III A A, Gordon S L 1982 Synopsis: workshop on idiopathic low-back pain. Spine 712:141–149

APPENDIX: CONTENT OF PAIN QUESTIONNAIRES FOR PATIENTS

MANCHESTER & SALFORD PAIN CENTRE *GREEN AREA*

Direct Line: 0161 787 4791   Fax: 0161 787 1929

Dear,

You have been referred to the Pain Centre. To help to provide the best service we can, we need to know if your wish to attend. If you do, please complete the enclosed questionnaires and tear off the slip at the bottom of this page and return them all to us in the enclosed pre-paid envelope. If you are willing to come to the clinic at very short notice, should there be a cancellation (this may be only an hour's notice), please let us have your work and home telephone numbers so we can contact you.

When we have received your completed questionnaires and the slip, we will then give you an appointment to be seen. We will notify you by phone or post of your appointment to be seen. If for any reason you are unable to come, please ring the clinic <u>as soon as possible</u> so we can give you an alternative date so that we do not waste clinic time.

If your do not reply within four weeks from the date of this letter, we are obliged to remove you from our waiting list.

Your sincerely,

Dr C.C. Spanswick
Clinical Director
Centre for pain Management

--------------------------------- --

I wish/do not wish* to attend the Pain Centre.
I am/am not* willing to come to the clinic at short notice if there is a cancellation.
*Delete as appropriate   Home Tel No ....
                                          Work Tel No ....
NAME ....   Hospital No ....

This is a confidential questionnaire which will be used only to help understand the type of pain from which you are suffering. It enables you to give detailed information and allows us more time for discussion and explanation at your clinic appointment. We are interested to know all about your pain, so there are many questions. It may take you some time to complete this questionnaire. Please do not feel you have to do this all at once; do a little at a time.
The pain you suffer may have had a bad effect on you and your family so please write down any information which you think may help us to treat your pain. Please try to answer all the questions and return the questionnaire in the envelope provided so that we are able to give you an appointment for assessment as soon as possible. If you need help completing the questionnaires please ring the clinic.

1. How and when did your pain problem start?
2. What does your pain feel like?
3. What makes the pain worse?
4. What makes the pain better?
5. Does your pain vary during the day? When is it at its best and worst?
6. Has the pain got better or worse over time, or is it much the same?
7. What tests or investigations have you had for the pain eg X-Rays, scans, blood tests or nerve tests? Give dates and Hospital if possible.
8. What treatment are you having for the pain *now?* Please give details. Do any of the treatments help?
   Medicines (please list name, dose and how many taken each day).
   Physiotherapy
   Other therapies: acupuncture, chiropractic, osteopathy, homeopathy or herbal treatment.
   Corset, splint etc.
9. What treatments have you had for the pain *in the past?* Were they helpful?
   Medicines
   Operations (give operation, surgeon and date if possible)
   Physiotherapy
   Other therapies: acupuncture, chiropractic, osteopathy, homeopathy or herbal treatment?
   Corset, splint etc.
10. Do you need help to look after yourself because of the pain? If so, please give details.
11. Do you need to use aids or appliances (wheelchair, crutches, walking stick etc.) because of the pain?
12. What have you had to give up because of the pain (job, friends, family commitment, social life etc.)?
13. Has the pain problem affected your financial situation? If so, by how much per year?
14. Are you receiving or in the process of claiming any state benefits (Unemployment, Invalidity, Disability or Mobility)? If so, please give details.
15. Have you in the past taken, or are you at present taking legal advice or made any claim on account of your pain problem? If so, please give details.
16. Do you suffer from any other medical condition not related to the pain, or are you receiving medical treatment, including medicines from your own doctor?
17. Are you waiting to see any other specialists or to have an operation because of the pain? If so please state the hospital and specialist.
18. What do you think is causing your pain?
19. What would you like to achieve by coming to the pain clinic?
20. What questions would you like to ask us about your pain?

PAIN QUESTIONNAIRE

PLEASE SELECT FROM THE LIST BELOW WORDS THAT YOU WOULD USE TO DESCRIBE YOUR PAIN (tick the appropriate column for each word);

	NONE	MILD	MODERATE	SEVERE
Throbbing	_____	_____	_____	_____
Shooting	_____	_____	_____	_____
Stabbing	_____	_____	_____	_____
Sharp	_____	_____	_____	_____
Cramping	_____	_____	_____	_____
Gnawing	_____	_____	_____	_____
Hot-burning	_____	_____	_____	_____
Aching	_____	_____	_____	_____
Heavy	_____	_____	_____	_____
Tender	_____	_____	_____	_____
Splitting	_____	_____	_____	_____
Tiring-exhausting	_____	_____	_____	_____
Sickening	_____	_____	_____	_____
Fearful	_____	_____	_____	_____
Punishing-cruel	_____	_____	_____	_____

MARK A CROSS ON THE LINE BELOW TO INDICATE THE INTENSITY OF YOUR PAIN;

(a) RIGHT NOW;

NO
PAIN |——| WORST
POSSIBLE PAIN

(b) AT ITS WORST IN THE LAST MONTH;

NO
PAIN |——| WORST
POSSIBLE PAIN

(c) AT ITS BEST IN THE LAST MONTH;

NO
PAIN |——| WORST
POSSIBLE PAIN

PRESENT PAIN INDEX;

WHICH OF THE FOLLOWING WORDS EXPLAINS YOUR PRESENT PAIN (tick one only);

0	NO PAIN	_____
1	MILD	_____
2	DISCOMFORTING	_____
3	DISTRESSING	_____
4	HORRIBLE	_____
5	EXCRUCIATING	_____

Pain Drawing

Mark the areas of your body where you feel the following sensations:

Numbness	Pins and Needles	Ache	Pain
= = = = =	O O O O O O O O	X X X X X X	/ / / / / /
= = = = =	O O O O O O O	X X X X X X	/ / / / / /
= = = = =	O O O O O O O O	X X X X X X	/ / / / / /

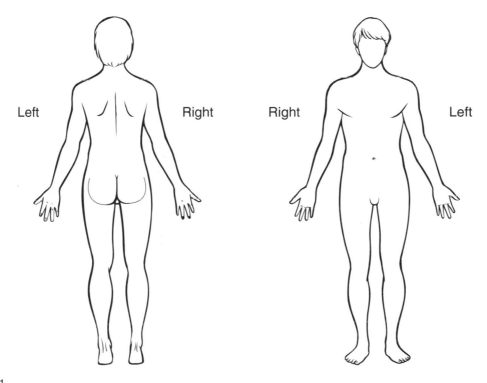

Fig. 7A.1

Pain diary

Please describe the type of activity, mood and medication for each hour of a typical day. Use the 0–10 scale for pain and indicate how the pain affects your activity and feelings. Record medication as name and number of tablets.

Time	Pain	Activity	Mood	Medication
6.00am				
7:00am				
8:00am				

Instructions for diary

Please write in the day and date at the top of the page.

Each hour (or as near the hour as is convenient) please write down what you have just been doing, how bad the pain is, where you feel the pain, any medication or tablets you have taken in the last hour and how you have been feeling.

For PAIN write a number from 0–10, depending on how bad it is:

0————————————————————————10

No pain   The worst pain you could possibly imagine e.g. 0 would be no pain; 1, 2 or 3 a little; 4, 5 and 6 moderate amount and so on.

For MOOD also write a number from 0–10:

0————————————————————————10

Not depressed   As depressed as you can imagine

So, 1, 2 or 3 would mean just a little depressed, and so on.

Example:

DAY AND DATE   Monday, 1st April

Time	Activity	Pain Amount	Pain Place	Medicine or Tablets	Mood
11.00 a.m.	Sitting by fire	7	Mainly head	One Aspirin	4

In this example, you filled in the sheet on Monday, 1st April. At 11.00 a.m. in the morning you were sitting by the fire, the pain was fairly bad (7), and you felt it mainly in your head, you had one aspirin in the last hour and you felt a bit depressed.

Please try to fill in as carefully as you can. Then, at the end of the day, write down the total number of hours you have spent lying down in the last 24 hours (including sleep).

Health status questionnaire (SF – 36)

(*Medical Care Research Unit, University of Sheffield Medical School.*)

The following questions ask for your views about your health, how you feel and how well you are able to do your usual activities. If you are unsure about how to answer any question, please give the best answer you can and make any comments in the space after question 10.

please tick one

1. In general would you say your health is:

Excellent	○
Very good	○
Good	○
Fair	○
Poor	○

2. Compared to one year ago,
how would you rate your health in general now?

Much better now than one year ago	○
Somewhat better now than one year ago	○
About the same	○
Somewhat worse than one year ago	○
Much worse than one year ago	○

HEALTH AND DAILY ACTIVITIES

3. The following questions are about activities you might do during a typical day.
Does your health limit you in these activites?
If so, how much?

Please tick one circle on each line

	Yes, limited a lot	Yes, limited a little	No, not limited at all
a. Vigorous activities, such as running, lifting heavy objects, participating in strenuous sports	○	○	○
b. Moderate activities, such as moving a table, pushing a vacuum cleaner, bowling or playing golf	○	○	○
c. Lifting or carrying groceries	○	○	○
d. Climbing several flights of stairs	○	○	○
e. Climbing one flight of stairs	○	○	○
f. Bending, kneeling or stooping	○	○	○
g. Walking more than a mile	○	○	○

h. Walking half a mile   ◯   ◯   ◯

j. Walking 100 yards   ◯   ◯   ◯

j. Bathing and dressing yourself   ◯   ◯   ◯

4. During the past 4 weeks, have you had any of the following problems with your work or other regular daily activities as a result of your physical health?

Answer yes or no to each question

	YES	NO
a. Cut down on time spent on work or other activites	◯	◯
b. Accomplished less than you would like	◯	◯
c. Were limited in the kind of work or other activities	◯	◯
d. Had difficulty performing the work or other activities (e.g. it took extra effort)	◯	◯

5. During the past 4 weeks, have you had any of the following problems with your work or other regular daily activities as a result of any emotional problems (such as feeling depressed or anxious)?

Answer yes or no to each question

	YES	NO
a. Cut down on the time you spent on work or other activites	◯	◯
b. Accomplished less than you would like	◯	◯
c. Didn't do work or other activities as carefully as usual	◯	◯

6. During the past 4 weeks, to what extent has your physical health or emotional problems interfered with your normal social activities with family, friends, neighbours or groups?

Please tick one

Not at all	◯
Slightly	◯
Moderately	◯
Quite a bit	◯
Extremely	◯

7. How much bodily pain have you had during the past 4 weeks?

Please tick one

None	◯
Very mild	◯
Mild	◯
Moderate	◯
Severe	◯
Very severe	◯

8. During the past 4 weeks, how much did pain interfere with your normal work (including work both outside the home and housework)?

Not at all   ◯

A little bit	○
Moderately	○
Quite a bit	○
Extremely	○

Health in general

9. Please choose the answer that best describes how true or false each of the following statements is for you.

Please tick one circle on each line

	Definitely true	Mostly true	Not sure	Mostly false	Definitely false
a. I seem to get ill more easily than other people	○	○	○	○	○
b. I am as healthy as anybody I know	○	○	○	○	○
c. I expect my health to get worse	○	○	○	○	○
d. My health is excellent	○	○	○	○	○

YOUR FEELINGS

10. These questions are about how you feel and how things have been *during the past month*. (*For each question, please indicate the one answer that comes closest to the way you have been feeling*).

How much time during the past month	All of the time	Most of the time	A good bit of the time	Some of the time	A little bit of the time	None of the time
a. Did you feel full of life?	○	○	○	○	○	○
b. Have you been a very nervous person?	○	○	○	○	○	○
c. Have you felt so down in the dumps that nothing could cheer you up?	○	○	○	○	○	○
d. Have you felt calm and peaceful?	○	○	○	○	○	○
e. Did you have a lot of energy?	○	○	○	○	○	○
f. Have you felt downhearted and sad?	○	○	○	○	○	○
g. Did you feel worn out?	○	○	○	○	○	○
h. Have you been a happy person?	○	○	○	○	○	○
i. Did you feel tired?	○	○	○	○	○	○
j. Has your shealth limited your social activities (like visiting friends or close relatives)	○	○	○	○	○	○

MSPQ

Please describe how you have felt during the PAST WEEK by putting
a tick (√) in the appropriate box.
PLEASE ANSWER ALL THE QUESTIONS
Do not think too long before answering

	Not at all	A little slightly	A great deal quite a bit	Extremely could not have been worse
Heart rate increasing				
Feeling hot all over				
Sweating all over				
Sweating in a particular part of the body				
Pulse in neck				
Pounding in head				
Dizziness				
Blurring of vision				
Feeling faint				
Everything appearing unreal				
Nausea				
Butterflies in stomach				
Pain or ache in stomach				
Stomach churning				
Desire to pass water				
Mouth becoming dry				
Difficulty swallowing				
Muscles in neck aching				
Legs feel weak				
Muscles twitching or jumping				
Tense feeling across forehead				
Tense feeling in jaw muscles				

MOD ZUNG

Please indicate for each of these questions which answer best describes
how you have been feeling recently

PLEASE ANSWER ALL THE QUESTIONS

	Never	Now and then	Quite often	Most of the time
I feel downhearted and sad				
Morning is when I feel best				
I have crying spells or feel like it				
I have trouble getting to sleep at night				
I feel that nobody cares				
I eat as much as I used to				
I still enjoy sex				
I notice that I am losing weight				
I have trouble with constipation				
My heart beats faster than usual				
I get tired for no reason				
My mind is as clear as it used to be				
I tend to wake up too early				
I find it easy to do the things I used to				
I am restless and can't keep still				
I feel hopeful about the future				
I am more irritable than usual				
I find it easy to make a decision				
I feel quite guilty				
I feel that I am useful and needed				
My life is pretty full				
I feel that others would be better off if I were dead				
I still enjoy the things I used to				

8

Medical assessment

Chris C. Spanswick
Raymond Million

INTRODUCTION

Medical assessment is essential prior to 'pain management' (Box 8.1). Both the pain management team and the patient need to be convinced it is physically safe to rehabilitate in the face of continuing pain and that there is no serious treatable underlying disease process. All reasonable treatment options for reducing and curing the pain should have at least been considered. There should be explicit reasons for not pursuing such treatments if they are to be discounted.

Assessment and management cannot be entirely separated, as has been discussed in the previous chapter. Management begins at the first contact with the patient. How patients are handled will influence how they behave, how open they may be to quite searching questions and even how they respond to physical examination. If patients perceive that they are not being taken seriously or that they are being treated dismissively they will

---

Box 8.1   Purpose of medical assessment

- Provide medical advice to the pain team
- Medical screening and exclusion of important treatable pathology
- Diagnosis, classification or clarification of pain problem
- Identification of medical barriers to rehabilitation
- Checking of adequacy of previous investigation and treatment
- Thorough general and specific medical examination
- Assessment for suitability for further medical/surgical treatment if required

not give credence to anything that is said to them. Patients are certainly very unlikely to partake in any treatment that is suggested unless they are convinced that they have been assessed carefully and completely, and that all of their questions have been answered (as far as is possible). Patients must also have an understanding of the reasons why some treatments are being offered and in particular why others are not.

THE EXPERIENCE OF THE DOCTOR

The medical assessment is therefore a vital part of the total assessment of the patient. The medical specialty of the doctors involved is less important than their understanding of the nature of pain management. Since doctors are primarily involved in medically screening patients for pain management programmes they should have a broad experience in general medicine as well as specialised training and experience in assessing and treating patients with chronic pain. Their experience should cover a wide range of medical and surgical problems. This should be at least as broad as the experience of a GP. In addition, however, it is important that they should have considerable experience in their own field, which should be relevant to the patient population being assessed. Their experience should include knowledge of allied specialities and disciplines that will also be involved in the treatment of this particular population of patients. Most pain clinics and associated pain management programmes are supported medically by anaesthetists although others including rheumatologists and orthopaedic surgeons may also be involved. Anaesthetists are well placed to provide medical support by the nature of their broad training and experience of medicine, surgery and all other specialties. In addition they are usually actively involved in the management of acute pain and the running of pain relief clinics. They therefore have a wide experience of assessing and treating a wide variety of pain conditions. The specific competencies required are discussed elsewhere (Ch. 16); however, they are mentioned here briefly simply to put the medical clinician's credentials in context.

THE NATURE OF MEDICAL ASSESSMENT WITHIN THE ASSESSMENT TEAM

There are two major problems that face doctors. The first relates to their previous method of working and the second to the nature of the patients they are assessing.

As already mentioned most pain clinicians come from an anaesthetic background. Many will have been involved in running pain clinics single handedly with little or no access to psychological services other than as a formal referral to a department of clinical psychology. Anaesthetists who are used to assessing the patient on their own frequently develop a style of assessment that is broader than most straightforward medical assessments. They frequently will ask questions relating to the psychosocial factors, and physical functioning. They may ask questions relating to the patient's beliefs, coping styles and strategies and the impact the pain has had on the patient. However, the doctor's job within the team requires a different approach and doctors must be focused almost entirely on the 'medical' issues. They are in effect acting as the medical advisor to the interdisciplinary team. This involves letting go of 'other issues' and allowing other members of the team to assess these issues, as they will be able to do this more skilfully and more effectively. Oddly enough the more 'pain management' orientated medical specialists have been in the past, the more difficult it may be for them to adapt to a new way of working. They may feel that they are returning to the 'old ways' of not enquiring about the psychological impact of the pain. Inclusion of non-medical items in the medical assessment is not only wasteful of time and resources but can act to confuse, frustrate or annoy patients if they are asked to give the same information to a number of different team members within a short space of time. What is vital, however, is that the physician focuses on a very careful and complete medical assessment.

The second is the nature of the patient. Most if not all pain clinics, and in particular those that offer a pain management programme, tend to attract patients who have seen a large number of different specialists and had a considerable amount of failed treatment. The veracity of their complaints has often been questioned by their previous medical advisors and it may have been implied that the pain is 'all in the head'. Some patients have been invited to seek psychiatric help. Not unreasonably patients tend to develop a sceptical view of doctors. Their previous experience will colour their interaction with all subsequent doctors. Doctors, therefore, often have to perform some repair work prior to any assessment to convince patients that their pain is being taken seriously. Physicians will have to take active steps to both assess patients' previous consultations and reassure them that their pain is taken seriously. Doctors may also have to explain why previous consultations have been less than helpful.

It is important that the medical assessment is very focused. The team will require a succinct medical appraisal of the patient. Only the important and relevant medical points should be made (Box 8.2, Case study 8.1). It is all too easy to be overinclusive of information that ultimately is redundant and not used in the decision-making process. Many centres, Salford included, have spent considerable time in developing a *minimum* medical data set. This chapter will discuss the major points of this medical data set and how best to gain this information. (An example of an aide memoir used in new patient assessment is given in the Appendix to this chapter, p. 159.)

PAIN HISTORY

Patients will expect an enquiry into their pain and a thorough medical assessment must include such an enquiry. In many cases it does not provide any evidence of cause or diagnosis, and it has often been well documented in the patient's previous medical file. However, patients should be allowed to explain what their pain feels like. They will have some beliefs as to attribution and if necessary these will need to be challenged. This area is best addressed by doctors largely because patients are likely to give more credence to their opinion. They will need to

---

Box 8.2   Major points of medical assessment

- Pain history, including primary pain, secondary pains, onset, possible causes
- Previous investigation, interpretation
- Previous treatments, responses to treatments, specialists, current treatments
- Concurrent medical problems
- Medication uses, current and past, including all substances (legal and illegal)
- Current level of benefits, medicals due, litigation
- Thorough physical examination, pain specific, general
- Behavioural responses to physical examination

Case study 8.1   Example of *important* medical data (for presentation to the team)

A 6-year history of severe pain in the left leg, following a trivial accident: the patient is unable to weight bear. The leg is swollen, cold, sensitive, painful and discoloured. The patient has already had a series of guanethidine intravenous regional blocks with minimal benefit. Lumbar sympathetic blocks have not been helpful despite being accurately placed. All appropriate medications have been tried to no avail. The patient is currently taking high dose morphine also to no effect.

There is no evidence of serious pathology (e.g. cancer). There are no other concurrent medical or surgical problems. All appropriate investigations have been completed and do not demonstrate any underlying cause. Examination has confirmed no neurological abnormalities.

Signs of complex regional pain syndrome are present.

---

explain carefully, with frequent checks to see if the information is understood, and in words that patients understand, why their attribution is incorrect (Case study 8.2).

Some of this information may be collected by questionnaires sent to patients prior to their attendance at the assessment clinic. This enables doctors to confirm points of history rather than tediously question patients at great length. Patients will have recounted their story many times before and the use of questionnaires enables doctors to be interactive in their style rather than inquisitorial. This will put patients at ease and allow them to discuss aspects of their history they might otherwise not mention. The use of questionnaires fundamentally changes the nature of the medical interview. More time can be devoted to explanation and exploring

---

Case study 8.2 Case example of major misattributions

John is 30 years old and has severe back pain. He is able to walk slowly and is extremely guarded in his movements. He has been referred for pain management by a consultant spinal surgeon. He has lost his job as a gardener. He has become very disabled and spends most of his time sitting or laying down.

He has seen a number of different specialists including two orthopaedic surgeons. The first surgeon showed him the X-rays of his spine and told him he had arthritis of the spine in an effort to try to explain his pain. No treatment other than painkillers was offered. While waiting to see the second surgeon John happened to find himself sitting next to an elderly woman in a wheel chair.

'What's wrong with you?' John enquired. 'Oh, I've got arthritis of the spine,' the woman replied. John explained at his assessment in the pain centre that seeing what had happened to the woman with the same diagnosis had a profound effect on him. He became ever more fearful of movement in case he should do more damage

and too end up in a wheelchair. He interpreted more pain as more damage to his spine. He gave up any thought of returning to work as he believed that would definitely damage him and he felt work had probably damaged his back in the first place.

By the time John came to the pain centre he was convinced his back was slowly crumbling. None of his previous doctors had asked what his opinion was nor corrected his misconceptions.

He was assessed carefully and in depth. His old X-rays had been obtained prior to the assessment. He was shown X-rays of other patients to demonstrate that the X-ray changes do not tell us about pain. It took some considerable time to explain why doctors use the phrase 'spinal arthritis' to describe degenerative changes and that degenerative changes are 'normal' and do not explain the pain. He ultimately did understand at the end of the assessment that his pain did not mean further damage.

---

patients' beliefs about their pain—an area that is a vital part of both assessment and treatment.

Onset of pain

It is important to trace the progression of the pain from onset to the present time: 'How long ago did the pain start? Has there been a more recent time when the pain has changed a lot?' The onset may have been gradual and insidious or sudden and associated with trauma or surgery. Patients may attribute the onset of the pain to a particular incident or accident. Doctors will need to check whether this is reasonable or not. Patients' understanding of the original cause and any continuing cause is important, as they may have adopted unhelpful behaviours as a consequence of those beliefs. The beliefs will need to be either confirmed or challenged.

Site of pain

The site or sites of the pain and its radiation or spread should be documented (e.g. using a pain drawing—see Appendix to Ch. 7, p. 133). This is sometimes helpful in classification or diagnosis. However, although the patient will expect the doctor to give a diagnosis, this is frequently not possible. Patients should be given an explanation

for their pain if at all possible. This is not necessarily a 'diagnosis' but is vital to aid communications with them. A clear explanation of the reasons why a 'diagnosis' may not be possible must be made where appropriate. Patients should be reassured that it is common not to be able to give a precise diagnosis to many of those attending a pain clinic. This is vital, in order to gain patients' confidence and give them an understanding that the fact they have pain is not in question. Doctors must give the impression of confidence and of having seen many of these problems before. They must convey the fact that if they cannot give a precise diagnosis this is neither unusual nor important, *provided an adequate assessment including investigations has been made*. They should, if appropriate, reassure patients that there is no sinister cause and that the ultimate cause is not necessarily of great importance in determining the management of their pain.

Patients' previous doctors may have given a strong message either verbally or non-verbally that they don't understand their patients' pain. Patients will consequently have lost confidence in doctors in general. This may have been compounded when doctors have said or implied the pain is 'all in the head' or emphasised 'there is nothing wrong' because they cannot make a diagnosis. It may therefore be best to say that we simply do not understand all about pain.

Factors affecting pain

In some cases it is perfectly possible to make a diagnosis. The details of the pain history, including site, radiation, variability, provocative and palliative factors, together with other points in the history lead doctors to be able to come to a conclusion. This is commonly not because a common diagnosis has been missed, but usually because the diagnosis is either difficult or not commonly seen in general medical practice. Explaining the reason for the lack of previous diagnosis may reduce patients' natural anger and frustration.

The case outlined in the Case Study 8.1 illustrates the problems of diagnosis of complex regional pain syndromes (CRPS) (previously known as reflex sympathetic dystrophies). All of these cases start with an initiating injury, however minor. The diagnosis is often not made until quite late for a number of reasons. These will include:

- complex regional pain syndromes are rare
- the initial symptoms overlap with the 'normal' symptoms following any injury
- the diagnosis is not easy to make owing to the considerable variability of symptoms and signs
- the syndrome is not understood well
- there are no known cures for the syndrome
- trainees in most specialties may have *never* seen a case

In the case outlined these problems delayed treatment considerably, in fact by 2 years. Even then all treatments did not seem to help. This made the patient very angry and suspicious of all subsequent doctors.

The patient's understanding

At the end of enquiring into the pain and its nature doctors should have a clear and accurate understanding of the pain problem and patients' understanding of the cause and meaning of their pain problem. Doctors must ensure that misconceptions are corrected so that both patients and

their team ultimately share the same understanding as to the cause of the pain (if it is known) and whether the ongoing pain is a sign of continuing damage, serious pathology or not. If there is any doubt on doctors' part they should explain that to the patient and institute further enquiry, examination, tests and even second opinion. The medical assessment is not yet complete, but explanations at this stage will give reasons for further enquiry and examination and give confidence to patients that the doctor is competent and takes the patient's pain problem seriously. This will enhance the patient's compliance with both further enquiry and examination.

PREVIOUS INVESTIGATIONS AND TREATMENTS

Extracting information from patients by direct questioning about previous investigations and treatments can be tedious and often leaves large gaps in the history. Some information may be obtainable in the hospital notes or from patients' GPs. However, GPs may not know about all of the previous treatment especially if it involves alternative therapies. The information in the hospital notes is often not in a format that allows a quick résumé of the past treatment. Frequently patients attending a pain clinic have been to several hospitals and may be consulting several doctors concurrently.

It is for these reasons that use of the questionnaires sent to patients' homes prior to the assessment clinic is very helpful. Patients can recall in their own time what has happened in the past. They can check with members of their families and they are unpressured. In the clinic setting patients may be anxious and nervous and will often not be able to recall details of previous hospital attendances and treatments.

Previous investigations

It is often possible to predict from patients' questionnaires what other records and investigation results may be required at the assessment. Obtaining these prior to the assessment and feeding the results back to patients in understandable

English will not only be a more efficient use of time in the assessment clinic, but enormously powerful in allaying patients' fears and correcting any possible misconceptions.

A thorough and meticulous review of previous investigations should be undertaken. It is essential that all appropriate and reasonable investigation should have been performed. The results of such investigations should be documented. If there is any uncertainty or dispute as to the results the test should either be repeated or a colleague expert in these areas should review the original results (e.g. X-rays, computerised tomography (CT) scans and MRI scans).

Purpose of obtaining investigation data

There are two important points to bear in mind. First, there should be enough information about patients to exclude reasonably any treatable pathology that will produce a worthwhile reduction in patients' pain and/or disability. Secondly, patients should have an understanding of the significance of the results of such investigations and the reason for their instigation.

No assumptions should be made about the adequacy of previous investigations. At the Salford centre we have regularly come across frank organic pathology that has been missed by previous specialists. Patients must be assessed fully and in depth once and for all so that a line may be drawn under the past. They can then address the issue of rehabilitation in the safe knowledge that all reasonable treatable causes have been excluded. Both patients and teams require confidence to continue with the rehabilitation process (which may increase the pain in the short term) in the knowledge that hurt does not mean harm. This simply cannot be done unless patients have been assessed and investigated adequately and convinced by the team that there is no other option for treatment.

The role of investigations in challenging patients' attributions

There will be occasions when a particular investigation is not clinically indicated, for example an MRI scan of the lumbar spine in chronic mechanical back pain with no radiation and all other tests normal. If, however, patients are convinced of 'something wrong' and the doctor is convinced that showing them a normal MRI scan will help them move on and address managing their pain rather than seeking a cure, then it is justifiable to do the test. There are two important points to be made. First, such tests are a double-edged sword. They can throw up red herrings, which may compound patients' fears. That may be a risk worth taking. Secondly, doctors must be explicit as to the reason for doing the test with both patients and radiologists. This will enable radiologists to interpret the scans in the light of patients' complaints and patients should understand clearly that the reasons for the tests are for reassurance and not in the anticipation of abnormal findings.

The interpretation of investigations for the patient

Frequently patients have been given no understanding of why particular investigations have been instigated. Even when the results are available these have usually not been interpreted for the patient. Doctors and others have a tendency to use medical jargon, which patients do not understand and often will find intimidating and frightening. Part of the review of the previous investigations, therefore, should include exploring patients' understanding of not only why certain tests were done but also what the results mean. In particular doctors must explore how patients' understanding of the results influences their understanding of their pain. Patients' understanding of the test results may lead them to conclude that they have a disease process that will be progressively disabling.

Patients' misunderstanding may be profound (see examples in Case studies 8.3 and 8.4). Doctors often know how patients can misinterpret what has been said to them and come up with ridiculous ideas. The doctors tend to write this off as a 'patient' problem. However, this is a 'doctor' problem, or a least a doctor–patient

---

Case study 8.3   Case example of misunderstanding of test results

Susan is 40 years old and has a long history of pain in a number of sites including back, neck, arms and some of the larger joints. She has been investigated thoroughly by a rheumatologist. All of the tests have been normal with the exception of one of the tests for rheumatoid arthritis, which was very weakly positive. Clinically she has absolutely no features of rheumatoid arthritis but she is now convinced that she has this.

Nobody has tackled her misconceptions about the test results. She thinks that if it is positive then she has the disease. She has seen what the disease can do to others and is now very protective of herself. This is reinforced by her husband whose mother had rheumatoid arthritis.

None of her doctors have explained that tests do not give black-and-white answers and they are not 100% accurate. It was not explained that tests are usually done to confirm or refute a 'clinical diagnosis'. Only an explanation from the rheumatologist in the team was able to challenge this lady's misconception successfully. She proved to have all the markers of primary fibromyalgia. She required further investigation to rule out other causes of myogenic pain, but was counselled carefully prior to testing.

Case study 8.4   Case example of misunderstanding of scan results

Lynda had a fall at work 4 years ago and has had severe disabling back pain ever since. She has been seen by a large number of specialists and had a considerable amount of conservative treatment. At a medicolegal assessment a doctor stated that one of the scans she had had showed that she has spina bifida occulta. No other abnormality has been discovered. Lynda is now convinced that her spinal abnormality is the cause of her pain and is seeking an operation to repair the defect.

None of Lynda's doctors had explained that the spina bifida occulta is unlikely to be the cause of all of her pain. Indeed Lynda had this minor abnormality prior to the accident and it was entirely asymptomatic.

---

communication problem, and doctors bear the greater responsibility for imparting knowledge to patients in terms the latter can understand.

The doctor's review of previous investigations must, therefore, include constant checking and rechecking with patients as to their understanding of the results of tests. Doctors must correct misconceptions as they arise. Patients must not be allowed to continue with either unrealistic expectations of the accuracy or validity of various tests or misconceptions about their interpretation. The advent of high technology scanning has lead both patients and doctors to tend to place undue emphasis upon structure. Patients must be taught to put the test results of structure into context. The function of the back, for example, is not explained only by the visualised bones, discs and nerves on an MRI scan. A time will be reached when the likelihood of further investigation revealing any treatable pathology is so small that a judgement has to be made whether to do it at all. This should be discussed openly with patients. Ultimately the investigation has to influence the decision regarding treatment to be worth while doing. If treatment will not change following a particular investigation, then it is debatable whether that investigation should be done at all.

Previous treatment

Most if not all patients have had a significant amount of previous treatment prior to referral to a pain centre, particularly if they are being referred specifically for 'pain management' as opposed to further physical intervention. By the nature of the patient's problem they will not have responded well to previous treatment and indeed may have been made worse by it. Even if they have not suffered any significant physical side-effects from failed treatment, it should be remembered that failed treatment is not innocuous. Failed treatment is demoralising, depressing and reinforces a sense of helplessness and hopelessness. Patients' hopes will have been raised, however carefully they may have been counselled prior to the procedure. Patients tend to be much more optimistic about the outcome of treatment than their doctors.

It is important to go into this area in some detail. Doctors must explore the detail of the previous treatments and patients' responses. Doctors should be confident that reasonable treatments have been performed properly and

---

Case study 8.5   Example of counselling re previous treatment

Mark is 45 years old and had had his back pain for several years. It came on following an injury in a game of rugby. Prior to his injury he was a keen sportsman and fitness fanatic. His previous specialist had given him a large number of epidural injections. These seemed to produce significant help for a number of weeks and helped him to return to almost normal levels of activity, although he had never played rugby again.

Mark was convinced that there was something specifically wrong with his back. This was reinforced by his response to epidurals. All he wanted was some form of treatment that could produce the effect of an epidural permanently. He didn't understand why this could not be done. There was certainly nothing 'psychological' about his pain!

When it was explained to him that epidurals commonly only produce short term benefit he became quite angry. Why was he given so many epidurals when they don't cure the problem? He had been wasting his time. He needed to find a doctor who could do something and knew what he is talking about.

It took some time and skill to calm him down. The following points were made for him to consider:

- all health-care professionals have their own specific skills
- doctors and others tend to offer the treatments they are good at
- doctors respond to patients' distress as well as their clinical problems
- doctors are just as susceptible to despair and pressure from patients as patients are themselves
- this may lead the doctor to at least try 'something' in desperation
- short term remedies may be all that is necessary
- the initial response naturally leads to further treatments
- now is the time to consider long term management in the face of the failure of short term treatments
- no blame should be attached to what has happened.

The purpose of the above is not to defend doctors but to explain to patients why doctors try some treatments that have a low chance of 'curing' the problem. By being non-judgemental about previous treatment doctors will be able to gain patients' confidence and help them to consider alternative methods of managing their pain.

---

the response charted accurately. For example, failure to respond to treatment may be due to inaccurately placed injections, and not to a lack of response on the patient's part. Such previous experience may give rise to a number of different emotional responses from depression to anger. Doctors must be prepared to ride this and take a careful history of previous treatments and their effects. They will have to provide answers as to why some treatments were performed and why they were not successful or why they produced only a short term benefit. Patients will often ask why can the treatment not be given in such a way as to produce a long term benefit or cure.

On occasions patients will become angry at being given a treatment that had little chance of producing long term benefit. It is not helpful in being openly critical of previous doctors. It helps neither teams nor patients and usually only serves to fire the patients' anger, thus diverting them from the task of dealing with now rather than the past. Doctors must be honest and explain the reasons behind why certain treatments are offered even if they have not been

shown to be very efficacious. Doctors must give patients an understanding of the helplessness of other doctors in such situations, especially when they are pressurised by very distressed patients (Case study 8.5).

FURTHER TREATMENT

Doctors must decide whether any treatments need repeating or any other treatments should be tried. They should explain the nature of the treatments and the expected long term as well as short term outcome together with the risks and complications. They should also explain why other treatments have been offered as well as why they have been ineffectual.

In many instances patients will have been sensitised against further treatment of any kind. Doctors must explain carefully the nature of any proposed further treatment, including further physical intervention if it is deemed necessary. A careful exposition of the expected outcomes and what is required of patients is vital. Doctors will need to constantly check patients' understanding of their treatments and outcomes of such treatments both past and current. Doctors must correct any misconceptions as they become evident.

Failed treatment is demoralising both for patients and therapists. The negative effect of failed treatment can be profound and this should be born in mind when further treatments and procedures are considered. There should be clear positive indications for further intervention with a substantial chance of major benefit if this is to be considered seriously.

Getting patients to change their model

If 'pain management' is likely to be considered doctors must begin to help patients consider looking at their problem in an entirely different way. They will need to help patients shift their stance from one of seeking a cure or respite from the pain to managing and mastering the pain and looking primarily at restoring levels of physical and social functioning.

The aforementioned may seem tedious in the extreme. However, it is vital as it represents one of the most important building blocks of pain management. The rehabilitation process will be simply impossible unless these issues are addressed specifically. On the pain management programme patients will be asked to ignore pain and other symptoms that they have interpreted as being an important reason for limiting activity. Patients will have interpreted pain as meaning further damage. Unless patients feel the doctor (team) has an understanding of their problem from their point of view they will not participate in treatment. If the patient's view is incorrect, then the doctor (team) must correct this, so that both the doctor (team) and the patient are working with the same model. Only then is there any likelihood of success.

CONCURRENT MEDICAL PROBLEMS

With regard to patients' fitness for attending a pain management programme, which entails a substantial amount of physical exercise and activity, doctors should satisfy themselves that patients do not suffer from any concurrent medical problems that would either substantially interfere with such activity or even be hazardous for the patient and put them at risk of harming themselves. The team must be able to be confident in ignoring illness behaviour on the pain programme. Doctors must, therefore, be as confident as possible that it is safe to ignore illness behaviour. The commonest cause of illness behaviour in the general population is organic disease. Mistakes will not only damage the individual patient but also can potentially destroy the confidence of the other members of the group and thereby ruin the progress they might otherwise have made. Indeed it may sensitise them against further attempts at rehabilitation.

A systematic enquiry must be made of past medical and surgical problems together with details of any concurrent medical problems and a 'review of systems'. This should include expected clinic visits and any anticipated treatments. Doctors not only have to convince themselves and the team that a rehabilitation programme is safe, they must also convince the patient. This can only be done by careful assessment and enquiry into all the medical aspects of the patient.

Not all of the medical problems that may interfere with a rehabilitation programme are absolute barriers to inclusion on such a programme Case study 8.6). Many problems will be relative exclusions and the decision to list for the programme or not is dependent on the team discussion following the advice of the doctor. This will put the medical problems into context.

If there are any doubts about the safety of rehabilitation, then further advice must be sought from the relevant specialist. Patients will ultimately have more confidence to have a go if they have been given permission to do so by a 'specialist'.

If patients are to be included on the programme with some medical problem that may interfere with the rehabilitation process (e.g. diabetes) then the team must be made aware of the problem and be given advice as to how the problem may affect performance and how these patients should be handled. Patients may need

---

Case study 8.6 Examples of potential medical barriers

1

Mrs Y. had a history of mild angina in addition to her back pain problems. She had been investigated by a cardiologist about 2 years ago. The results of investigation did not demonstrate severe coronary artery disease that required surgery. Her symptoms were well controlled with regular medication. She very rarely suffered any chest pain. In fact she had not used her glycerin trinitrate (GTN) spray for months despite moderate exercise.

It was felt that Mrs Y.'s mild angina was not a barrier to the physical aspects of the programme. She could safely exercise and it was felt that an increase in her fitness would be beneficial. This was explained to Mrs Y. who accepted it. If there had been any reservations on either doctor's or patient's part a final review by a cardiologist would have been arranged prior to inclusion on a programme. The medical problems were recorded in the patient's records to give all the team members confidence in managing any problems that might arise during the programme.

2

Mr A. is 58 years old and has a small amount of osteoarthritis (OA) in some of his joints as well as his back pain problem. The OA effects largely the joints of his fingers. He has some minor problems with other small joints but it does not affect his lower limbs to any great extent. He is mildly asthmatic, having developed this later in life. He has had no major problems with his asthma that had required admission to hospital and his symptoms are fairly well controlled on inhaled steroids and bronchodilators as necessary.

Although Mr A. had some minor physical restrictions due to concurrent medical problems, these were not regarded to be at a level that would represent a major restriction to activity on a rehabilitation programme. It was also felt that the programme would not make Mr A's symptoms of asthma or OA worse and would not represent a major risk.

3

Mr B. is 48 years old and has had significant back pain for 15 years. He has not worked for 25 years. He was retired on medical grounds following major surgery for non-malignant gastrointestinal problems. His postoperative period was stormy and he spent 6 months in intensive care. He has had recurrent problems with abdominal wall hernias, with multiple attempts at repair. He is a diabetic and occasionally has problems when he has bouts of vomiting making control difficult. He has migraine, which also makes his diabetes difficult to manage when he vomits. He is desperate with his back pain and has difficulty in coping. He knows there is no specific answer to the pain, but painkillers make his gastrointestinal problems worse.

Mr B. has multiple problems, which preclude his being included in a group pain management programme. His other symptoms are too unpredictable to enable him to attend all of the sessions. He might easily develop significant medical problems unrelated to his back pain. If he had to drop out this might adversely affect the morale of the group. In addition his symptoms related to his other problems could be made worse by the programme. He really requires some individual work with the team. The doctor will provide continuing support and supervision of the other problems, calling for help from other specialists as required.

---

specific advice during the programme and the rest of the patients on the programme may need to be given an understanding if it is relevant to their own problems and providing it does not breach patient confidentiality. The patient's permission must, of course, be given in such a case.

MEDICATION

The problem

There are two major reasons for patients resorting to medication. First they will naturally seek an effective analgesic. This obviously occurs during the acute phase of the pain problem and, indeed, the analgesics may well be very effective initially. Secondly, patients with persistent pain commonly suffer significant sleep problems as a consequence of pain. Either they have problems getting off to sleep, or they are woken by their pain and are unable to get back to sleep. Some patients will have had sleep problems prior to their pain problem and the pain will have compounded the problem.

Patients commonly resort to two different types of medication in order to provide help with pain and sleep. These usually include an opioid or an opioid-containing analgesic and some form of sedative to help with sleep. It is still common for benzodiazepines to be prescribed, although tricyclic antidepressants are also commonly used to provide night sedation.

Many patients with chronic pain experience some difficulties with medication (Box 8.3). Usually this is in the form of lack of efficacy or at least a falling off in efficacy. Patients often continue

> **Box 8.3** Main problems with medication
>
> - Opioids seem to be less effective with time in most chronic pain states of benign origin
> - Many patients develop a habit of tablet taking
> - Many patients seek stronger tablets in the face of decreasing efficacy
> - A substantial minority of patients take tablets in excess of the recommended dose without benefit
> - Multiple medication is common
> - Patients (and their doctors) become increasingly desperate in their search for analgesia
> - Side-effects are common, particularly with combinations of medicines
> - Patients, their family and doctors worry about addiction
> - Most patients do not like being reliant upon tablets

to take such medication in the belief that at least they are doing something. They will frequently seek stronger and stronger tablets in the search of pain relief. They may be given stronger analgesics, but usually these too become ineffective or produce significant side-effects. The night sedatives do not seem to help with their sleep either. In desperation patients may resort to other substances both legal (e.g. alcohol) and illegal.

Disclosure of sensitive information

One of the most important issues for physicians to address is patients' use of medication. A significant number of patients with chronic pain fail to obtain relief of their symptoms with medication. They often continue to consume tablets despite the lack of effect. Small but significant numbers of patients not only continue to take medication but do so in excess of the maximum recommended doses. This frequently produces a number of side-effects, most of which are well documented in the literature and are well known to most general practitioners. Some of the side-effects, however, are subtle and not well known to either patients or their general practitioners or even some specialists.

Many patients feel guilty about their use of tablets. They may have been sensitised by their previous consultations with doctors. In addition their family may well express their disapproval of overdependence on tablets. Patients may feel bad about their use of medicines and over-reliance upon them.

When taking a drug history, it is important to be non-judgemental in technique. This must apply to both verbal and non-verbal communication. It must be made explicitly clear to patients that no blame is attached to either patients or their doctors. Often using the techniques of 'blaming' the pain or giving examples of 'other' patients is a useful way of 'allowing' patients to disclose the amount of medication and other substances that they are taking. Reinforcing the fact that most patients have problems will allow patients to drop their guard and disclose more information. An example of the technique is given in Box 8.4.

Identifying the problem

It can be seen from the above example that non-threatening questioning techniques allow patients to admit a higher level of drug consumption than they might normally wish to. By implying that the blame lies with the pain and not the patient, patients will feel more comfortable in revealing their true level of tablet consumption. Aggressive questioning or even just open questions may lead patients to become defensive and therefore unwilling to reveal their true drug usage. Many patients have been sensitised either by members of their family or by accusations of being an addict by other doctors. It is not surprising that they become defensive when directly questioned. Considerable skill must be used in carefully extracting details while still retaining patients' trust. It may be necessary to state specifically that no blame for the current level of drug use lies with patients or their doctors; it is just something that happens when patients become desperate and doctors feel helpless.

It is important to gain the confidence of patients if they are to feel able to admit and reveal some facts about their problems, which perhaps they would rather not have to face up to. Many of a patient's previous consultations will have been with clinicians who do not come across clinical problems with drug misuse very often. They will not, therefore, have developed

---

Box 8.4 Medication use interview: non-judgemental interviewing

Dr: 'Do you take any painkillers to help with the pain?'
Patient: 'Yes, but they don't help very much.'
Dr: 'Which ones do you take at the moment?'
Patient: 'Tylex.'
Dr: 'I expect that they are not as helpful now as they were when you first went on them.'
Patient: 'I did ask my GP for something stronger, but he wouldn't give me anything.'
Dr: 'Do you take the Tylex everyday?'
Patient: 'Yes.'
Dr: 'How many do you normally take.'
Patient: 'I try to take as few as possible.'
Dr: 'Are there some days when you don't need to take any?'

Patient: 'No I have to take them every day.'
Dr: 'How many do you take on a good day?'
Patient: 'I don't have any good days.'
Dr: 'OK, what is the least number of capsules you might take?'
Patient: 'Well, it may be 6 or 7.'
Dr: 'When the pain is at its worst how many does it make you take?'
Patient: 'When it's really bad I sometimes have to take three at a time.'
Dr: 'Some of our patients tell us that they have to take 10 or more capsules a day.'
Patient: 'Well, yes sometimes I have to take as many as 10 or 12 in a day.'

Box 8.5 Medication use interview: predicting patients' response to medicines

Dr: 'What painkillers do you take?'
Patient: 'I think they are called dihydro something.'
Dr: 'I expect that they are dihydrocodeine.'
Patient: 'Yes. That's it. I remember now, Dihydrocodeine.'
Dr: 'Many patients tell me that the painkillers seem to lose their effect over time.'
Patient: 'Yes. When I first went on dihydrocodeine it seemed to work quite well.'
Dr: 'That's very common. The painkillers seem to work quite well to start with. By the time they get to see me they tell me the painkillers at best only "take the edge off the pain" and sometimes "don't seem to work at all".'
Patient: 'Yeah. Sometimes I wonder if they are worth taking at all.'

---

the skills of interviewing such patients and will often have difficulties in relating to the problems that such patients have. The end result of such consultations is that patients are made to feel guilty about something, that is not entirely within their control. People (including doctors) are often unsympathetic and 'blame' patients for their failure to improve and the apparent 'addictive behaviour'. This is not only not helpful to patients but also sensitises them to admitting to problems with medication to new doctors whom they fear may take the same unhelpful stance. It can be seen that doctors in this situation are already working at a potentially significant disadvantage. Any technique that enables

doctors to gain patients' confidence will be invaluable.

One of the most effective ways of gaining patients' confidence is to predict to patients how they feel, what problems they may have encountered and even how other doctors may have reacted to this. This immediately gives patients the feeling that 'this' doctor has seen this problem before and understands it. Immediately patients feel more comfortable in agreeing with the doctor's predictions and may volunteer some additional details of other difficulties they have had. With regard to medication use, predicting the loss of effectiveness of opioids and the patient's need to increase the dose to get the same effect is a useful non-threatening lead into the problems of drug use. A typical opening of an interview is given in Box 8.5.

It can be seen that this interaction contains very few questions—in fact only one. The doctor is using open-ended statements, which the patient may comment on if wished. The doctor is carefully searching out what the patient feels and how the medication is being taken almost without the patient realising. This is done by discussing 'other' patients rather than the patient in front of the doctor. Patients are then free to agree (if they identify with the 'other' patients) or not as necessary. Open-ended statements are often more helpful than direct questioning in gaining an understanding of patients' problems. Direct questioning is appropriate indeed essential for some issues, but clearly sensitive issues are best tackled in a more subtle way. It is important to develop a number of interviewing skills so that the appropriate skill may be used in the varying situations as they arise. If necessary swapping from one style to another may be necessary if one tack does not seem to work.

Getting patients to consider a different strategy

Having established a good rapport and gained the patient's confidence it is possible to build on this by further use of open-ended statements to gain more information about patients' use of medication, which will help establish an appropriate management plan (Box 8.6). Using this technique patients will feel confident in the advice given as they are more likely to follow this if they feel their doctor has a full understanding of their problem.

Obviously the conversation with the patient in the example in Box 8.6 does not stop there. But this snippet illustrates how to build on the confidence the patient has with the doctor. It is important that patients understand that *this* consultation is not the same as all of the others and they will not be treated dismissively. Patients should understand that they will be taken seriously and the doctor has seen many similar patients and will guide the patient in the right direction.

Other medicines

Emphasis so far has been placed on the use of opioids or opioid-containing medication. Although this is an important group of medicines adequate enquiry of other tablets and medicines must also be made. Similar non-threatening techniques may need to be used with the enquiry regarding tranquillisers, night sedatives and perhaps antidepressants, but in general such enquiry is not so fraught with problems as is that about the opioid drugs.

This point in the assessment is often a useful time to begin management. Lecturing patients on their misuse of medicines is unlikely to produce change. Indeed it may well lead to patients 'digging their heels in' and may ruin any chance of helping patients to make changes in the future. At this stage it is best to get patients to consider simply whether the medicines really help much at all—in other words, to get patients to 'consider' an alternative strategy. Doctors should offer the opportunity for further consultations to go through methods of how to get the best out of medicines at a later date.

Drug withdrawal

Drug withdrawal is an option, but not the only option. Any withdrawal of medicines must be done carefully. Patients must be fully aware of the consequences and have plans for how to manage any withdrawal symptoms. In addition

---

Box 8.6   Medication use interview: changing patient's expectations

Dr:	'You told me that the dihydrocodeine seems to have lost its effect.'
Patient:	'Yes.'
Dr:	'And sometimes you feel that the tablets are a waste of time.'
Patient:	'Yes. I have tried stopping them.'
Dr:	'Many patients, like you, don't like taking tablets and try to stop them. The problem is that although the tablets don't seem to help, the pain increases dramatically when they suddenly stop them. They sometimes feel very ill if they suddenly stop them and are then forced to continue taking them.'

Patient:	'How can I get off them?'
Dr:	'Well, first you shouldn't feel guilty about being stuck on these tablets. It happens commonly. We can show you a successful way of reducing them and ultimately coming off them altogether. I don't doubt you are motivated to do this; we simply need to teach you the skill and offer you some support while you make the necessary changes.'
Patient:	'Won't my pain get much worse again?'
Dr:	'Yes, if we suddenly stop the tablets. That's happened to you before. Not if we help you do it much more slowly and carefully.'

> **Box 8.7** Initial advice to patients for drug withdrawal
>
> - Do not make any sudden changes to your current level of medicines and tablets
> - Work out how many tablets you take a day and then divide them evenly throughout the day
> - Stabilising and regularising your tablets is the first step to reduction
> - Try to start taking your tablets at regular times of the day rather than only when the pain is bad
> - Do not underestimate the number of tablets
> - Keep the length of time between each tablet much the same
> - Break the pain–pill habit
> - If you are on tablets for other conditions *do not* change these at all without speaking to your GP
> - Explain to your GP that you wish to begin to reduce your painkillers
> - Write down how your take your tablets and bring it with you next time
> - We will help you plan your reduction at your next visit

patients' GP must be informed and given advice if necessary. This must be tackled at a separate time from the assessment. Patients should be advised to make no changes in their medication use unless they are in danger of harming themselves with toxic doses, but to begin to take their medication on a time-contingent basis rather than only in response to the pain (Box 8.7).

The need for a careful and detailed drug history cannot be overemphasised. It is important to make it explicit to patients that they may ask questions about their medication, and answers should be provided in order to help them adopt a more rational approach to medication use. Some patients become very angry when they realise that they 'have been prescribed' unhelpful or even inappropriate medication. Care must be taken in explaining the rationale for the use of various drugs in different situations. It is not helpful just to be critical of other doctors. The prescription of any medication has to be put into its original context, which may be entirely different from the situation in which patients now find themselves.

Non-pain medicines

Great emphasis has so far been placed on pain-related medicines. A thorough history of all medicines should be taken, both pain related and non-pain related. Patients will often forget medicines taken for other problems (e.g. high blood pressure). This will give doctors a chance to cross-check other concurrent medical problems. In addition doctors must emphasise that some medicines should never be stopped and must be continued indefinitely (e.g. antidiabetic tablets, asthma treatments).

Other substances

Finally, an inquiry into patients' use of recreational substances both legal and illegal should be made. This is relevant as alcohol and other substances do have the potential for dependence and can interfere with cognitive function. Illegal substance use is relevant to the patient's assessment. This is a very delicate topic. It is probably best to enquire about legal substance use (tobacco and alcohol) first. Again this should be done in a way that allows patients to admit their helplessness without feeling too vulnerable, using similar techniques to those described above. This is a useful way of leading patients to disclose their use of illegal substances. Doctors should be non-judgmental. If patients are to be included on a pain management programme they will have to abide by the rules of the group, which will include regulation of all medications and substances. The team needs, therefore, an accurate pretreatment assessment of the use of all medication and other substances.

CURRENT LEVEL OF BENEFITS AND LITIGATION

Many patients attending pain clinics are in receipt of state benefits. Some of these benefits are given on the basis of the patient's reported and observed level of disability, usually following medical examinations at the request of the Benefits Agency (in the UK).

If patients are to make any progress with regard to rehabilitation they must be made aware of the consequences of improvements in physical functioning, performance of activities of daily living and potential for work. These consequences may include loss of benefits and a reduced amount from litigation. Benefits may be at such a level that they steal away the urgency with which patients address the question of return to work. As a consequence they may become rapidly more unfit, disabled and less able to return to work.

Benefits

Careful documentation of all financial benefits should be made. This should include all of the list in Box 8.8. The list will need constantly updating as legislation changes from time to time. Enquiry about other sources of income related to disability should also be made.

Patients must be made aware that they may lose benefit if they are included on a pain management programme. They must be aware of the financial consequences and must be prepared to 'take the risk'. Similarly the team must be aware of all of the benefit issues in order to help patients address them. As in litigation patients may be asked to 'prove' their disability repeatedly. The assessments and physical examinations are often very stressful and demeaning. Patients frequently say they have been hurt

---

Box 8.8   Benefits that may be claimed by patients with pain-associated disability in the UK 1998

Statutory sickness pay
Incapacity benefit:
— short term
— long term
Disability living allowance:
— care needs
— mobility
Invalidity allowance
Attendance allowance
Invalid care allowance
Severe disablement allowance
Industrial disablement benefit
Disability working allowance

Other potential sources of income dependent on proven disability
Criminal injuries compensation
Job-related pension (early retirement)
Private permanent health insurance
Company insurance schemes

---

during physical examinations. This may lead to a sense of injustice and anger with the system.

Litigation

Although the presence of litigation (either a civil compensation case or for medical negligence) should not preclude admission to a programme the litigation process does have an influence on outcome. Patients may well have been labelled as 'malingerers' by others either explicitly or implicitly. It is not uncommon for treatments to have been denied on the basis that the patient is involved in litigation. Patients may, therefore, have become sensitised to questioning about their level of benefits and seeking compensation. Considerable skill and tact is required when making enquiries in this area. Doctors should be open and honest. They should show that they understand how patients feel about the whole litigation process and how stressful and threatening it can be. They should explain the need for enquiry into benefits and litigation and should reassure patients that these do not influence the decision to offer treatment, providing patients are willing to risk losing benefits and reducing the amount of their legal claim. Patients usually respond well to honesty; it is easier for them to make decisions when they are in possession of all of the facts and there are no hidden agendas. When litigation is an important issue then patients must be made explicitly aware that they need to convince the team they are willing to sacrifice any financial incentive for remaining disabled if they are to be taken on to a programme.

There is an important risk of which doctors should make patients aware. If patients are involved in litigation and decide to take up the offer of a place on the programme but drop out before the end of the programme, it will look very bad in court and may be used by the defendants as an indication of lack of motivation. So once on the programme patients must complete the course. The advantage to patients of completing a programme and doing well is often used to encourage patients to accept treatment as it may be used as a marker of good motivation. However, the risks are not always spelled out.

Finally, all of these benefits, including the litigation process, require patients to 'prove' their disability from time to time and sometimes on a regular and protracted basis. This usually takes the form of 'medical assessments' but also includes private surveillance companies videoing patients without their knowledge. The team must have an understanding of where the litigation process is up to and if there are any anticipated medical assessments due either for litigation purposes or for benefits. Patients may ask for help in establishing the 'reality' of their pain and associated disability. The team members should desist from becoming embroiled in the process as they will be asked to do the impossible task of supporting disability while trying to improve it.

PHYSICAL EXAMINATION

A full and thorough examination of patients is essential. This should include an examination of all the other systems that are not involved in the pain problem as well as those that are. This enables doctors to put the disability due to the pain problem in the context of any other abnormalities that may be detected. Doctors have the responsibility of ensuring the safety of patients and reviewing the whole of a patient's health. It is likely that this will be the first time this has been done for patients and will be profoundly beneficial for the doctor and the rest of the team. Patients will gain a sense of seriousness and completeness about the assessment and will be much more likely to take notice of what is said to them. The converse is certainly true. If patients perceive that they are being 'fobbed off' or not taken seriously they will not take part in any treatment plan suggested, especially if it does not involve a cure or attempted cure.

This means paying attention to every single physical or medical problem that patients raise and addressing that in history and examination. This can be very tedious with some patients as they may raise a whole number of apparent red herrings; however, if this is not done the patient may well be repeatedly distracted by various minor problems that they feel nobody has taken

seriously. Such problems may just be relevant. Certainly patients will feel so until they receive specific reassurance.

It is not appropriate to go into the details of how to examine a patient. There are other texts available covering such matters in detail (Table 8.1). The doctor should be competent in general examination techniques and also demonstrate skill in the relevant specific areas (Ch. 16). Doctors should develop their skills and be able to identify when to refer on for second opinions. There are, however, a number of important issues that should be born in mind when examining a patient.

Reassuring patients

Many patients may have been physically hurt during previous medical examinations, particularly if they have been performed by doctors who are assessing them in relation to some form of compensation claim, whether it be for state benefits or in the process of litigation. Patients may, therefore, have been sensitised to physical examination and indeed be quite fearful of being hurt during examination or suffering considerably for days after the examination.

It is as important to put patients at their ease with regard to the examination as it is to do so for the interview. There is nothing to be gained from hurting patients during examination. It reveals little if any additional information. Patients should be specifically reassured on this point. Some patients are apologetic for not being in bad pain at the time of examination, almost as if the doctor had some particular way of seeing their pain. As with the interview the doctors must disabuse patients of erroneous beliefs and explain that doctors cannot see pain; neither does it help the examination if patients are in severe pain, and indeed the examination may be more difficult.

Behavioural responses to examination

Patients will commonly display 'behavioural responses to examination'. These may be quite bizarre and will often make the eliciting of

Table 8.1 Differing medical problems and their assessment

Medical problem	Key issues in medical assessment	Specific examination techniques	References
General issues (for all patients)	• Screening for clinical 'red flags' • Exclusion of important serious pathology • General health check • Review of previous investigations and treatments	• Complete general examination	Clinical examination (eds) Macleod J, Munro J, 7th Edn 1986. Churchill Livingstone, New York
Musculoskeletal pain	• Screening for rheumatological disease • Screening for orthopaedic problems	• Careful survey of joints, muscles and connective tissues • Initiate or check appropriate blood tests	Clinical examination in rheumatology Docherty M, Docherty J 1992. Wolfe Publications. New York
Non-specific low back pain	• As for general issues *plus* • Screening for clinical 'red flags' for low back pain	• Check for structural abnormalities • Neurological examination of lower limbs	Assessment of severity of low back disorders Waddell G, Main C J 1984. Spine 9: 204–208 The back pain revolution Waddell G 1998. Churchill Livingstone, New York, chs 2 and 8
Neurogenic pain problem (including CRPS)	• Screen for other neurological disorders • Screen for other contributory problems (e.g. orthopaedic)	• Check for structural abnormalities • Full neurological examination	Neurological differential diagnosis John Patten 2nd edn 1996. Springer-Verlag, London Reflex sympathetic dystrophy: a reappraisal (eds) Janig W, Stanton-Hicks M. 1996. IASP External validation of IASP diagnostic criteria for complex regional pain syndrome and proposed research diagnostic criteria Bruehl S et al 1999. Pain 81: 147–154
Unexplained multisite pain	• As for general issues *plus* • Screening for rheumatological disorders	• Careful survey of joints, muscles and connective tissues • Initiate or check appropriate blood tests • Survey of 'tender points'	Myofascial pain & dysfunction: the trigger point manual, Travell J G, Simons D G, 1983. Williams & Wilkins, Baltimore. Wolfe F et al 1990 The American College of Rheumatology Criteria for the Classification of Fibromyalgia Arthritis and Rheumatism 33(2) : 160–172.

specific organic signs very difficult if not impossible on occasions. It is important not to be 'thrown' by such responses, but to concentrate carefully on the organic findings. Behavioural signs and organic findings are not mutually exclusive; nor are behavioural findings a sign of faking or malingering. They correlate with patients' levels of distress and are their physical expressions of this distress. They should be noted (and scored if, for example, the patient has back pain) and the doctors' behaviour and demeanour should be such as to ignore them and

not reinforce them. Patients may ask specifically why, for example, their whole leg is numb. Doctors should be honest and explain that it does not indicate a physical problem with the nerves but that it indicates the level of the patient's distress. If necessary the doctor should explain that medicine does not entirely understand the phenomenon but that this is seen very frequently in many patients in the pain centre.

Finally doctors should ask patients if there is anything that has not been addressed that the patient feels is important. Doctors should check that there are no unanswered medical questions. It may be necessary to address these at the feedback, but doctors must feel confident that they have all of the necessary facts to advise the team.

Examples of pain problems have been outlined in Table 8.1 to illustrate the differing types of medical problems that may be encountered and how they should be assessed. The reader is directed to other texts for the specific methods of assessment and examination. Doctors should be able to screen patients for serious disease, examine the patient thoroughly and (if necessary seek further advice) advise the pain management team on the cause, diagnosis and medical treatment of the patient.

RECOMMENDATIONS TO THE TEAM

Prior to the feedback session to patients, and their partners if present, the team meets to exchange information (Ch. 12). All members of the team are responsible for presenting the relevant data from their assessments. The doctor's responsibility to the team is to determine three major issues.

First, is there serious underlying pathology that requires specific medical or surgical intervention?

Secondly, is this patient fit, in the medical sense, for a rehabilitative pain management programme? If the patient is not, the doctor should outline the medical barriers and indicate whether any of these barriers are surmountable. For example a final test may be all that is required to reassure the patient and the team. It may be that further active physical treatment is required. Nevertheless the team must be able to feel that either the patient may be considered for a pain management programme or that this decision needs to be postponed pending either further investigation or treatment. If the patient will never be fit medically for a programme (e.g. because of severe asthma) then the team will have to address the problem of considering an alternative strategy.

Thirdly, the doctor must act as a team member in identifying whether the patient is ready for

pain management. In other words, is the patient convinced that all the tests, investigations and treatments are completed? Doctors may be satisfied, but if patients are not convinced then they will not accept the plan of treatment offered. The nature of the feedback session will, therefore revolve around changing patients' beliefs.

FEEDBACK TO PATIENTS

The doctor's role in the feedback session is to address the medical issues specifically. Only the doctor can give the patient 'permission' to stop seeking cures and to begin actively to seek restoration of function in the face of continuing pain. It is the doctor who can give the patient the confidence that it is safe to ignore the pain; that pain does not mean harm (if that is indeed the case). To some extent the doctor legitimises the whole process of team assessment and pain management rather than cure. Therefore doctors must act in a supporting role when they have finished explaining to the patient that there is no further treatment required. Doctors should not dominate the conversation, but make it clear they are but one member of the team.

If there are remaining doubts about further investigation or treatment in the patient's mind at the end of the session the doctor must address these. This may require a further visit and investigation in order to allow patients to let go of cure seeking behaviour and begin to face up to the future realistically.

CONCLUSION

Assessment cannot be entirely separated from management. The nature and quality of the assessment, in particular the quality of the communication, may have a profound effect on the willingness of patients to disclose information and partake in treatment and its outcome.

All of the factors outlined in the previous chapter are relevant to this chapter. Doctors to the team must possess all of the general skills required to be a team member in a pain management team. In addition they must have general medical skills and the skills of their specialty.

Doctors must be prepared to work within a team and allow their opinion to be affected by the information gathered by others. Only then can the team function in a way in which the boundaries between the disciplines blur and the members almost act as one. This is a very powerful tool in managing the most difficult patients with the most difficult problems. Ultimately it is very rewarding for all team members, but it requires that the doctor and all team members possess and retain the highest level of skill within their own discipline.

KEY POINTS

- Thorough medical assessment is essential prior to pain management.
- The doctor should medically screen patients for serious pathology.
- The medical assessment should be focused in order to provide a succinct medical appraisal of the patient to the team.
- The assessment should include enquiry into: the pain, previous treatment and investigations, concurrent medical problems, medication, benefits, litigation and a physical examination.
- Patients should be made aware that acceptance of treatment may affect benefits and litigation.
- The medical assessment should enable the doctor to advise the team if the patient is medically fit for rehabilitation and if the patient is ready for rehabilitation.

APPENDIX: NEW PATIENT ASSESSMENT FORMS (MANCHESTER & SALFORD PAIN CENTRE ©)

NEW PATIENT ASSESSMENT

Name :_____   D.O.B. _____   Hosp. No.:_____

Referred by :_____   Date :_____   Team :_____

Outcome of assessment/Plan

Primary pain complaint/presenting symptoms

Pain history (i.e. insidious/traumatic/accident onset etc? claim ongoing)

Aggravating factors   **Easing factors**

Past investigations/patient's perception of findings

Past treatments for pain (including surgery) and outcome

Current treatments including current medication

Treatments or investigations pending? (not necessarily just for pain)

Concurrent medical problems. Past medical problems (incl. Surgery)

Concurrent medical problems. Past medical problems (Incl. Surgery).

Systems review

Gen Health   Appetite   Wt   Bowels   Cardioasc

Chest   GUS   CNS

Social history

Work status/work history

Benefits

24 hour day

Aids/appliances/household adaptations

Perception of pain problem

Expectations of the centre

MANCHESTER AND SALFORD PAIN CENTRE NEW PATIENT ASSESSMENT PLAN OF ACTION

Patient name :_____   Hospital number :_____
Staff names :_____   Date :_____

Problems identified

Plan of action

Further information needed for the next appointment

Physical examination

Functional tests

	Time	Comments
Timed 20-metre speed walk (s):		

	Number	Comments
Step-ups in 30 seconds:		

	Score	Comments
Transfers: on/off floor		
Transfers: sit-stand		
Transfers: on/off bed		

Score: I = Independent / H = With the help of someone else / A = With the assistance of supports/aids

Summary of info in pain questionnaire booklet

PHYSIOTHERAPY: NEW PATIENT ASSESSMENT

Name :_____   Hosp No _____   Dob _____

Date of assessment :_____   Referred by :_____   Team :_____

Assessment Decision

Primary pain complaint : ——————————————————————————————

Patient's perception of
problem at assessment: _____

Physio when what what effect	
Other	

Pending   _____

Current   _____

Current Co-morbidity
Do you have any other health problems which interfere with your activities?

A   CHD   DM   OP   Epi   COPD   HyperT   Stroke

Previous injuries/accidents
Have you had any injuries or accidents in the past

Aggravating factors	**Easing factors**

Regularly lie down   YES / No
because of pain?   *If yes, how much?*

Aids or household adaptations :	

Typical day	Difficult with	Help needed with .....
a.m.		
p.m.		
eve		

Pacing :
What is the difference between a good and bad day? When you start a job do you have to finish it before you go
onto something else or do you tend to break it up? How do you decide when you've done enough of any one job?

Hobbies

Now	Prior to pain onset

Family / household:

Patient's goals	
Patient's expectations of the centre	

9

Assessment of pain, disability and physical function in pain management

Paul Watson Helen Parker

INTRODUCTION

Although a reduction in the patient's pain report following intervention is reported by many pain management rehabilitation programmes, it is not one of the declared primary aims of pain management. Patients are not encouraged to expect a reduction in their level of pain and the focus is on the management of the pain and disability, thereby helping them to manage the intrusive nature of their pain. Nevertheless, a reduction in the level of pain is a desirable characteristic of pain management rehabilitation and so measurement of pain should be conducted. Measurement of the level of pain also describes the patient population. It allows comparison between programmes for audit and research purposes. It is not intended to give a detailed account of the measurement of pain in its various forms in this chapter; the reader is directed to specific texts on the subject such as the excellent book by Turk & Melzack (1992). A brief review based on the observations by Price & Harkins (1992) and others is given in the appendix at the end of this chapter.

ASSESSMENT OF PAIN

Pain characteristics

Pain may be described by its intensity, affective component and location. Each requires investigation. Other pain states such as hyperalgesia or allodynia may be evident only on testing and would not be amenable to most self-report measures. The assessment of such states will not

---

> **Box 9.1** The three domains of pain intensity
>
> 1. The autonomic nervous system
> 2. The motor domain
> 3. The verbal domain

> **Box 9.2** Criteria for pain measurement (Price & Harkins 1992)
>
> - Have ratio scale properties
> - Be relatively free of biases inherent in different methods
> - Provide immediate information about the accuracy and reliability of the subjects' performance of the scaling responses
> - Be useful for both experimental and clinical pain and allow for reliable comparison between both types of pain
> - Be reliable and generalisable
> - Be sensitive to changes in pain intensity
> - Be simple and easy to use in pain patients in both clinical and non-clinical settings
> - Separately assess the sensory intensive and affective dimensions of pain

be addressed in this chapter and the reader should investigate specialist texts on this subject (e.g. Boivie, Hansson & Lindblom 1994).

Pain intensity

Classically, pain intensity has been assessed in three domains as shown in Box 9.1. They comprise: the effect on the autonomic nervous system (evidenced by an increase in heart rate, skin sweating and blood pressure), effect on the motor domain (in terms of reflexive responses, adoption of pain-relieving postures or alteration in movement), and effect on the verbal domain (patients' self-report).

- Assessment of the autonomic responses to pain (heart rate, skin sweating and blood pressure) is difficult to perform accurately outside of the laboratory and so is of little use in clinical practice and will not be addressed here.
- The assessment of motor activity (including reflexive responses, adoption of pain-relieving postures or alterations in movement) can be monitored by surface electromyography in the laboratory or the clinic setting. In the clinic the systematic observation of pain-associated motor behaviours is more useful and this is discussed later under the assessment of pain behaviours.
- The most popular method, and perhaps the most valid measure of pain, is patients' own self-reports. This is the easiest information to collect but can be the most misunderstood and misused.

Those with chronic pain almost invariably report that their pain, although continuous, is of a variable quality and intensity. It varies throughout the day and changes depending on whether the patient is active or at rest. This makes the snap-shot of the pain that we measure on initial assessment and at follow-up rather a blunt instrument in pain assessment. Our assessment needs to

reflect different dimensions of the pain experience. However, we first must identify the criteria for good pain measures. Price & Harkins (1992) have identified the criteria for pain assessment measures very clearly. They give eight key criteria for pain measures (Box 9.2). It must be stated that almost all commonly used pain measures fail to satisfy all of these criteria, but an understanding of why they fail can help in the evaluation of the relative usefulness of different measurement instruments.

For the purposes of this chapter it is not essential that all the above points are considered in detail and only those aspects that are most important in the clinical setting will be dealt with here. (The implications for experimental pain and comparisons between experimental and clinical pain will not be discussed.)

Pain affect

Pain has been described as a sensory and an emotional experience. Patients in pain not only make some judgement about the intensity of the signal but also respond to the sensation with differing degrees of emotional reaction, affording it a degree of unpleasantness or intrusiveness. This is termed the 'affective dimension' of the pain experience. However, an assessment of intensity does not necessarily address the intrusive nature of the pain. People may endure pain and not allow it to intrude into their lives to the point of limiting their activity. A reduction in the intensity of the pain following a pain management programme may not be achievable but a reduction in the intrusive nature or unpleasantness of the pain *is* a realistic aim of pain management programmes.

Pain location

The localisation of pain can be ascertained by use of a pain drawing (see the Appendix to Ch. 7, p. 133).

Scaling properties

Pain measures ideally should have ratio scale properties. A pain measure should start at zero and the distance between each of the points on the pain scale should be equal, the change in intensity between one and three should be equal to the change in intensity between three and five and five and seven, and so on. This confers a linear relationship between an increasing intensity and an increase in pain report. Experimental evidence suggests, however, that the relationship between increasing scores on pain instruments or verbal report for pain are non-linear. A fall in pain rating from nine to seven may represent a different reduction in intensity than from five to three. Verbal rating scales relying on adjectives describing the pain are particularly prone to this phenomenon of non-linearity. The data collected on such scales are categorical and do not have ratio scale properties. The difference in intensity between 'mild pain' and 'moderate pain' may not be the same as the perceived difference between 'moderate pain' and 'severe pain'. This is very important when dealing with the data statistically and makes nonsense of statements such as: 'The patient group reported a mean reduction of 30% in their pain'. Categorical scales such as these can only tell us that the pain increased or decreased; they cannot give meaningful information about the importance of the change in pain. Evidence from experimental evidence suggests that scoring systems such as visual analogue scales (VAS) are less prone to this phenomenon. However, they can be used as ratio data only if they have a zero starting point (i.e. are anchored by 'no pain' at one end). Verbal rating or verbal descriptor scales are particularly prone to distorted scaling.

A further distortion can arise if attempts are made to quantify responses to descriptive scales by converting them into numerical ratings and assigning them the status of ratio or interval data. The Short Form McGill Pain Questionnaire or SF-MPQ (Melzack 1987) requires subjects to report the level of intensity of different descriptors of pain in both the sensory and affective domains. This is then ascribed a number and the sensory component is assumed to give an indication of the intensity of the pain. It may be argued that this is a qualitative measure of pain rather than a quantitative measure. A patient may only describe their pain as having only one descriptive sensory component (e.g. throbbing) but report it as being severe, while another patient may report mild pain on more than three descriptors and the scores would be the same.

Influences on pain rating

The way in which the measure is introduced to the patient can unwittingly introduce a bias in the measure. Social desirability in a patient wishing to demonstrate to a clinician that a treatment is having an effect may influence the reporting of pain. It is very difficult to control for this. Similarly subjects on initial presentation with painful conditions are unlikely to make light of their pains for fear that the clinican may not take their conditions seriously.

The presentation of the instrument to the patient by the clinician can similarly influence the results. A measure that requires minimal explanation to the patient is desirable. Scales such as the VAS may require significant explanation for some people. Despite this, even with appropriate explanation some subjects still find them difficult to understand.

Influences of language

Many self-report measures depend upon the use of descriptive words. Patients are presented with a list of words and are required to choose a word or words that best describe their pain. Such measurement instruments are biased against those who have poor educational attainment or whose first language is not the same as the language of the questionnaire. Communication problems such as those occurring following stroke likewise threaten the validity of such questionnaires.

Some patients find their pain hard to describe. Patients with chronic regional pain syndromes in particular have been demonstrated to have difficulty in identifying their pain with the words on commonly used standardised pain questionnaires.

Practical considerations

Pain measures used in the clinical setting should be relatively simple to administer and to score, especially if patients are expected to complete them regularly. Few pain management centres will have research assistants to administer and check all the responses. Complex measures with complicated scoring systems are more susceptible to scoring errors. This presents us with the age-old problem of looking for measures that are simple but give sufficient information to allow us to represent patients' pain and monitor change adequately.

Validity across patient groups

It would be advantageous to have pain measures that could be used to describe mixed groups of patients. Pain management programmes take patients with a variety of conditions, some of which are better represented in numbers than others. The validity and generalisability of pain measures determine the relative confidence in the measure to produce the same results for a given intensity within individuals as well as within and between different patient groups. Can we assume that the intensity of the pain and the affective component are generally the same in different pain populations? This is probably not the case. Differences in the magnitude of the affective and sensory components have been demonstrated between different pain conditions. Well-established measures such as the VAS and the MPQ have demonstrated differences in report of pain in the intensity and affective scales in patients with different medical diagnoses (Price & Harkins 1992).

Sensitivity to change

The scaling of the measure determines its sensitivity to change. The most popular pain measures utilise scales from 5 (Present Pain Intensity, or PPI—Melzack 1997) to 101 (VAS) reference points. The more choices patients have the more likely the scale is to detect change. Scales relying on fewer points, such as four-point scales of no pain, mild, moderate and severe pain, are less discriminative than those with a greater number of points. Patients may have moderate pain at the beginning of the programme and may report a reduction in pain on direct questioning but may still class their pain as 'moderate'. Hence, the pain measure has failed to detect the change.

Problem of non-linearity

It has been demonstrated in experimental research that there may not be a direct relationship between the stimulus intensity and report of pain when using conventional clinical pain measures. If the relationship between the rise in the stimulus and the increase in pain report is variable then the sensitivity to change of the measure used will vary also. It is therefore highly likely that this is also the case in clinical pain. This means that changes, for example, in the upper intensity scores may be easier to detect that those at lower levels of intensity.

Importance of the affective component

In pain management, a change in the intensity of the pain is not the focus of treatment but a reduction in the intrusiveness or the emotional component of the pain should be expected. For this reason it is recommended that the affective component of pain is evaluated. (This is available on both the long and the short forms of the MPQ. A simpler method is the affective VAS. A brief more specific account of these measures is given at the end of this chapter.)

ASSESSMENT OF PHYSICAL FUNCTIONING: THE CONCEPTUAL BASIS

Key goals of a pain management programme are reduction of incapacity and an increase in physical function to the maximum achievable. As a declared outcome it becomes incumbent upon the clinician to monitor and measure the level of function and disability. It is worthwhile to define the terms used in the measurement of patient performance and discuss their relevance to the various measurements that may be employed in pain management.

The concept and classification of impairment, disability and handicap is outlined in the 1980 World Health Organisation's International Classification of Impairments, Disabilities and Handicaps (ICIDH). This classification can be seen in Figure 9.1.

The ICIDH model starts with the assumption that there is an initial disease or dysfunction as the root cause of the handicap; this may be due to a disease process, trauma or a congenital abnormality. Impairment is defined as the loss or abnormality of the anatomical, psychological or physiological function of the body. Disability refers to the restriction of ability to perform functions as a result of that impairment. The handicap is the disadvantage resulting from the inability to perform those functional tasks to a level considered normal for a person of the same age, sex and culture. In this respect the handicap refers to the socially defined roles rather than the individual's function. In this model the handicap may be related to the social environment. It cannot be adequately evaluated without reference to external factors, for example the attitudes of employers to those with a long history of work loss due to musculoskeletal pain.

Impairment

The relationship between a disease process and the resulting physical impairment is clearly not as linear as the above model suggests. In many persistently painful conditions, especially those arising from the musculoskeletal system, the precise diagnosis of a causal pathology may be very difficult or even impossible. This has proved to be particularly true in chronic low back pain where there may be no obvious cause of the pain. Patients may report extreme pain and demonstrate gross physical impairment, loss of range of movement and weakness of muscle action, with little actual identifiable pathology. Pain-free subjects may demonstrate evidence of considerable abnormality (e.g. degenerative changes on X-ray of the spine) but have excellent measurable function.

Influence of restriction

Continued restriction of activity and function, which frequently accompany chronic painful conditions, may further complicate matters by producing a varying degree of secondary physical impairment. These include physical deconditioning and loss of cardiovascular fitness, reduced exercise tolerance, muscle wasting, restricted range of joint motion and loss of extensibility of soft tissues though the development of guarded movements. These in themselves may also contribute to the painful condition. Reduced paraspinal muscle endurance has already been implicated in the possible generation and elevated resting muscle action in the back has also been identified as a contributor to back pain. This demonstrates that the development of disability is not linear but a dynamic process, which is interrelated to other factors. The development of disability is discussed specifically in Chapter 5.

Quantification of impairment

All of the above discrepancies become even more apparent when attempting to quantify the

"Disease" ⇒ Impairment ⇒ Disability ⇒ Handicap

Figure 9.1   ICIDH model of disability and handicap.

physical impairment. When measuring physical capacity in this context it should be understood that the measurement is one of human *performance* rather than *physical capacity*.

Physical capacity and physical performance

Physical capacity refers to the actual performance that would be predicted by the physiological parameters. The maximal force developed by the contraction of a muscle would be predicted by, amongst other factors, the length–tension relationship of the muscle, the coordination, type and size of motor units recruited, the cross-sectional diameter of the muscle, fibre arrangement, the type of contraction and the velocity of the contraction (Rothwell 1987).

Influence of psychological factors

When assessing the pain patient the performance of a test is modified by motivational and cognitive factors, which render the assessment of true capacity difficult if not impossible. Measures of physical impairment cannot be seen as true measures of physical capacity; they are psychophysiological measurements and should be interpreted as such. All performance measures are likely to be perceived by patients in terms of their relationship with the immediate or anticipated environment, for example access to treatment or anticipated pain (Watson 1999). A summary of the key features of physical capacity and physical function is shown in Box 9.3.

Box 9.3   Key points: physical capacity vs physical function

- Physical capacity is determined by physiological parameters
- Physical performance is determined by physiological *and* psychological parameters
- Patients' performance is affected by their perception of the possible consequences of that performance

---

Disability

The measurement of disability relies on the assessment of performance, particularly performance of social roles. It is at this point that the poor relationship between the disease state, pain and performance becomes apparent. Research into various painful conditions has repeatedly commented on the lack of a direct relationship. The ICIDH model omits the important internal and external influences, which are so potent in the development of disability. Disability is now recognised as a multidimensional phenomenon (Ch. 5).

Psychological influences

Internal processes may be described as psychological attributes and coping styles adopted by individuals in response to the disease state. Those who develop low self-efficacy beliefs or who are very fearful of activity because of distorted beliefs about the nature of their condition are more likely to demonstrate poor function and higher levels of disability. (These factors have already been discussed in Ch. 2.)

Social and environmental influences

External influences include a large number of factors from the social and physical environment. The role of the family or significant others can serve to reinforce or reduce disability. Those with over solicitous partners are more prone to reducing their social role when compared with those with non-solicitous partners. Access to employment is frequently limited for persons with chronic pain and retraining or work experience placements for such people are rarely if ever available. (These factors are discussed more fully in Ch. 4.)

Handicap occurs when individuals interact with their environment. For example people in wheelchairs may be able to perform all the functions of daily living in their home environments that has been adapted for their needs. They are not disabled in this environment. Once they go outside of their homes, however, access to transport and into buildings, including the provision of ramps, lifts and disabled toilets, handicaps them from participating in society to a full extent. The environment not the condition is the limiting factor. Patients with back pain may be unable to remain at work because there is no provision in the work task for changing position regularly, chairs are unsuitable for them or work stations are badly designed to meet their needs.

IMPORTANT CONSIDERATIONS IN MEASUREMENT

Although studies have failed to demonstrate a strong relationship between measures of physical function, functional limitation (impairment) and disability in the broadest context, the assessment of physical and functional measures serves several different functions in chronic pain management other than simply that of attempting to infer cause and effect. The main purposes of assessment are shown in Box 9.4.

Despite significant limitations these measures are useful. They will help in describing the population being observed. Such data may be used for research purposes provided the measures are standardised. They also serve as a baseline, which will aid goal setting with individual patients. Finally they may be used as outcome measures for audit (Ch. 17).

Reliability

All measures must have a known degree of reliability and repeatability. The reliability and repeatability of many of the physical function tests normally performed on chronic pain patients have frequently been established on

---

Box 9.4 Purposes of assessment of physical incapacity, functional limitation and disability

- Population description (case mix)
- Pretreatment baseline for goal setting (treatment)
- Potential outcome measures (audit)

---

normal controls or on other patient groups (i.e. acute or subacute conditions). It is not wise to assume that measures tested on one group of subjects will necessarily be appropriate for another. Many simple and well-used measures have accumulated a large database for comparisons to be made between populations. (This may not be true of new measures based on equipment that may be marketed well in advance of the development of a wide database of normal subjects and may have no database for chronic pain subjects.)

The importance of reliability

The inter- and intratester reliability must be known for particular tests and users of these tests should subject themselves and their coworkers to scrutiny and not rely solely on the results of other studies to provide them with information on reliability and repeatability. The complexity of the measurement task and the amount of training required to achieve competence will inevitably affect the results. (The issue of reliability is discussed further in the context of psychological tests in Ch. 10, p. 185.)

Validity

The measure should be accurate enough to measure what it is designed to measure. The influences of extraneous activity of joint and muscle groups other than those to be tested should be minimised. Furthermore, the test must be limited by pain and dysfunction that accompanies the chronic pain condition.

Appropriateness for the population studied

Chronic pain management programmes vary in their referral patterns. The majority of patients are referred to pain management after seeing a variety of clinicians. This creates a filtering and refiltering process, which may mean patients with the same diagnoses differ substantially on many parameters between centres. Wise researchers will endeavour to develop their own comparative database.

Ability to discriminate

Physical function tests must also differentiate the patient from the normal age- and sex-matched healthy controls and be relatively independent of exaggerated pain behaviour. There are very few tests that successfully meet all these criteria. Such a series of tests have been produced for the examination of chronic low back pain patients (Waddell 1992) but to date there has been a relative paucity of studies to investigate measures in other chronic pain conditions.

Clinical relevance

The measures should ideally be generalisable to everyday function. Changes in a physical performance measure should, therefore, reflect an increase in levels of physical activity. Not only should the measures relate to function but they should also be sensitive to changes that may occur following a rehabilitation programme.

Relationship with outcome

The relative usefulness of physical function measures at outcome is a poorly researched area. Many reported rehabilitation schemes rely on self-report of pain and disability as outcome measures rather than physical function measures. The relationship between measures of physical function and self-report of physical activity, however, has not been established. (The issues are discussed further in Ch. 17.)

(Validity is discussed further in the context of psychometric tests in Ch. 10, p. 190.)

MEASURES OF PHYSICAL FUNCTION AND IMPAIRMENT

Measures of physical function used in pain management should be easy to use, familiar to the patient (to offset the effect of learning), require a minimum of equipment and reflect activities that would be performed in everyday life.

Range of motion

The range of motion of the affected area can be measured by goniometry, or other means such as the modified Schoeber's test for spinal movement using a tape measure. The reliability, reproducibility and validity are generally good for most measures if careful attention is paid to the isolation of the particular joint action. Many measures of range of motion fail to be valid, however, because they are composites of different joint ranges. This is exemplified in the measurement of lumbar spinal movement. Fingertip distance from the floor for the lumbar spine is often used. This is an inaccurate measure of lumbar spinal movement as it is a composite of lumbar spine and hip motion. Similarly the angle of the humerus in relation to the trunk as a measure of the shoulder activity is a composite of all the shoulder girdle complex not the glenohumeral joint alone.

The importance of normative data

Many of the normal values for range of motion are for general populations and there are few modified for age and gender. It is insufficient for those measuring range of motion to assume that a particular measure is repeatable and reliable in their clinic before they have established the fact. All clinicians who intend to rely on such measurements must satisfy themselves of this before they can draw conclusions on outcomes.

The influence of psychological factors

Ranges of joint motion rarely appear to be related, in chronic low back pain, to the degree of disability (Gronblad, Hurri & Kouri 1997) and have been reported as being significantly influenced by exaggerated illness behaviour and fear of movement. It is therefore important to be aware of the other factors that may influence these measurements by having measures of the other factors.

Muscle strength

The Oxford scale

Muscle strength is often recorded as a measure of outcome. Measures such as the Oxford scale classification are not useful in patients on pain management programmes. The Oxford scale has only a five-point classification and is sensitive to only very gross changes.

Objective measures

Objective measures of muscle strength usually require the use of sophisticated machines such as isokinetic or isometric muscle-testing machines. These require training and expertise to give meaningful results. They usually have a known level of reliability, reproducibility and validity and have been used extensively in clinical research. Most have published normative databases for comparison but these are on a normal general population and not specifically matched to a sedentary group. There is some experimental evidence to suggest that degree of underperformance of a test can be identified by analysis of the variance in repeated performances of the test (Mayer et al 1994).

Limitations of objective measures

Such machines have a number of disadvantages in the pain clinic or pain management programme. They are expensive to purchase and to maintain. The machines are designed to test specific joint and muscles necessitating the purchase of different machines if different joints or range of motion measurements are required. There is a considerable learning effect with repeated testing and this is greater in patients than in controls (Newton et al 1993). Patients may be daunted by the machine. The machines by their nature are large and look very threatening. The context in which the measurement takes place may represent a great challenge to the patient. Finally, patients with low self-efficacy beliefs perform less well than do those who are more confident about their ability to perform the task required (Estlander et al 1994; Lackner, Carosella & Feuerstein 1996). Results from such machines therefore should be interpreted with considerable caution (Main & Spanswick 1995).

Muscular endurance

In recent years the role of the endurance or 'fatigability' of muscles in the maintenance or generation of painful conditions has received attention. The evaluation of muscle endurance as a measure of physical performance or limitation has, therefore, been established.

The nature of muscle endurance

Muscle endurance can be termed central (as a result of the subject's willingness to maintain the contraction and identified by the number of action potentials recorded from the muscle on electromyography) or peripheral. The changes in the type of muscle fibre activity (a reduction in fast twitch activity and an increase in slow twitch activity) within the muscle, which occurs as a result of physiological fatigue, may be recorded by electromyography. This relatively new branch of measurement has the advantage of being (presumably) entirely objective. It appears to discriminate a physiological event from a psychological one (Roy et al 1995).

The role of endurance

The role of endurance in chronic low back pain is, at present, the only area with sufficient data to establish cause and effect. The reliability and repeatability for the most sophisticated methodologies appear to be very good (Roy et al 1997). Whether increases in endurance as assessed by median frequency measures are changed after specific exercise programmes and whether these are accompanied by a reduction in pain and incapacity has not been demonstrated. This type of assessment requires sophisticated equipment and a high level of expertise to operate reliably and is unlikely to be appropriate for the average pain clinic.

Clinical measures

A simple measure of general, non-specific, activity endurance without electromyography holding the arms aloft at 90° to the body, has been used and found to be reliable, reproducible and sensitive to change following pain management (Harding et al 1994). Other endurance measures that may be used are sitting and standing tolerance. These performance measures are highly correlated with measures of pain behaviour and are interpreted as such by some authors (Vlaeyen 1991). No statements can be made about physiological muscular endurance from these tests.

Cardiovascular fitness

Utility

Cardiovascular fitness is commonly measured in chronic pain management programmes. Many patients with chronic pain suffer secondary deconditioning as a result of limited activity. An assessment of cardiovascular fitness can help to quantify the degree of deconditioning and may be used to monitor progress. The utility of cardiovascular fitness testing in assessing adherence to an exercise regimen and to monitor increased fitness at follow-up appears an attractive proposition, but to date there are no valid studies on this in the pain management field. There is a considerable database on normal, healthy age- and sex-grouped cardiovascular responses to exercise testing for use as a comparable database. However, these are gathered from normal active individuals and so may not be comparable to pain patients with restricted function and sedentary lifestyle.

Assessment

Cardiovascular testing may be performed using treadmill or bicycle ergometers. There is no physiological advantage in either method of testing.

The ability to tolerate each test may depend upon the specific functional limitation (i.e. location of the pain problem). It has been reported that patients with chronic low back pain, particularly those with spinal stenosis, tolerate the bicycle ergometer much better than the treadmill. Improvements in ergometer tolerance times and increases in physical fitness have been reported following pain management programmes.

Submaximal testing

Submaximal testing should be used for considerations of safety and standardised protocols for cardiovascular testing exist. A target rate of age-related maximal heart rate (usually 75 or 85%) is predetermined and the work rate is increased gradually until the target rate is achieved. The baseline heart rate, the time taken to reach the target, work performed during the test and the target (or maximum rate achieved) is recorded. Anticipation of the exercise task and its performance may be psychologically stressful for some subjects and cause a stress/anxiety-related tachycardia thus affecting the reliability of the results. Desensitisation through familiarisation with the task and a low level practice run with the equipment may assist in the establishment of a more representative baseline.

Timed tests

A number of studies have described using timed physical function measures. Many of the timed measures have good reliability, reproducibility and have been shown to be sensitive to change in back pain and general pain groups (Gronblad et al 1997, Harding et al 1994, Simmonds et al 1998). The correlation between each of these measures appears to be very high. It is debatable, therefore, whether they individually contribute anything unique to the assessment of the patient or may be substituted for by a single measure alone. Investigations on general pain populations have not usually attempted to identify differences in performance by site of pain other than by upper and lower body pain.

Timed walk

The time taken to complete a fixed distance for walking or the distance walked in a set time has been used in many pain management studies. These vary in length from a 20-metre timed test to a measure of the distance walked in a fixed time (which can range from 1 to 10 minutes). A timed 20-metre walk test has the advantage of being relatively quick to perform. A distance is marked out on a flat corridor and the patient is asked to walk the distance as fast as possible and is timed over the course. Normally this is performed without walking aids. The reliability, repeatability and sensitivity to change of the 20-metre, 10-minute and 5-minute walk tests have been demonstrated to be very good. These tests appear to correlate highly with each other so the assessor should decide if the extra length of assessment time is necessary, particularly if many physical measures are to be tested in a short time. One disadvantage of the shorter walk test is that there is likely to be an uneven distribution of the scores particularly in the less-disabled patient group.

Psychological influences.   The relationship of timed walk with disability and illness behaviour once again is not well established and requires further research. Differences in performance should also be expected between patients with upper and those with lower body pain.

Stair climbing

The subject is asked to climb up and down a set of stairs as many times as possible in one minute. The measure demonstrated excellent interrater reliability and is sensitive. A highly significant correlation has been demonstrated between tests of differing length, suggesting that 1 minute is sufficient to give good data and will tire the person less.

Sit-ups

The performance of sit-ups in a timed period has been suggested by some authors, but the skewed distribution of performances in task performance has been shown to be a problem. In a study by Harding et al (1994) 52% of subjects scored zero prior to pain management suggesting poor patient compliance and low acceptability of the test. None the less it has been demonstrated to have moderate test–retest reliability and is sensitive to changes following interventions. One minute is the recommended test period (it correlates highly with longer test periods).

Other physical measurements

A whole battery of physical assessment measures has been used in research but these are generally poorly described. This has not allowed standardisation amongst research projects. Grip strength, peak flow and performance of a general exercise or functional task circuit have all been employed. Subjects are often required to complete an exercise circuit and the time taken to perform the whole circuit or the number of exercises performed (or both) is recorded. Generally the reliability of these measures has been mixed and they have not proved to be particularly sensitive to change. This may be due to the variability inherent in broad-ranging exercises or the mixed nature of the groups studied. A number of key considerations in the use of physical function tests are presented in Box 9.5. (Their usefulness as outcome measures is considered in Ch. 17.)

MEASURES OF DISABILITY

There are a number of self-report disability scales from which the clinician can choose. However,

---

Box 9.5   Key points: using physical function tests

- Is the test a valid measure?
- Has the reliability and validity of the test been established for this group of patients?
- Is there a reliable and comparable, normative database?
- Is the test acceptable to the patients–will they comply?
- What may be the effect of performing large batteries of physical tests on the performance of the patient?
- Establish which tests are to be used as outcome measures and which are to be used for goal setting.
- Determine, and periodically check, your own intra- and interrater reliability

many are disorder specific. The Roland and Morris Disability Questionnaire (Roland & Morris 1983) for example is designed for the assessment of low-back-pain-associated disability. Others have been used in a wide variety of chronic pain conditions and therefore will be briefly reviewed here. They vary greatly in length, a factor that may be important if there are constraints in terms of time or patient compliance (as when patients are requested to complete large numbers of questionnaires). The obvious advantage of the longer questionnaires, however, is that they give a more comprehensive appraisal of the chronic pain problem (and often incorporate measures of pain, coping and adaptation into their structure), though these may be less sensitive and reliable than instruments designed specifically to look at these constructs. The same considerations with regard to reliability, validity and reproducibility discussed earlier of course still apply. A careful review of the literature is recommended before the clinician opts for one instrument over another.

Sickness impact profile (SIP)

The Sickness Impact Profile (Bergner et al 1981) is a well-researched, wide-ranging and comprehensive assessment of disability, physical and social functioning. It is split into three major sections covering all areas of activity including physical activity, psychosocial, recreational and work activities and has 12 specific category scores. Normative data is available for healthy controls and subject groups with differing conditions including chronic pain groups. It was developed for use with people with chronic illness and not specifically for those with chronic pain. It has been demonstrated to have good reliability in chronic pain patients and correlates with avoidance of activity in low back pain subjects. It has been demonstrated to be sensitive to changes following cognitive–behavioural interventions in a group of general chronic pain patients and low back pain patients (Follick, Smith & Ahern 1985, Harding et al 1994, Williams et al 1996). Some observers have suggested (Deyo & Inui 1984) that it may be a more appropriate measure of deteriorating health rather than improvement. The major disadvantage of the SIP is its length (136 items), making it possibly the longest disability measure. Other workers have produced shortened disability measures based on the SIP categories for specific patient groups (e.g. Roland & Morris 1983).

Short form 36 (SF36)

The Short Form 36 (Ware & Sherbourne 1992) has eight subcategories covering the areas of physical functioning, role-physical, role-emotional, bodily pain, general health, vitality, social functioning and mental health. These scales can be summarised into physical and mental health scales. Normative data sets graded by age and sex are available and population norms have been developed for chronic pain and chronic illness groups. It must be pointed out that the inclusion and exclusion criteria for the subjects in these population norms are very broad and rather vague. They relied heavily on patients' reports of physician diagnoses. It has an advantage of being relatively short and easy to score when compared with other measures. It has demonstrated very good reliability and repeatability in both normal population and chronic illness groups. It has been recommended as a generic outcome measure for use in a variety of conditions. To date its use in the assessment of outcome following treatment intervention in chronic pain patients has not been widely reported.

Chronic illness problem inventory (CIPI)

The Chronic Illness Problem Inventory (Kames et al 1984) addresses all problem areas associated with chronic illness. It has 19 individual scales including scales for physical limitation, psychosocial functioning, health-care usage and marital changes. It is still a formidable length (65 items) but is shorter and more easily scored than the SIP. It has been demonstrated to be reliable in a variety of chronic diseases including chronic respiratory and chronic pain patients (Kames et al 1984) and differentiates these groups from healthy controls. The responses are graded from 0 (not at all) to 4 (very much) allowing an insight into the degree of perceived disability as well as the perception of the existence of a problem. This is not possible with some of the dichotomous 'yes/no' responses in some disability questionnaires. In a study by Romano et al (1992) the CIPI was sensitive to changes following a pain management programme and it correlated highly with the SIP in chronic low back pain patients and was demonstrated to correlate with pain report, reclining time and overt pain behaviours. However, the group in this study were moderately disabled and demonstrated low levels of overt pain behaviour and the relationships between the variables may be different in a more disabled group. To date few studies have reported using the CIPI to judge its usefulness in a wide variety of pain conditions.

Pain disability index (PDI)

The Pain and Disability Index (Pollard 1984) was designed to be a short and quick-to-use multidimensional measure of disability. It is divided into seven categories requiring the respondent to chose responses on a Likert scale scored from zero to ten. The test–retest reliability was demonstrated to be only modest in a relatively small group of chronic pain patients. It has been seen to correlated highly with other limited measures (also Likert scales) of self-report of disability (downtime, stopping activity) but did not correlate significantly with observed downtime (Tait, Chibnall & Krause 1990). Interestingly the scores for the PDI were significantly correlated with patients self-scoring their own pain behaviour suggesting that the scores on the PDI are related to the communication of pain behaviour. Comparisons with a wide variety of observed physical activity data are not available to confirm this, however. Although the PDI is short and easy to score it has not been compared with other more established measures of dysfunction and disability to assess its validity.

Multidimensional pain inventory (MPI)

Developed by Kerns, Turk & Rudy (1985) as the West-Haven Yale Multidimensional Pain Inventory (Ch. 5), this was an attempt to identify not only the impact of patients' pain on their function but also the response of others to this pain, the level of distress associated with the pain and a gross assessment of the coping style (adaptive coping subgroup) and perceived control. As such it is not purely a measure of disability or functional interference. It was developed from a cognitive–behavioural view of disability hence the assessment of factors that influence disability as well as measures of functional interference. Responses to the questionnaire have been clustered into three groups (dysfunctional, interpersonally distressed and adaptive copers). It is a relatively brief instrument and has been used widely in a broad range of pain-associated conditions and has demonstrated excellent reproducibility since its original development.

OCCUPATIONAL OUTCOME

As will be discussed in Chapter 17, assessment of outcome is difficult not only because of the wide range of possible measures (such as pain severity, impaired functioning, distress, health-care usage and return to work) but because different stakeholders may differ in the importance they give to the alternative outcome measures.

The pre-eminence of occupational variables as outcome measures for pain management in North America, for example, is a direct consequence of the socioeconomics of health care where there is an important relationship between the provision of health insurance, the workplace and employer through the Workmen's Compensation Board schemes (Ch. 5). Satisfactory return to work in this situation is considered to be the main criterion of success of treatment programmes since they are usually established and funded with the specific aim of enabling people to return to work.

Treatment programmes in the UK, however, frequently include patients who are unemployed and may have been so for a considerable time. Richardson et al (1994) reported that in a group of general pain patients recruited on to a pain management programme 74% of the subjects were unemployed. At 1-year follow-up 30% of the unemployed group had found employment. Waddell (1994) reported that 46% of persons claiming sickness and invalidity benefit for back pain were not employed at the commencement of benefit. Such patients frequently do not feature in North American programmes.

Outcome data in terms of work status may not therefore be comparable. It has to be recognised that post-treatment work status is determined not only by response to pain management but also by the availability of work and marketable job skills (Ch. 14). None the less, as far as many patients are concerned, staying at work or returning to it is of prime importance and, although traditionally this has not been targeted as the principal objective of rehabilitation, recent initiatives by the UK government specifically encourage partnerships between employers, the Department of Health (DoH) and the Department of Employment (DoE) (Health and Safety Executive, or HSE). (Further implications of these new changes in the context of secondary prevention are discussed in Chs 17 and 19.) Fundamental to evaluation of the impact of any such changes will be the assessment of work status and work capacity.

Work status

The impact of rehabilitation on work has to be considered in the context of *previous* work status, and also in the context of job availability. High levels of unemployment make it particularly difficult for individuals with a history of musculoskeletal pain or injury to obtain work. Increase in litigation requires consideration of the degree of risk of further injury facing a potential employer in considering employing or re-employing someone with a history of injury. Studies into the success of rehabilitation have varied in their definition of successful outcome. Outcome has to be measured against the goals for the individual and the objectives of the

---

Box 9.6 Occupational outcome following rehabilitation
1. Full return to previous job at long term follow-up (1–2 years?)   2. Obtaining new job and remaining at work at long term follow-up (1–2 years?)   3. Returning to old job (temporarily on a part-time basis)   4. Returning to old job (but with restricted duties)   5. Return to only part-time work   6. Sheltered work (on a full- or part-time basis)   7. Not working (assuming availability of work)   8. Medically retired

programme (Ch. 6). There may be several 'stake-holders' all having different criteria for successful outcome. For those not intending to adopt paid employment following treatment (such as housewives, the elderly or schoolchildren) working status may not be an appropriate outcome measure.

A possible general classification in terms of paid employment is shown in Box 9.6. Clearly, a wide range of classifications with varying amount of detail is possible.

Readiness for work

There is no universally agreed system for assessment of readiness for work although the most systematic approach is probably the Functional Capacity Evaluation, or FCE, of Mayer & Gatchel (1988). They adopt a sports medicine framework for the assessment of work capacity in a rehabilitation setting and have developed a highly quantified assessment system with emphasis on muscle strength, task performance and endurance measured in response to a range of ergonomically designed tasks and endurance measures. They incorporate psychological counselling and vocational advice within their programme, but appear to place much less emphasis on psychological obstacles than on performance criteria. Despite their stated claims of an extremely impressive return-to-work rate, to be accepted for the programme patients not only have had to complete a 'preselection' programme, and usually have to have available a job to them as well as a considerable financial incentive to return to work or disincentive to fail. Their system of assessment (and treatment programme) requires expensive computerised equipment and is not therefore a practical proposition for most pain management programmes, even if doctors considered the sports medicine approach to be relevant to their clinical population.

None the less, as will be discussed in Chapter 19, combining traditional pain management with specific occupational rehabilitation seems a promising extension for pain management programmes. In a study of a group of chronically unemployed people (mean time unemployed 45.3 months) with low back pain Main & Watson (1995) demonstrated a 60% positive outcome in terms of return to work or commencement of workplace retraining or education 3 months after a pain management programme integrated with vocational counselling and advice.

For programmes not established with the specific objective of return to work, it may be important none the less to appraise the patient status at the end of the pain management programme in terms of a number of general characteristics that might have an influence on future employability. They are shown in Box 9.7.

(As mentioned in Ch. 4, however, success in return to work will be dependent also on factors outside the control of the individual or the pain management programme team, such as job availability, re-employment policy and attitude of employer and colleagues to musculoskeletal injury.)

In conclusion, while it would appear that for most clinically oriented pain management programmes it is unrealistic, and probably unnecessary, to undertake highly sophisticated FCA, job aptitude or specific fitness for work assessments, consideration might usefully be given to the factors outlined above.

MEASUREMENT OF PAIN BEHAVIOUR

The conceptual basis

The reduction of pain-associated behaviours is frequently cited by pain management programmes as a desired outcome. The theoretical basis of pain behaviour has already been presented in Chapter 2, but it is worth reviewing some of the key features in the context of physical assessment.

It is important to understand that the demonstration of pain behaviour is *normal* when people experience pain. We communicate the experience of pain to others by means of pain behaviours. It is possible to identify a wide range of individual pain behaviours but it is perhaps helpful to distinguish between behaviours that can be observed, and those that are not observed but reported (Box 9.8). It is important none the less to remember in the context of clinical assessment that whereas pain or pain behaviour may be *reported* only pain behaviour can be *observed*.

Pain behaviour is influenced by experiences of pain from the past, sometimes specific pain

---

Box 9.7 Appropriateness to undertake active job seeking or return to work

- Level of fitness
- Strength
- Range of movement
- Tolerance for exercise or sustained posture
- Vigilance and concentration
- Medication use
- Psychological obstacles to return to work (yellow and blue flags)

Box 9.8 Types of pain behaviour

Observed
- Facial grimacing
- Sighing
- Groaning/verbalising
- Limping
- Touching and rubbing affected area
- Bracing—reluctance to move affected area
- Inappropriate reaction to examination
- Behavioural signs on examination
- Unnecessary use of supports and equipment

Reported
- 'Downtime'
- Medication usage
- Alcohol abuse
- Amount of physical activity
- Behavioural symptoms

memories, and is therefore influenced not only by the perceived intensity of the current sensation, but also by the previous consequences that followed from it. Sometimes the only way to try to make sense of apparently bizarre pain behaviour is to understand it in a historical sense (in the context of prior learning).

Although associated with aspects of physical examination, including medical status, number of surgical interventions, disability status, duration of pain and reported pain intensity, pain behaviour can also be distinguished from them (Waddell et al 1980, 1984) and is specifically predictive of outcome of treatment in its own right.

As mentioned in Chapter 3, pain behaviours are influenced by their social context. Researchers have shown that pain behaviour is influenced by the presence of an over attentive or oversolicitous spouse. In medicolegal contexts the demonstration of pain behaviours in response to clinical examination has sometimes been used as an indicator of exaggeration or even malingering. Pain behaviour on activity or examination may also be heavily influenced by the patient's level of fear of injury and harm. If patients suffer an injury or a worsening of symptoms on performing a particular exercise then they may be more reluctant to perform such activities in the future. Research from our own laboratories has demonstrated that guarded movement in patients with chronic low back pain is closely related to their fear injury as a result of activity and their perceived ability to function despite pain. Previous medical examinations may have been painful to patients and this will influence their behaviour on subsequent examinations. They may be more likely to report pain in order to prevent an exacerbation of their condition by the palpation or passive movements performed by the clinician. During a physical examination patients may well assume that the demonstration of the pain will assist the clinician in diagnosis. Patients may exaggerate their responses in order to convince the clinician of the genuineness of their symptoms and gain access to treatment. The interpretation of responses to physical examination has been highlighted in a recent review (Main & Waddell 1998).

Self-report measures

One of the simplest measures of pain behaviour is the pain and activity diary (see Appendix to Ch. 7, p. 133) (Follick, Ahern & Laser-Wolston 1984). Patients are required to record their pain and activity levels on a daily basis. The major advantage this has over all other measures is simplicity of administration. There is evidence that this is a valid and reliable method of data collection. It has the added advantage of assessing the patient's cooperation with the treatment protocol. A patient who is unwilling to participate in the completion of a pain/activity diary is unlikely to comply with the more rigorous demands of a pain management programme. Wide research into this method of assessment has demonstrated good levels of agreement with patient self-rating, electronic assessment and with spouse reports of activity. The obvious draw back is the individual variability and accuracy in the completion of the diaries. Willingness (or not) to comply with simple diary assessments can be a useful contributor to the decision as to whether or not to offer pain management (Chs 10 and 12).

Observational rating scales

The University of Alabama—Birmingham Pain Behaviour Scale (Richards et al 1982) was designed to be used in a naturalistic setting by trained observers. It relies on a list of behaviour not dissimilar to the Behavioural Observation Test (see below) with additional rating for vocalisation of complaints, body language, activity levels, use of supports and medication. With adequate training it demonstrates good inter- and intra-rater reliability. It does require an environment where a representative sample of behaviour can be obtained over a period of time such as an in-patient or day-care setting. For these reasons it is not suitable for use in many out-patient settings. In the initial development of the tool it did not demonstrate any correlation with pain report prior to pain management but did so on the completion of a pain management programme. It did correlated strongly with degree of self-reported disability. Electronic recording of patient activity can be used to measure the time the patient spends lying down (Sanders 1983). These recorders are attached to the patient's bed and record the total amount of time spent in 'downtime' lying down versus 'uptime' sitting, standing or moving around. By their very nature they can be effectively used only in the hospital in-patient setting and so are of limited use. Results demonstrate a close relationship between 'downtime' self-reported disability and self-report of activity level.

Videotaped assessments

The Behavioural Observation Test by Keefe & Block (1982) is probably the best researched of all the observational measures. It was originally developed for use with chronic low back pain patients but has since been used successfully in patients with rheumatoid arthritis, osteoarthritis of the lower limbs and cancer pain. Patients are videoed during a 10-minute standardised series of movements including walking, standing, lying and sitting. The observer then rates the presence of a number of key behaviours associated with the communication of pain. These are facial grimacing, guarded movement or bracing of the affected area, rubbing the affected area, sighing/groaning. Scoring requires trained observers and constant retraining and rescaling to ensure reliability. With such training this method has demonstrated very good reliability and correlates with a high number of physical findings on examination. This system has also been demonstrated to correlate with the patient's self-ratings of pain in some studies although the relationship is by no means robust, and also with naïve observers' ratings of the patients' pain. It has been show to discriminate pain patients from pain-free individuals and is sensitive to changes in pain following treatment interventions.

Apart from the difficulty in scoring, the test has been criticised for using tasks that are easier to perform rather than everyday functional tasks. Its simplicity does make it appropriate for use with all but the most severely disabled but it may not be sensitive to pain behaviours specific to functional tasks (e.g. housework or occupation-related activity). Chronic pain patients may report pain at rest but demonstrate little pain behaviour until they are asked to become active. Thus, pain behaviour in some patients at least may reflect the increase in pain due to activity rather than a measure of usual pain. Furthermore, their performance may be more closely related to patients' self-efficacy beliefs, their belief in their ability to perform tasks and their ability to be active despite the pain than to report of pain (Buckelew et al 1994).

A functional task-orientated pain behaviour measure was developed by Watson & Poulter (1997) this was based on the aforementioned measure but involved a greater number of functional tasks. Although currently underdeveloped it demonstrated high correlations with other measures of magnified illness presentation and high pain behaviour scores were significantly related to exaggerated fear-avoidance beliefs, low self-efficacy and increased disability but did not demonstrate a significant correlation with pain self report.

A facial action coding system (FACS) of pain behaviour has been developed by Ekman & Freisen (1978). Facial activity of subjects is videotaped and the activity of the facial muscles is coded. This system is also very time consuming and requires intensive, specialist training. It has been demonstrated to correlate with reported pain in a wide variety of situations and has been reported to discriminate faked pain expression from genuine and identify suppressed expression. Much of the research into facial pain has examined severe, phasic or transitory pain rather than chronic pain. The plastic nature of responses means that responses to pain adapt to reflect an increase in intensity of the painful stimulus over and above the base level. Chronic pain patients do not constantly demonstrate a facial expression for pain although they may report constant pain. Therefore a chronic pain patient may not demonstrate facial responses during the 'normal' pain state but only when the pain state increases above that level. The system none the less has been an extremely important research tool, particularly in the study of neonates.

Responses to clinical examination

Assessment of magnified illness behaviour in low back pain patients was developed by Waddell and colleagues (Waddell et al 1980, 1984). This consists of a number of signs and symptoms considered inappropriate to the disease state. They were developed by examination of the literature and by assessment of the experiences of orthopaedic surgeons. The occurrence of seven signs and seven reported symptoms considered inappropriate to the anatomical and physiological pattern of the disease of low back pain was tested in a large group of low back pain patients. They have been demonstrated in studies to predict outcome of treatment, return to work. The advantages of the test is that they have been demonstrated to have good reliability, and are well known and widely used. They can be administered during a routine assessment by any clinician experienced in the examination of patients with low back pain. They were originally demonstrated to be closely associated with levels of psychological distress; the relationship of the inappropriate signs with the fear of pain or harm during the examination has not been clearly established. One study has described a strong relationship between disease conviction measured by the presence of a serious underlying, undiagnosed disorder and high scores on both the physical signs and symptoms. As aforementioned, they are often used in the context of medico-legal assessment although their interpretation is controversial (Main & Waddell 1998).

Overview

The recognition of the behavioural component in the context of illness has revolutionised our understanding of the management of pain. Clinical recognition of the phenomenon by Fordyce in the early 1960s and the production of his textbook (Fordyce 1976) has stimulated 30 years of research and rehabilitation. The concept of pain behaviour is both simple and subtle. A range of approaches to the assessment of pain behaviour have been discussed in this chapter. Highly sophisticated research tools are available, but require careful use following appropriate

---

Box 9.9 Pain behaviours – an overview
• Pain behaviour is at the core of pain management • Pain behaviours can be reliably assessed • They can be assessed with varying degrees of sophistication • They are associated with, but distinct from, the self-report of disability • They are associated with, but distinct from, the self-report of pain • They change in response to pain management and are therefore important outcome measures for pain management • Pain behaviour measures may be better viewed as the effect of pain on the individual rather than as an expression of pain intensity per se

---

training. In chronic pain management we are mostly treating variants of pain behaviour rather than nociception or pathology. Pain behaviour needs to be understood as the way in which patients respond to their pain and communicate it to the outside word. The importance of this conceptual framework cannot be overstated. A summary of the key features of pain behaviour is presented in Box 9.9.

REASONS FOR SYSTEMATIC ASSESSMENT

Assessment is fundamental to pain management. Without careful assessment, it is impossible to arrive at a competent clinical decision about treatment. However complex the ultimate formulation of a patient's set of problems, it is important to recognise that the patient presented initially with pain and pain-associated incapacities. Assessment of pain, reported disability and physical functioning is therefore absolutely fundamental. The reasons for systematic assessment are summarised in Box 9.10.

The assessment of the psychological factors that influence pain, disability and physical functioning is addressed in the next chapter.

CONCLUSION

The assessment of pain, disability and physical function is fraught with pitfalls. It is important to

---

Box 9.10   Reasons for systematic assessment of pain, disability and physical functioning

- Initial evaluation of the significance of the pain problem
- Appraisal of the relative importance of various aspects of the patient's difficulties
- Correcting any iatrogenic confusion or misunderstanding
- Alleviation of iatrogenic distress and anger

- Identification of possible treatment objectives
- Decision about specific treatment strategies
- Monitoring of change
- Evaluation of outcome

KEY POINTS

- Measurements of pain, disability and physical function should conform to minimum scientific criteria.
- There are clear distinctions amongst impairment, physical capacity, physical performance and disability.
- Measurement tools should be chosen with care and be dependent upon their intended use.

- Self-report measures have significant limitations and should be chosen according to their intended use (e.g. case mix, outcome measures).
- Occupational outcome may be of particular importance but has been shown to be difficult to quantify.
- The context of the measurement of pain behaviour will dictate which measure should be used.

---

use measures that are clinically relevant and suitable for the purpose. For example, measurement of outcome must be made with a tool that is not only sensitive to change but must also describe the population being treated accurately. It is wise to use a number of measures of differing types in order to ensure a broad and accurate assessment of the patient group.

REFERENCES

Bergner M, Bobbitt R A, Carter W B, Gilson B S 1981 The Sickness Impact Profile: development and final revision of a health status measure. Medical Care 19:787–805

Boivie J, Hansson P, Lindblom U (eds) 1994 Progress in pain research and management vol 3. Touch, temperature and pain in health and disease mechanisms and assessments. IASP, Seattle

Buckelew S P, Parker J C, Keefe F J, Deuser W E, Crews T M, Conway R 1994 Self efficacy and pain behavior among subjects with fibromyalgia. Pain 59(3):377–384

Deyo R A, Inui T S 1984 Towards clinical applications of health status measures: sensitivity of scales to clinically important changes. Health Services Research 19:275–289

Ekman P, Freisen W V 1978 Facial action coding system: a technique for the measurement of facial movement. Consulting Psychologists, Palo Alto, CA

Estlander A M, Vanharanta H, Moneta G B, Kaivanto K 1994 Anthropometric variables, self-efficacy beliefs and pain and disability ratings on the isokinetic performance of low back pain patients. Spine 19:941–947

Follick M J, Ahern D K, Laser-Wolston N 1984 Evaluation of a daily activity diary for chronic pain patients. Pain 19:373–382

Follick M J, Smith T W, Ahern D K 1985 The Sickness Impact Profile: a global measure of disability in chronic low back pain. Pain 21:67–75

Fordyce W E 1976 Behavioural methods for chronic pain and illness. C V Mosby, St Louis MO

Gronblad M, Hurri H, Kouri J-K 1997 Relationships between spinal mobility, physical performance tests, pain intensity and disability assessments in chronic low back pain patients. Scandinavian Journal of Rehabilitation Medicine 29:17–24

Harding V R, Williams A C, Richardson P H et al 1994 The development of a battery of measures for assessing physical functioning of chronic pain patients. Pain 58(3):367–375

Kames L D, Naliboff B D, Heinrich R L, Schag C C 1984 The Chronic Illness Problem Inventory: problem-oriented psychosocial assessment of patients with chronic illness. International Journal of Psychiatry in Medicine 14:65–69

Keefe F J, Block A R 1982 Development of an observational method for assessing pain behavior in chronic low back pain. Behavior Therapy 13:363–375

Kerns R D, Turk D C, Rudy T E 1985 The West-Haven Yale Multidimensional Pain Inventory (WHYMPI). Pain 23:345–356

Lackner J M, Carosella A M, Feuerstein M 1996 Pain expectancies, pain and functional self-efficacy expectancies as determinants of disability in patients with chronic low back disorders. Journal of Consulting and Clinical Psychology 64(1):212–220

Main C J, Spanswick C C 1995 Functional overlay and illness behaviour in chronic pain: distress or malingering conceptual difficulties in medico-legal assessment of personal injury claims. Journal of Psychosomatic Research 39:737–753

Main C J, Waddell G 1998 Spine update: behavioural responses to examination; a reappraisal of the interpretation of the 'non-organic signs'. Spine 23:2367–2371

Main C J, Watson P J 1995 Screening for patients at risk of developing chronic incapacity. Journal of Occupational Rehabilitation 5:207–217

Mayer T, Gatchel R J 1988 Functional resoration for spinal disorders: the sports medicine approach. Lea & Febiger, Philadelphia

Mayer T, Tabor J, Bovasso E, Gatchel R J 1994 Physical and residual impairment quantification after functional restoration. Spine 19:389–394

Melzack R 1987 The Short-Form McGill Pain Questionnaire. Pain 30:191–197

Melzack R 1997 Present Pain Intensity

Newton M, Thow M, Sommerville D, Henderson I, Waddell G 1993 Trunk strength testing with iso-machines, part 2: experimental evaluation of the Cybex II back testing machine in normal subjects and patients with chronic low back pain. Spine 18:812–824

Pollard C A 1984 Preliminary validity study of the Pain Disability Index. Perceptual and Motor Skills 59:974

Price D D, Harkins S W 1992 Psychophysical approaches to pain measurement and assessment. In: Turk D C, Melzack R (eds) Handbook of pain assessment. Guilford, New York, pp 111–134

Richards J S, Nepomuceno C, Riles M, Suer Z 1982 Assessing pain behaviour: the UAB pain behavior scale. Pain 12:393–398

Richardson I H, Richardson P H, Williams A C, Featherstone J 1994 The effects of a cognitive–behavioural pain management programme on the quality of work and employment status of severely impaired chronic pain patients. Disability and Rehabilitation 16:26–34

Roland M, Morris R 1983 A study in the natural history of back pain. Part I: development of a reliable and sensitive measure of disability in low-back pain. Spine 8(2):141–144

Romano J M, Turner J A, Freidman L S et al 1992 Sequential analysis of chronic pain behaviours and spouse responses. Journal of Consulting and Clinical Psychology 60:777–782

Rothwell J C 1987 Control of human voluntary movement. Croom Helm, London

Roy S H, De Luca C J, Emley M, Buijs R J C 1995 Spectral electromyographic assessment of back muscles in patients with low back pain undergoing rehabilitation. Spine 20:559–564

Roy S H, DeLuca C J, Emley M et al 1997 Classification of back muscle impairment based on the surface electromyographic signal. Journal of Rehabilitation Research and Development 34:405–414

Sanders S H 1983 Automated versus self monitoring of 'uptime' in chronic low back pain patients: a comparative study. Pain 15:399–406

Simmonds M J, Olson S L, Jones S et al 1998 Psychometric characteristics and clinical usefulness of physical performance test in patients with low back pain. Spine 23:2412–2421

Tait R C, Chibnall J T, Krause S 1990 The Pain Disability Index; psychometric properties. Pain 40:171–182

Turk D C, Melzack R 1992 Handbook of pain assessment. Guilford, New York

Vlaeyen J W S 1991 Chronic low back pain: assessment and treatment from a behavioural rehabilitation perspective. Swets & Zeitlinger, Amsterdam

Waddell G 1992 Biopsychosocial analysis of low back pain. Ballières Clinical Rheumatology 6:523–557

Waddell G 1994 Clinical Standards Advisory Group epidemiology review: the epidemiology and cost of back pain. The annex to the Clinical Standards Advisory Group's report on back pain. HMSO, London

Waddell G, McCulloch J A, Kummel E, Venner R M 1980 Non-organic physical signs in low-back pain. Spine 5(2):117–125

Waddell G, Bircher M, Finlayson D, Main C J 1984 Symptoms and signs: physical disease or illness behaviour? British Medical Journal 289:739–741

Waddell G, Main C J, Morris E W, DiPaolo M, Gray I C M 1987 Chronic low back pain, psychological distress and illness behaviour. Spine 11:712–719

Ware J E, Sherbourne C D 1992 The MOS 36-item short-form health survey (SF-36). I. Conceptual framework and item selection. Medical Care 30(6):473–483

Watson P J 1999 Non-physiological determinants of physical performance in musculoskeletal pain. Pain 1999—an updated review. IASP, Seattle, pp 153-159

Watson P J, Poulter M E 1997 The development of a functional, task-orientated assessment of pain behaviour in low back pain patients. Journal of Back and Musculoskeletal Rehabilitation 9:57–59

Williams A C, Richardson P H, Nicholas M K et al 1996 Inpatient vs. outpatient pain management: results of a randomised controlled trial. Pain 66(1):13–22

APPENDIX: A BRIEF REVIEW BASED ON THE OBSERVATIONS BY PRICE & HARKINS (1992)

MEASURE	DESCRIPTION	COMMENTS
Visual Analogue Scale	Patients mark a point on a 10cm line indicating their level of pain between two "anchors" such as "no pain" to "pain as bad as it could be" for intensity and "not at all bad" to "the most unpleasant feeling possible" for affective assessment. Operator measures the distance from the zero anchor in millimetres.	Can be considered to have ration scale properties. Scored quickly to give feedback to clinician Sensitive to treatment effects. Good evidence for reliability and repeatability for both affective and intensity scales. Good evidence for discrimination between affective and intensity domains. Explanations to patient need to be clear and may influence rating. Elderly people, drowsy patients, and people of low intelligence find them less easy to use than other measures.
Numerical Rating Scale	Patients are asked to verbally rate their pain on a scale of either 1-10 (NRS 11) or 1-100 (NRS 101) between two anchor points as described in the VAS.	Can be considered to have ration scale properties. Rating is instant and does not have the potential for measurement error in the VAS. NRS 101 offers a large number of response categories and so is sensitive to change. NRS 11 is not as sensitive to change as the VAS. NRS for affective change is poorly researched, requires explanation and may still not be understood by elderly or drowsy patients.
Verbal Rating Scales	Lists of words are presented to the patient to assess either the intensity or the affective domain. Patients are asked to chose from the list one that best describes the intensity or the affective component of their pain. Scores are assigned to the words in increasing levels of intensity or affect. Current scales use 5, 6 or 15 point scales.	Represent ordinal data Rating is instant Requires a level of understanding and reading ability not necessary in other measures Allows a choice of only one word which may not fit the patients own description Reliability may not be as good as other measures.
Picture Scale (Pain Faces scale)	Line drawings of eight faces representing a person experiencing different level of pain intensity are presented to the patient and they choose the one which best represents their pain. The response is scored from 0 to 7.	Data is ordinal. Intended for the assessment of intensity but may more closely represent the affective domain. Easy to use and score. Useful in those who are unable to understand other measures (does not rely on understanding written instructions). Little data on the validity. Limited evidence for sensitivity to treatment. Limited 8 point scale.
McGill Pain Questionnaire (MPQ)	Consists of 20 subclasses of grouped words; a categorical evaluation of the pain (the PPI) which uses a no pain anchor and 5 affective descriptive words and a pain drawing with description of the nature of the pain. The following are calculated: responses from the 20 subclasses are scored, based on their ranked value in the subgroup, into sensory, affective, evaluative and miscellaneous domains and summed to give a total score. A PPI categorical evaluation provides an additional score. The number of words chosen is also recorded.	Multidimensional instrument assessing all areas of pain response and intensity. Frequently used as ration data but may be more representative of ordinal data. Complex scoring does not give immediate feedback and may result in errors. Widely used with very good evidence on validity, repeatability and reliability in a wide range of conditions. Sensitive to change in affect and sensory components. Discriminated the affective and sensory components. Reliance on descriptive words-some of which may be unfamiliar to many patients. Unsuitable for use in those with difficulty reading or low educational level. Responses differ between clinical groups.
Short from MPQ (SF-MPQ)	Patients are required to chose from 15 descriptive words (11 sensory and four affective) those that best describe their pain and rank the intensity of that word from none to severe. A VAS scale for intensity and the PPI scale are also included.	Assesses the multidimensional aspects of pain. Frequently used as ration data but may be more representative of ordinal data. Less complex than the MPQ. Scoring errors may occur. Evidence for reliability, repeatability and validity in wide number of conditions. Some evidence for differential responses from different clinical groups. Unsuitable for use in those with difficulty reading or low educational level. Demonstrates sensitivity to changes in the affective, sensory and intensity domains.

10

Psychological assessment

Helen Parker Chris J. Main

INTRODUCTION

In Chapter 7 some of the general issues relating to the assessment were discussed; this chapter will look at the assessment of the presenting psychological characteristics and the psychological mechanisms that can influence the perception of pain. (See Ch. 2 for a discussion specifically of psychological mechanisms.)

Initially some of the general issues relating to the nature and relevance of psychiatric factors will be addressed. The major focus of the chapter, however, will be on the assessment specifically of psychological features in the patient with chronic pain. (The assessment of psychosocial, economic and occupational factors in the context of clinical decision making will be discussed in Ch. 11.)

THE ASSESSMENT OF PSYCHOPATHOLOGY

The sort of assessment appropriate for a particular clinic will depend in part on whether there has been any 'filtering' of patients who have been referred to the clinic. With open access to health care, particularly with a 'fee-for-service system' such as used to be the norm in the USA, there may have been no clinical decision as to the suitability of the patient for pain management. In the newer system of managed care, treatment is rationed. Treatment providers have to pay careful attention to the selection of patients since treatment outcome is used in marketing to attract new business. Since arguably the screening carried out by HMOs (health maintenance organisations) is more financially than clinically based, many treatment providers will carry out some sort of psychological screening. In consideration for pain management, screening focuses primarily on the identification of primary psychological disorder, defined in terms of either axis I clinical disorders or axis II personality (character) disorders in terms of psychiatric illness

There are four circumstances in which formal psychiatric evaluation may be indicated:

- identification of primary psychiatric illness requiring treatment in its own right
- consideration for conjoint psychiatric care
- consideration of suitability for pain management
- identification of possibly compensable 'psychological injury' in the context of litigation.

Proper psychiatric diagnosis requires formal assessment according to established criteria such as in the fourth edition of the Diagnostic and Statistical Manual of Mental Disorders or DSM-IV (1994). There are two structured psychiatric interviews that produce reliable and valid psychiatric diagnoses based on the DSM-IV criteria. These are the diagnostic interview schedule (DIS) and the Structured Clinical Interview for DSM-IV (SCID).

The DIS has some advantages in that there is computer software available, whichs allow patients to self-administer the interview in the clinician's office. This software also allows the clinician to assess the patient's responses according to DSM-IV criteria and thus obtain a record of the patient's lifetime psychiatric history. It is not appropriate at this juncture to consider psychiatric diagnosis in detail, but a brief comment will be made on each of the major categories highlighted above.

DSM-IV distinguishes clinical disorders (axis I) from personality disorders (axis II). Although the distinction is not absolutely clear cut, in assessment of pain patients the presence of axis I disorders principally affects decisions about which type of treatment is likely to be most appropriate. The presence of axis II disorders has

---

Box 10.1 Axis I diagnoses most commonly ascribed to pain patients
• Generalised anxiety disorder • Anxiety due to a general medical condition • Adjustment disorders • Somatiform disorders • Conversion disorder • Hypochondriasis • Depression • Post-traumatic stress disorder • Pain disorder

more of a bearing on *whether* to offer treatment at all.

Axis I psychiatric disorders

The most commonly found psychiatric diagnoses among pain patients are found in Box 10.1 They are described in more detail with a brief commentary on their relevance in the context of chronic pain in the Appendix to this chapter (p. 203).

In summary, anxiety and depression seem to be the most relevant of the distinct psychiatric axis I disorders in patients with chronic pain problems. Identification of *clinically significant* anxiety or depression may be important in consideration for primary or conjoint psychiatric treatment. In the context of chronic pain, however, anxiety is usually characterised by specific fears or concerns and depression is usually secondary to pain and its disabling effects (and as such is most appropriately 'treated' by pain management).

If a patient presents with a clinical history suggestive of long-standing ill health affecting a variety of symptoms, then assessment of somatisation disorder may be indicated. If the patient has been injured in an accident, however, then assessment of post-traumatic stress disorder should be considered.

Identification of axis II personality or character disorder

A personality disorder is defined as (DSM-IV 1994, p. 629): 'an enduring pattern of inner experiences and behaviour that deviates markedly from the expectations of the individual's culture, is pervasive and inflexible, has an onset in adolescence or early adulthood, is stable over time and leads to distress or impairment'.

The major types of personality disorder are shown in the Appendix to this chapter (p. 209). A much fuller description of each of these syndromes is presented in DSM-IV (1994). The ascription of personality disorder is not without controversy. It could be argued that the concept of personality disorder is as much a cultural as a clinical concept. In the prospective Boeing study into the development of chronic low back pain (Bigos et al 1991), no *specific* personality disorder was found to predict chronic incapacity, but whether or not an individual had *any* personality disorder was found to be predictive. Since a major characteristic of individuals is (arguably) poor coping styles and strategies, in practical terms it would seem more useful to consider the influence of personality in terms of behaviours or attitudes likely to compromise individuals' suitability for treatment, their likelihood of benefiting from treatment or their likelihood of compromising the treatment of others. As part of clinical decision making (Ch. 12) it will be important to consider issues of substance abuse, likelihood of successful engagement in self-help and probability of being able to benefit from and contribute to group-based rehabilitation.

In conclusion, Gatchel (1996) has observed that when patients reach the more chronic stages of pain there is usually some significant psychopathology that needs to be dealt with. It might be argued that psychopathology in terms of distress, fear, mistaken beliefs and dysfunctional coping strategies is an inherent component of the chronic pain syndrome. Indeed, the management and modification of such features is at the heart of interdisciplinary pain management. High rates of psychopathology alone in pain patients does not have to interfere significantly with their rehabilitation (Gatchel et al 1994). Although recognising therefore that adoption of a psychiatric perspective may be appropriate for the identification of primary psychiatric disorder and personality disorder, the authors suggest that most patients should be evaluated from a psychological perspective.

PSYCHOLOGICAL ASSESSMENT: THE GENERAL CONTEXT

Psychological assessment is carried out in order to obtain information that can be used for a number of purposes; these are summarised in Box 10.2.

This chapter will focus on the initial evaluation of psychological factors to be carried out by a clinical psychologist working as a member of the pain management team. (i.e. area three of this list). Chapter 17 will deal with the issue of outcome measurement. A summary of the specific aims of the initial evaluation is presented in Box 10.3.

There are three main methods used in the initial evaluation:

- psychometric tests
- the clinical interview
- behavioural observation.

Whenever possible the assessment of psychological factors should not rely simply on information obtained from only one source but should be the product of a combination of these methods. A

Box 10.2 General purpose of psychological assessment

1. As a screening measure
2. To aid diagnosis
3. To facilitate treatment planning
4. To facilitate description of the population studied for use in research and/or clinical audit
5. To evaluate the outcome of treatment

Box 10.3 Specific aims of the initial psychological assessment

- Evaluation of presenting psychological characteristics
- Evaluation of mechanisms influencing the perception of pain and disability
- To identify any psychological barriers to treatment
- To identify whether further psychological treatment is required prior to embarking on pain management

discussion of psychometric assessment and the clinical interview follows (behavioural observation was detailed in Ch. 9.)

PSYCHOMETRIC ASSESSMENT

It is of great importance that any psychological measures selected should be reliable and valid (Ch. 9, p. 168) and that they have been standardised for use with the patient population. Thus a measure standardised for use with chronic low back pain may well not be appropriate for use with neck pain. In order to evaluate whether psychometric measures chosen meet the above criteria it will be necessary for the clinician to refer to the relevant research literature. The following section provides an overview of the concepts of reliability and validity; there are a number of standard texts on the subject that will provide the reader with fuller information on all the areas below.

Reliability of measures

Within the assessment of chronic pain there are three main types of reliability measures that will be of concern to the clinician in the selection of appropriate assessments: the coefficient of stability, the coefficient of internal consistency and the interrater reliability.

Coefficient of stability

Also known as test–retest reliability, this measure assesses the stability of the results of a test over time. The test is administered to the same group of individuals on two separate occasions and the results are correlated. The closer the correlation coefficient approaches to a score of one the more reliable the measure can be said to be. Williams (1988) indicates that reliability coefficients above 0.85 are generally regarded as high and those between 0.6 to 0.85 as being moderate.

When selecting measures consideration should be given to the size of the test–retest interval (in general the shorter the interval the higher will be the reliability coefficient). Very short intervals give some cause for concern as it is probable that those taking the test may well have recalled their previous responses and these memories will influence their responding on the second test occasion. A further consideration is that for a number of measures it is probable that the construct being measured will not be stable over time and that this will lead to lowered test–retest reliability levels. For example, use of coping strategy may alter over the passage of time, which would lead to a reduction in test–retest reliability. Changes in the underlying disorder giving rise to pain may also lead to reduction of test–retest reliability. For example, if a measure of depressive symptomatology is being assessed in a disorder such as rheumatoid arthritis (in which pain levels can fluctuate over time) a low test–retest reliability coefficient may be a reflection of changes in pain levels rather than being indicative of any inadequacies of the measure being used.

Coefficient of internal consistency

This is a measure of the consistency of content sampling and examines whether each item in a particular scale is measuring the same thing as the other scale items. The most common method of assessing internal consistency is by use of Cronbach's alpha coefficient. Generally coefficient sizes range from 0 to 1; the higher the coefficient the higher is the internal consistency of the scale. Todd & Bradley (1996) indicate that for a 10-item or more scale coefficients of 0.7–0.8 are acceptable. Excessively high values (e.g. 0.9 and above) generally indicate redundancy of scale items and those lower than 0.7 indicate that the scale is too diffuse a measure.

Interrater reliability

Within pain assessment this type of reliability is most commonly used in the evaluation of behavioural observation methods. The most appropriate method for assessing interrater reliability is Cohen's kappa statistic. Simple percentage agreement figures are a poor substitute for the kappa statistic as they can lead to over-inflated estimates of reliability. Values of kappa can range from –1 to +1 with higher ratings indicating increased agreement. Landis & Koch (1977) indicate that values of 0.41–0.60 can be considered as moderate, 0.61–0.80 as substantial and 0.81–1 as almost perfect.

Validity of measures

The validity of a test gives an indication as to how well a particular test measures what it is that it claims to measure. For example, does a test of depressive symptomatology actually measure this or is it measuring symptoms that are related to pain? Four types of validity are of importance in evaluating measures: face validity, content validity, criterion-related validity and construct validity.

Face validity

Face validity is not validity in the true sense of the word but refers to what a test appears to be measuring. Face validity can be of particular importance in assuring patient cooperation and motivation to complete tests. This is of particular importance if questionnaires are sent by post and the clinician may not have the opportunity to explain the reason for the use of certain tests. The higher the face validity the more likely it is that the patient will cooperate in completion of the test. Measures such as the MPQ will have high face validity for the majority of pain patients.

Content validity

This will determine whether the items of a particular test cover a representative sample of the area that is being measured. For example, a measure of depression should not be limited to questions relating only to appetite and sleep and a measure of pain behaviour should not be limited to the evaluation of only grimacing.

Criterion-related validity

Criterion-related validity will indicate how well a test is able either to predict a person's behaviour in specific situations (predictive validity) or to diagnose an existing state (concurrent validity). When concurrent validity is being evaluated the test will generally be compared with a 'gold standard' (i.e. the currently available best method for assessing the particular area); for example, a measure of depressive symptomatology may be compared with a DSM-IV diagnosis of depressive disorder.

Construct validity

This is a measure of the extent to which a test measures hypothetical constructs or traits—for example, constructs such as beliefs about the understandability of pain. There are a number of methods used to examine this aspect of validity. Factor analysis is often used with multiscale tests (e.g. the Pain Beliefs and Perceptions Inventory, or PBPI, p. 197) to confirm the presence of discrete subscales.

Discriminant and convergent validity

Both discriminant and convergent validity are forms of construct validity. In discriminant validity the aim is to demonstrate that the test does not correlate with other measures of dissimilar constructs and in convergent validity the aim is to demonstrate that the measure correlates well with other measures of similar or the same constructs.

Common problems encountered in the use of psychological tests

Inadequate psychometric properties

An example of this is that the reliability and validity of the test may not have been adequately investigated for the patient population for which the test is used. In certain cases, although investigators report reliability and validity information on a test, the sample used is either inadequately described or is comprised of a sample heterogeneous for type of pain, or both. For example, the sample may be comprised of patients suffering cancer pain, headache and low back pain.

Confusion between psychological symptoms and physical limitations

This problem is most commonly encountered when measures originally developed for use with, and standardised on, psychiatric populations are used with patients with chronic pain as a number of symptoms of certain psychiatric disorders and pain are common to both. The most commonly encountered tests that fall into this category are personality tests (e.g. Minnesota Multiphasic Personality Inventory, or MMPI), screening tests for psychopathology (e.g. Symptom Checklist, or SCL-90, General Health Questionnaire, or GHQ and measures such as the Beck Depression and Anxiety Inventories (BDI and BAI). Such tests frequently include items relating to physical factors that may lead to the production of 'false positive' errors as patients may endorse such items as a consequence of their pain not as a consequence of any underlying psychopathology. For example the SCL-90 psychoticism scale contains the item 'The idea that something serious is wrong with your body'. Obviously this item may well be endorsed by the patient with chronic pain as a consequence of their medical problems (or their beliefs about what is wrong with them) rather than being indicative of psychotic thinking.

Lack of comparability between groups of patients studied

Even if adequate psychometric properties have been demonstrated for one type of pain it cannot be assumed that the test will be reliable and valid for another pain type. For example, it cannot be assumed that a test developed and standardised for use with patients with arthritic pain will be either reliable or valid, or both, for patients with chronic low back pain.

Lack of normative data

A surprising number of articles describing the development of tests specific for pain patients fail to give basic statistical information regarding the means and standard deviations of scores obtained. This makes it impossible to evaluate the significance of an individual's score.

The administration of psychometric tests

The purpose of the assessment will dictate to a large degree the type of tests selected. Each test must have a specific role to play in the evaluation process. There is little use in administering a large battery of tests only to have these languishing in the back of the patient's notes unscored and unevaluated.

Our experience at the Salford Pain Management Programme is that patients rarely object to completing psychometric tests once they have understood their importance; indeed they would appear to regard such tests as a 'sign' that their problems are being taken 'seriously'. Refusal to complete tests may be an initial indicator of the patient's ambivalence about the whole assessment process.

Problems may be encountered if patients are of limited intellectual abilities and/or have problems with reading. Frequent questions and enquires from patients as to the meanings of words/phrases used on the measures and/or writing answers rather than checking the appropriate place on the questionnaire, and/or being asked by the patient what should they put for their answer, should alert the clinician to these problems. In these circumstances clinicians should use their experience to decide whether to continue with assessment. Problems with reading may be overcome by the clinician reading the questions out aloud to the patient although it must be noted that this may have an effect on the psychometric properties of the test and the clinician must resist the attempt to 'prompt' or answer for the patient.

In the Salford Pain Management Programme a limited number of psychometric measures are sent to the patient's home for completion and return to the unit prior to the triage process to decide if the patient is suitable for assessment and if so the type of assessment required (see Ch. 7). This method of administration has a number of advantages and disadvantages.

The advantages are: patients can complete the measures without feeling that there are any time constraints being placed on them nor any of the stress that may accompany attendance at hospital. It is probable that as clinicians we underestimate the degree of stress that may be generated in the patient attending for an initial appointment. The initial appointment may generate stress for a number of reasons; for example, patients may have high expectations of the assessment (e.g. hoping it will produce the 'cure' that they have been waiting for so long), or be concerned that they will be physically examined and that this will exacerbate their pain. Such factors may well act to produce a transitory increase in certain types of symptomatology, particularly those related to anxiety.

The disadvantages are that patients may omit (either intentionally or unintentionally) questionnaire items (if too many items are omitted this will mean that it is not possible to score the test or to obtain much meaningful information from it), they may ask for help from family members in completing the assessments and finally it is not possible to ascertain whether patients have completely understood the questionnaire instructions. Our experience has shown that sometimes, for example, although questionnaires may indicate that they should be filled in with respect to how the patient has been feeling, over a certain time period patients will ignore these instructions and complete the questionnaires with reference to how they were feeling when they had a particularly 'bad spell' of pain. This may occur for a number of reasons, which include: a fear that if they do not appear 'bad enough' that they will be denied treatment, failure to read instructions or a feeling that providing information as to how patients are during a bad episode will be of more value to the clinician.

If patients complete psychometric assessments in the clinic the advantages are that the importance of the measures can be stressed, any misconceptions cleared up, completed questionnaires can be checked for omitted items and clinicians can ensure that the questionnaires have been completed without outside assistance. The disadvantage is that the patient will have to attend for a longer period of time.

Prior to completing any psychometric tests it is important to stress to patients the routine nature of the use of such tests and that they are not to 'worry' if certain test items do not appear to be of relevance to them. Their attention should be drawn to any 'time limits' (e.g. certain tests require the patient to fill them in on the basis of how they have been feeling in a given time period such as in the past week) and procrastination should be discouraged by asking the patient not to spend too much time in answering the test items.

The majority of tests can be scored by clerical staff. Computer scoring programmes are ideal (particularly for measures such as the SF36, which is complex to score) and have the advantage that results can easily be incorporated on to a database and are therefore accessible for purposes such as research and audit.

Overview

There are a number of key questions to consider when selecting psychometric tests:

- What is the purpose for which I wish to use the test?
- Has this test been standardised for use with the particular patient population that I wish to employ it with?
- Is the test both reliable and valid for the purposes for which I wish to use the test?
- Are there adequate norms for the test?
- If selecting a test battery, how many different measures can I reasonably expect the patient to complete?
- Who will administer the tests, where will they be administered and who will score the tests?
- Who will interpret the test results?

THE CLINICAL INTERVIEW: GENERAL ISSUES

The clinical interview should be carried out by a clinical psychologist experienced in working with patients with chronic pain using a cognitive–behavioural approach (see Ch. 13 for a discussion of the specific skills required). It is strongly recommended that a semi-structured interview is used, first to ensure that the interview is consistent across patients (particularly if more than one psychologist is involved in the pain management team), secondly to make sure that all relevant areas are covered in the interview and thirdly to allow for easier access to information for audit and/or research purposes. There are a limited number of published structured and semi-structured interview schedules (see Bradley, Haile & Jaworski 1992 for a review of this area); however, such schedules are infrequently used in clinical work and reliability and validity information on them is scarce.

The precise format of the interview will be dependent on factors such as the type of pain problem being evaluated and needs to take into consideration which areas are being addressed by other members of the team. For example, in Chapter 8 the areas covered in the medical assessment were discussed and it would be of little value to duplicate them within the psychological interview. Duplication of enquiries can lead to the patient becoming confused, irritated or annoyed and wastes both the patient's and the team's time.

The semi-structured interview used in the Salford Pain Management Programme is reproduced in the Appendix to this Chapter (p. 211).

In order to cover all the areas discussed below it is probable that an interview of approximately 30–45 minutes will be sufficient for the majority of patients. However, certain patients, particularly if there is a complex history, may require considerably longer.

As the psychological interview occurs as part of the initial assessment process patients may well at this stage in their assessment be still adhering to a dualistic concept of pain and may be concerned that the role of the psychologist is to 'prove' in some way that they are either mentally ill or that their pain is 'all in the mind'. A small proportion of patients may be overtly hostile at the start of the assessment. It is

therefore vital that in the early stages of the interview the psychologist attempts to explain the purpose of the interview in terms that can be easily understood by the patient. It is important to stress that the psychological interview is a *routine* part of the assessment process, that the patient's pain is taken *seriously* and that no one believes their pain is 'all in the patient's mind'. It can be of great value to stress the 'normality' of distress in chronic pain. Finally, as many patients are confused about the difference between psychiatrists and psychologists, it can be worth while to spend a short period of time explaining the differences between the two professions. The introductory paragraphs of the clinical interview used in the Salford programme (see Appendix to this chapter, p.) will provide a starting point for those wishing to either develop or to refine their own introduction to the clinical interview.

THE ASSESSMENT OF PRESENTING PSYCHOLOGICAL CHARACTERISTICS

It is important to consider specifically certain features of the patient's presentation.

Anxiety and depression

In patients with chronic pain, psychological distress commonly presents in the form of depressive symptomatology and heightened somatic awareness of physiological events. The occurrence of higher rates of depression and depressive symptomatology in patients with chronic pain when compared with non-pain populations is now well documented. In the literature depressive symptomatology has been associated with increased pain report, increased pain behaviour, poorer response to treatment and impaired psychosocial functioning.

Tests

A wide range of tests have been used in the assessment of depressive symptomatology, anxiety and somatic awareness. These fall into

---

Box 10.4 Commonly used assessments for anxiety and depression

---

Batteries
The MMPI
GHQ
SCL-90

Single measures
BDI
Center for Epidemiological Studies Depression Scale (CESDS)
ZDS
BAI
Spielberger State/Trait Anxiety Inventory (STAI)
Modified Somatic Perception Questionnaire (SPQ)

---

two main categories: those tests that address only one area (e.g. depressive symptomatology) and screening batteries; these are summarised in Box 10.4.

The majority of these questionnaires were initially developed for use with, and standardised on, psychiatric populations. As discussed above, this creates difficulties when they are applied to the assessment of patients with chronic pain. It is recommended that if such measures are used then the results should be interpreted with caution.

There have been few psychometric tests that have been developed to specifically assess psychological distress in chronic pain. The exceptions are the Modified Somatic Perception Questionnaire, or MSPQ (Main 1983) and the Modified Zung Depression Scale, or ZDS (Main & Waddell 1984). Both these tests have been standardised for use with patients with chronic low back pain and normative data are available for the interpretation of the abnormality of scores obtained. In addition to identifying patients who are distressed the two scales can be used in combination to identify those at risk of becoming psychologically distressed (Main et al 1992).

Assessment of anxiety and depression in the clinical interview

There are a number of standard texts available that describe approaches to the assessment of mood and anxiety in the clinical interview (e.g. Hawton et al 1989). (The use of psychiatric interviews based on DSM-IV has already been discussed.) Usually patients are not psychiatrically ill, but they may be distressed, angry and fearful. The *focus* of these emotions must be identified.

Any competent clinical assessment will include an evaluation of premorbid psychological functioning. Specific inquiry should be made concerning treatment for any psychological or psychiatric disorders in the past.

If the source of pain is due to an accident there is a possibility that post-traumatic stress disorder (PTSD) may be present; this possibility should be explored by asking about the nature of the accident, any 're-experiencing' of the phenomenon, avoidance, numbing of responsiveness and symptoms of increased arousal (although some of these latter problems such as sleep problems may be difficult to distinguish from problems due to pain and/or depressive problems). A proportion of accident victims will be claiming compensation and this in itself can act as a considerable source of stress. It is possible to carry out a formal diagnostic assessment (see above), or ask the patient to complete a test such as the Impact of Events Scale, or IES, but a number of focused questions during the interview should be sufficient to decide whether specific psychological intervention is indicated. It is also of great importance to enquire into the presence of any non-pain-related stressors (both concurrent and in the past) which could be contributing to the patient's level of anxiety or depression, or both. Such stressors include recent bereavements or unresolved bereavement reactions, forensic problems and a history of physical and/or sexual abuse.

Psychological disorders most likely to interfere with the treatment process and require treatment in their own right are PTSD, unresolved bereavement and abuse. The patient should be referred on to the relevant agency for treatment prior to rereferral back to the pain centre for reassessment. Case study 10.1 is an example.

Case study 10.1 Post-traumatic stress disorder

Jack was a customer in a bank where there was an armed robbery. He was pushed to the floor in the raid, sustaining an injury to his back. He had never discussed his reactions to the raid as he feared that doing so would in some way indicate that he was unmanly. However, he actively pursued treatment for his back disorder, which had become chronic. At interview the psychologist elicited from Jack a number of symptoms indicative of PTSD; for example, he had frequent nightmares about what had happened, he had frequent intrusive thoughts, was unable to go into crowded shops, avoided talking about what had happened and had an exaggerated startle response. It was felt that although Jack would benefit from pain management that he would be unable to cope with the programme owing to his PTSD and was referred to specialist services for counselling prior to a reassessment at the pain centre.

Box 10.5 Assessment of distress

- If psychological assessment does indicate high levels of distress then this does not mean that the pain is 'psychological' in origin. As discussed in Chapter 2 such a dualistic conceptualisation of chronic pain, that pain is either 'organic' or 'psychological', is outmoded and has no place in modern pain management
- Factors unrelated to pain can also be a source of distress
- A high score on a measure of distress is not equivalent to a psychiatric diagnosis; thus an elevated score on the BDI is not diagnostic of the presence of depression
- If psychometric measures are used that have not been specifically standardised for use with patients with chronic pain then results should be interpreted with caution

Summary

A number of the key points in the assessment of distress are presented in Box 10.5.

Anger and hostility

Anger, hostility and passive aggressiveness are not infrequently encountered by the clinician working with chronic pain patients. The importance of these areas is a relatively new area of investigation (see Fernandez & Turk 1995 for a review). It is probable that inhibition of anger (i.e. the suppression of angry feelings) will impact on mood and pain levels and that the expression of anger will impact patients' relationships with others (including clinicians), compliance with treatment and their suitability for certain types of pain management (particularly group programmes). Our experience of running group programmes has shown that including those with high levels of expressed anger and hostility in a programme can have a highly disruptive effect on the group dynamics.

The use of psychometric tests in the assessment of anger and hostility

The main measures used to assess anger and hostility in chronic pain are the Spielberger anger scales (Spielberger 1988) and to a lesser extent the anger/hostility scale from the Profile of Mood States, or POMS (Nair et al 1971). Neither test has been specifically standardised for use with chronic pain.

Assessment of anger and hostility in the clinical interview

When a patient presents as particularly angry or hostile this obviously needs to be dealt with prior to continuing with the interview. The source and direction of the anger and hostility must be evaluated. Box 10.6 shows some of the sources and reasons for anger that may be encountered and would form a useful starting point for investigation into this area in the interview. Following this it is of importance to attempt to make an evaluation of the impact of anger on patients' lives in general and on their pain experiences in particular.

Psychological aspects of the evaluation of pain report and pain behaviour

The assessment of pain and pain behaviour has been reviewed in Chapter 9, but it is important to emphasise further the impact that psychological factors can and do have on ratings both of pain and of pain behaviour. It would be naïve to

Box 10.6 Attributions about objects of anger and appraisals about reasons for anger among chronic pain sufferers

Agent (object of anger)	Action (reason for anger)
Causal agent of injury/illness	Chronic pain
Medical health-care providers	Diagnostic ambiguity; treatment failure
Mental health professionals	Implications of psychogenicity or psychopathology
Attorneys and legal system	Adversarial dispute; scrutiny and arbitration
Insurance companies; social security system	Inadequate monetary coverage or compensation
Employer	Cessation of employment; job transfer; job retraining
Significant others	Lack of interpersonal support
God	'Predetermined' injury and consequences; ill fate
Self	Disablement, disfigurement
The whole world	Alienation

From Fernandez E & Turk D C 1995 Pain (61) 165–175 The scope and significance of Anger 1995, Elsevier Science, reproduced with permission.

assume that ratings of these areas can be completely separated from aspects of patients' functioning such as their level of distress, the demands of the situation in which pain is rated or that the pain has emotional qualities. For example, patients tend to report higher levels of pain to a medically qualified person than to those with psychological qualifications. Patient ratings of the intensity, sensory and affective qualities of their pain need to be interpreted with reference to patients' current levels of distress.

For example, the Pain Drawing test (Ransford, Cairns & Mooney 1976) undoubtedly has high face validity for patients and is a frequently used measure in clinical practice. Early research seemed to indicate that if certain factors were present (e.g. unreal drawings showing poor anatomical location) then this was indicative of psychological distress. However, further research has indicated that, although highly abnormal pain drawings are associated with distress, a significant proportion of highly distressed patents produce 'normal' pain drawings leading to

unacceptably high levels of false negative results (Parker, Wood & Main 1995). The pain drawing should not be used, therefore, as the only screening measure for psychological distress.

The relationship between psychological factors and pain behaviour has been shown to vary across different diagnostic groups. Thus depressive symptomatology has been found to be associated with pain behaviour in chronic low back pain but not in rheumatoid arthritis or fibromyalgia. An understanding that such differences can occur is of importance in assessing the patient with chronic pain and serves to highlight the dangers of assuming that a relationship that has been found to occur in one diagnostic group will 'hold true' across other groups.

Assessing the influence of personality characteristics and personality disorder

As previously discussed, an evaluation of such features is important not from the point of view of offering some sort of psychological intervention in order to address them but because they may prove to be powerful obstacles to compliance with treatment and therefore be a key perspective in clinical decision making.

The use of psychometric tests in the assessment of personality disorder

The MMPI has been used to identify abnormal personality profiles. In Chapter 2 some of issues surrounding its construction, use and interpretation have been highlighted. To our knowledge no psychometric measure has been specifically validated for use with chronic pain patients and a standardised interview incorporating a careful clinical history would seem to be preferable by far.

Assessment of personality disorder in the clinical interview

Structured interviews (using DSM-IV criteria for diagnosis) for the presence of axis I and II disorders are available, but in general these are rarely used in the assessment of chronic pain. A detailed review of DSM-IV based interviews in chronic pain is offered by Gatchel (1996). Such interviews are time consuming and furthermore may serve to alienate patients with chronic pain (who may already fear that they are seeing a psychologist because people believe that the pain is 'all in their mind'). As discussed at the beginning of this chapter, the frequency with which patients present at a pain assessment with frank personality disorders will depend in part on the mechanisms by which patients are referred to the programme. Thus it is likely that the incidence will be higher in self-referral programmes than in those where referrals are mainly from secondary sources. In practical terms, it is probably sufficient to rely on a number of pointers that may lead the clinician to suspect the presence of a personality disorder (Box 10.7). If such a disorder is present then it is important to evaluate the potential impact that this may have on treatment.

COGNITIVE FACTORS

Beliefs and attributions

Clearly the examination of clinical history and presenting psychological characteristics will have relied in a large measure on the patient's attitudes and beliefs. As illustrated in Chapter 2, however, the advent of cognitive–behavioural approaches to care has led to a much more focused investigation into beliefs, attitudes, adjustment to pain or disability. According to DeGood & Shutty (1992, p. 215): 'Problematic

beliefs about pain and its management we feel should not be viewed as mere artifacts of the chronic pain experience that will disappear once a correct diagnosis and treatment is found. Rather such cognitions can lie at the heart of the chronic pain experience.'

A number of studies have examined the effect of beliefs about pain, self-efficacy beliefs and locus of control beliefs on psychological distress and coping. The findings, however, are not entirely consistent—possibly because of differences in the nature of the pain populations studied. A consistent finding nonetheless is that in chronic pain, beliefs are not related simply to *duration* of pain (as was previously surmised). Studies including locus of control measures have indicated that certain beliefs about control are associated with increased distress, with the use of maladaptive coping strategies and with poorer outcome of treatment. (There are indications that treatment outcome is more favourable when the patient has high internal control beliefs.) Degree of confidence (in terms of self-efficacy) is also positively associated with actual performance and negatively related to pain intensity and disability. The few studies that have examined the relationship between self-efficacy and coping strategies indicate that positive strategies are associated with higher self-efficacy ratings and negative strategies with lower ratings.

The importance of mistaken beliefs about hurting and harming has already been highlighted, particularly in the development of disability (Ch. 5). Research has indicated that avoidance (which is often a consequence of mistaken beliefs about hurting and harming) does not, as many patients may well believe, lead to pain reduction in either the short or the long term. The importance of a systematic assessment of beliefs about pain and disability prior to embarking on pain management can hardly be overemphasised if one considers the key points summarised in Box 10.8 and Case study 10.2.

The use of psychometric tests

Over the past decade a number of psychometric tests have been designed to measure beliefs

Box 10.7 Pointers for suspecting a personality disorder	
• Relationship problems	e.g. estranged from family, multiple short-lived relationships, absence of social relationships, mistrust and suspiciousness of others
• Forensic problems	e.g. history of prosecution for antisocial acts, theft, drug or alcohol-related activities
• Work problems	e.g. inability to maintain consistent work record, frequent changes in occupation, absenteeism

---

Box 10.8   Influence of beliefs about pain

- The beliefs that a patient holds about pain and its treatment will have an influence on both behavioural and emotional functioning. For example, patients who strongly believe that hurt = harm will have the behavioural response of avoiding any activities that they perceive will cause hurt; patients who believe that their pain will be constant and they will obtain no relief from it may react by becoming depressed
- Beliefs may influence the coping strategies that patients use, which in turn will have an impact on their psychological adjustment
- Beliefs held by the patient about their pain may effect compliance with treatment and thus have an impact on outcome. Thus the hurt = harm belief may mean that the patient will be unlikely to comply with an exercise programme

- Beliefs are frequently the main target area of the cognitive–behavioural approach to treatment; therefore an accurate initial assessment of beliefs will allow for the measurement of change in beliefs during and after treatment
- Whilst patients may have no inappropriate beliefs about their pain and understand that hurt does not equal harm they may still engage in few activities if they hold low self-efficacy beliefs about their ability to carry out that particular activity. This will have implications for treatment in that such patients may fail to comply with treatment owing to the fact that they do not believe that they are capable of producing the behaviour necessary to produce the desired outcome (see Dolce 1987 for a review)

Case study 10.2 Mistaken beliefs about pain

Frank was a 37-year-old man who had suffered from chronic low back pain for 5 years following an accident at work. During his initial treatment he was told by one of the doctors that he might have a disc problem. Although subsequent investigations failed to confirm this, Frank firmly believed that his pain was due to a 'slipped disc' and that the only treatment possible was an operation to 'remove' the disc, which he felt would alleviate all his pain. Frank further believed that if he exercised he risked damaging his back further; this belief was reinforced by the fact that when he did take even minimal exercise his back pain increased. As a consequence of his beliefs he had failed to cooperate with conventional physiotherapy courses as he believed that the exercises would damage his back and he regularly attended his general practitioner to ask for referral to a surgeon.

---

about pain (see DeGood & Shutty 1992 for a review). Some of the more commonly used measures are mentioned below. (As with all the psychometric measures, readers should refer to the research literature to determine whether the test has been adequately standardised and validated for the population that they wish to use it with.)

Composite measures of beliefs.   The Survey of Pain Attitudes, or SOPA (Jensen, Karoly & Huger 1987), is comprised of 24 items providing measures on five scales: pain control, solicitude, medical cure, disability and medication. A number of revisions of the scale have subse-

quently been produced, including a 57-item version, which also includes emotional and harm scales (Jensen et al 1994). Tait & Chibnall (1997), however, failed to verify the seven-factor structure of the 57-item test and have developed a brief seven-scale 35-item version (the SOPA-B) based on factor analysis of the original 57-item scale.

The Pain Beliefs and Perceptions Inventory, or PBPI (Williams & Thorn 1989) is a 16-item measure. Initially Williams and Thorne described the inventory as being divided into three scales: time, mystery and self-blame. The time scale was related to beliefs about the temporal stability of pain, the mystery scale to beliefs that pain is mysterious and a poorly understood experience and the self-blame scale to beliefs about self-blame for pain. Subsequent research (e.g. Strong, Ashton & Chant 1992), however, supports a four-factor solution in which the time scale is divided into two scales: permanence (i.e. the belief that pain will be long standing and will not change in the future) and constancy (i.e. the belief that pain will be present all the time). There is conflicting evidence regarding the relationship between the scales, measures of psychological distress and coping strategy use.

Measures of beliefs about functioning.   The Pain and Impairment Rating Scale, or PAIRS, (Riley, Ahern & Follick 1988), is a 15-item measure of the belief that pain necessarily leads to a limitation in functioning. However, as the scale provides a measure of only one particular area of belief about pain it is of limited use.

Measures of Locus of Control. The Multidimensional Locus of Control, or MHLC (Wallston, Wallston & DeVellis 1978), is an 18-item measure comprised of three scales: internal control, control by 'powerful others' (e.g. doctors) and chance. A number of more specialised scales have been developed from the MHLC; these include: the Pain Locus of Control, or PLC (Main & Waddell 1991), a 20-item questionnaire comprising two scales relating to pain control and responsibility for pain (shown in the Appendix to this chapter, p. 219), and the Back Pain Locus of Control scale, or BPLC (Vakkari 1990), a 12-item measure comprised of three scales: internal control, chance and control by others, each containing four items.

Measures of self-efficacy beliefs. There are, as yet, few specific measures designed to evaluate self-efficacy beliefs (Dolce 1987). However, the SOPA and CSQ (see below) both contain 'control' scales, which provide limited measures of self-efficacy.

The Arthritis Self-Efficacy Scale, or ASES (Lorig et al 1989), is a 20-item questionnaire that provides three measures: self-efficacy for function (e.g. walking and dressing abilities, nine items), self-efficacy for controlling other symptoms (e.g. frustration and fatigue, six items) and self-efficacy for pain (five items). The scales have been demonstrated to have adequate internal consistency, construct and concurrent validity, however the scale is obviously limited to use with patients with chronic arthritis. The Chronic Pain Self-Efficacy Scale, or CPSES (Anderson et al 1995), was developed from the ASES. The scale is comprised of 22 items, which provide three measures: self-efficacy for pain management (five items), self-efficacy for physical function (nine items) and self-efficacy for coping with symptoms (eight items). Although its use is only reported in one study (which unfortunately does not include normative data for the three scale score) and a heterogeneous sample was used, the scale has shown good internal consistency and some support for its concurrent and construct

validity. In particular all three scales were significant predictors of depressive symptomatology.

Measures of fear and avoidance. The Fear–Avoidance Beliefs Questionnaire, or FABQ (Waddell et al 1993), provides a measure of patients' beliefs as to how physical activity and work affect their pain. The FABQ has good statistical properties but to date its use is limited to chronic low back pain. The questionnaire is comprised of 16 items (of which five relate to physical activity and seven to work). The authors found a strong relationship between the fear-avoidance beliefs about work and both work loss and disability in activities of daily living.

The Tampa Scale of Kinesiophobia, or TSK (Kori et al 1990), is a 17-item measure addressing patients' beliefs about the relationship between fear and injury. It has been used both for the assessment of responses to experimental pain and in the evaluation of clinical pain. (Recent evaluation of the instrument in the Manchester and Salford Pain Centre would suggest that there may be two distinct scales: a 'fear of (reinjury' scale and a 'negative speculation' scale.) It would seem to merit further consideration.

Assessment of beliefs in the clinical interview

DeGood & Shutty (1992) identified four main categories of beliefs that are most regularly encountered in treatment settings. These are summarised in Box 10.9. All these are areas that need to be addressed in the clinical interview. It is of value to enquire about what patients have been told about the cause of their pain; this may reveal that patients have been given several 'diagnoses'

Box 10.9 Beliefs about pain encountered in treatment settings

Aetiology of pain	e.g. pain is due to a 'slipped disc'
Diagnostic expectations	e.g. I should have an X-ray or a scan; this would find out the cause of my pain
Treatment expectations	e.g. the belief that they need medication to control their pain
Beliefs relating to outcome goals	e.g. the belief that their pain can be cured

leading to confusion and erroneous beliefs as to what is wrong with them. It is also of importance to enquire about any 'mismatches' in beliefs about pain between what patients believe and what they have been told as this may have an impact on acceptance of the pain management model.

Key questions in the assessment of beliefs

These include the following:

- What are patients' beliefs regarding the cause of their pain?
- Do patients believe that previous investigations have been adequate?
- What are their beliefs about treatment and outcome?
- Do patients believe that they have control over their pain?
- Who do patients see as having responsibility for their pain, themselves or others?
- What activities are patients avoiding for fear of pain and has this avoidance increased over time?

Coping strategies

The importance of coping strategies in adjustment to pain and in the development of chronic incapacity has already been addressed in Chapter 2. In that chapter, however, catastrophising was discussed as an type of appraisal; in the following section of this chapter it will be discussed as a type of coping strategy. The modification and implementation of coping strategies is at the heart of pain management. The more behaviorally oriented pain management programmes place particular emphasis on behavioural strategies. The more cognitively oriented programmes place more emphasis on cognitive strategies. It now seems well established that individuals who report that they use catastrophising as a coping strategy and perceive themselves to be ineffectual in controlling pain are more disabled and depressed. This has been a consistent finding in a number of different pain conditions ranging from chronic low back pain to sickle cell disease (Jensen et al 1991). It may be that successful

coping with chronic pain is more the result of *avoiding* the use of certain negative strategies (i.e. catastrophising) rather than *adopting* positive strategies such as diverting attention. More research is needed, but it is clear nonetheless that coping strategies are of critical importance to the understanding and management of chronic pain and should be assessed systematically.

The use of psychometric tests in the assessment of coping strategies

There are a number of psychometric measures that have been designed to measure coping strategies (see DeGood & Shutty 1992 for a review of this area). Currently available measures tend to focus on cognitive methods of coping (e.g. using coping self-statements) rather than behavioural coping methods. The review that follows discusses some of the more commonly used tests for the assessment of coping strategies.

The Coping Strategies Questionnaire, or CSQ (Rosenstiel & Keefe 1983), is probably the most commonly used measure of coping strategies and has been used in a wide variety of chronic pain problems such as: phantom limb pain, fibromyalgia, sickle cell disease, osteoarthritis and chronic low back pain. There are two versions of the scale, containing 44 and 50 items respectively. Both scales yield measures of seven categories of coping strategies: six cognitive and one behavioural. The cognitive measures are: coping self-statements, catastrophising, diverting attention, ignoring pain sensations, praying/hoping and reinterpreting pain sensations; the behavioural measure is increasing activity levels. There are a further two items on the scale that measure perceived ability to control and perceived ability to decrease pain using coping strategies. The 50-item scale yields a further measure of pain behaviours; however, this scale is rarely used owing to poor internal consistency. In general, coping self-statements are the most commonly used strategy and reinterpreting pain sensations the least used. There is a considerable body of literature that supports the reliability and validity of the CSQ, the relationship between catastrophising and psychological distress being particularly robust across different pain types. Factor-analytic studies of the CSQ have produced results that are somewhat inconsistent both amongst different types of pain and across different studies. For example, some studies have identified a two-factor solution and others a five-factor solution with different scale items loading on different factors from study to study. It is advised therefore that individual scaled scores, rather than factor scores, are used for the interpretation of the scale. Use of the individual scaled scores would appear to give a better understanding of the specific coping strategies used by a particular patient. The questionnaire is shown in the Appendix to this chapter (p. 220).

The Vanderbilt Pain Management Inventory, or VPMI (Brown & Nicassio 1987), was developed specifically to assess coping strategies in rheumatoid arthritis. The scale is comprised of 18 items divided into two scales: active and passive coping. Snow-Turek, Norris & Tan (1996) found that the active and passive scales were not significantly correlated, which would imply that they represent two different constructs and are not simply the opposite ends of the same continuum. However, comparing the VPMI with the CSQ they concluded that the latter was a more psychometrically sound measure of active and passive coping strategies.

The Pain-Related Self-Statements and Pain-Related Coping Strategies questionnaires (PRSS/PRCS—Flor, Behle & Birbaumer 1993) provide measures of situation-specific cognitive coping (PRCS) and general attitudes to pain (PRSS). The PRSS is comprised of 18 items divided into two scales: catastrophising and coping; the PRCS is comprised of 15 items divided into two scales: helplessness and resourcefulness. It has so far been used in only a relatively small number of studies.

Coping strategy inventories have been criticised for including items that reflect both cognitive and behavioural measures of coping in one inventory. One relatively new measure designed to evaluate behavioural coping strategies is the Chronic Pain Coping Inventory, or CPCI (Jensen et al 1995). This scale also has the advantage of having a 'significant other' version. The scale is comprised of 65 items divided into 11 subscales. The subscales are grouped into three areas: illness-focused coping (guarding, resting, asking for assistance, opioid medication use, non-steroidal medication use and sedative hypnotic medication use), wellness-focused coping (relaxation, task persistence, exercise/stretch and coping self-statements) and other coping (seeking social support). Unfortunately the scale was developed on samples that were heterogeneous for type of pain and no normative data are given in their article for any of the scales.

The above measures all evaluate strategies for coping with pain. If the clinician is interested in evaluating more general coping efforts for stressors other than pain then the Ways of Coping Checklist, or WCCL (revised version, Vitaliano et al 1985), is a test that evaluates coping strategies for a stressor specifically identified by the patient. The test is comprised of three parts: part one is a list of common stressors (e.g. financial) from which patients must select the current major stressor in their life; part two comprises 42 items that form five scales measuring the coping strategies of problem focusing, wishful thinking, seeking of social support, self-blame and avoidance; part three comprises 14 items relating to beliefs about the stressor.

Assessment of coping strategies in the clinical interview

Initially patients may be resistant to the notion that anything that they do can alter their pain. When this is the case then it can be of value to attempt to introduce the concept of coping with pain by starting off by enquiring about what seems to make the pain worse. This can lead on to enquiry about any particular activities etc. that patients have noticed appear either to improve their level of pain or to help them cope better with the pain and its effects. Enquiries should also be made of any strategies used in the past that have been abandoned and the reasons for this. For example, patients may have started on an exercise programme but abandoned this for fear that the pain they experienced meant they were harming themselves.

By virtue of the fact that they are attending for assessment for pain management, patients will be coping ineffectively with their pain and it is probable that during the interview the types of strategies that will be reported will be passive strategies (e.g. resting, avoiding activity, use of pain-contingent medication) and/or maladaptive (e.g. catastrophising) in nature. Once the strategies that patients commonly use to cope with their pain have been elicited it is then important to attempt to obtain an indication from patients as to the effectiveness of these approaches.

Key questions in the assessment of coping strategies

These include the following:

* What coping strategies do patients use?
* Do these vary according to pain severity, environmental factors, etc.?
* How are patients' choices of strategies related to their beliefs about the nature of pain and disability?
* How effective do patients believe their coping strategies to be?

CONCLUSION

Assessment of the psychological features associated with chronic pain is an essential, and possibly the most important, aspect of clinical decision making whether with a view to individualised psychological therapy or to a comprehensive pain management programme. Chronic pain is a psychologically mediated disorder. Unfortunately, psychological assessment in the field of pain is still a relatively young science. Although recent conceptual advances have offered a better understanding of chronic pain and its development, assessment of the psychological impact of pain still represents a formidable challenge. There are different approaches to assessment using a range of techniques incorporating direct observational techniques, systematic structured interview and self-report questionnaires. Unfortunately many psychometric instruments are as yet inadequately constructed and insufficiently validated. Some of the newer instruments nonetheless have potential. Systematic assessment is key to a better understanding of the psychological processes underpinning the development of chronicity. Only with improved understanding will better treatment result.

We recommend that each clinic develop a systematic assessment including a standardised interview (including the assessment of 'readiness to change', iatrogenic distress and iatrogenic misunderstandings) and a small psychometric battery, designed to assess (as a minimum) pain, pain behaviour, distress, beliefs and coping strategies.

KEY POINTS

* Psychological assessment can be employed for a wide variety of purposes.
* Assessment will usually include the use of psychometric tests, some sort of behavioural observation and a focused clinical interview.
* Originally psychometric tests were used principally for the identification of psychopathology.
* Now a much wider range of tests are available focused more specifically on pain and treatment outcome.
* Tests must be adequately validated for the purpose in hand and on the clinical population concerned.
* Further research is needed on the usefulness of the tests in the prevention of chronic incapacity.
* Behavioural observation is important but specific training may be needed to obtain the degree of assessment accuracy required in clinical appraisal.

REFERENCES

Anderson K O, Dowds B N, Pelletz R E, Edwards W T, Peeters-Anderson C 1995 Development and initial validation of a scale to measure self-efficacy beliefs in patients with chronic pain. Pain 63:77–83

Bigos S J, Battie M C, Spengler B M et al 1991 A prospective study of work perceptions and psychological factors affecting the report of back injury. Spine 16: 1-6

Bradley L A, Haile J M, Jaworski T M 1992 Assessment of psychological status using interviews and self-report instruments. In: Turk D C, Melzack R (eds) Handbook of pain assessment. Guilford, New York, ch 12, pp 193–213

Brown G K, Nicassio P M 1987 The development of a questionnaire for the assessment of active and passive coping strategies in chronic pain patients. Pain 31:53–64

DeGood D E, Shutty M S 1992 Assessment of pain beliefs, coping and self-efficacy. In: Turk D C, Melzack R (eds) Handbook of pain assessment. Guilford, New York, ch 13, pp 214–234

Dolce J J 1987 Self-efficacy and disability beliefs in behavioral treatment of pain. Behavior Research and Therapy 25:289–299

DSM-IV 1994 Diagnostic and statistical manual of mental disorders, 4th edn. American Psychiatric Association, Washington DC

Fernandez E, Turk D C 1995 The scope and significance of anger in the experience of chronic pain. Pain 61:165–175

Flor H, Behle D J, Birbaumer N 1993 Assessment of pain-related cognitions in chronic pain patients. Behaviour Research and Therapy 31:63–73

Gatchel R J, Polatin P B, Mayer T G, Garcy P D 1994 Psychopathology and the rehabilitation of patients with low back pain disability. Archives of physical medicine and rehabilitation 75: 666-670

Gatchel R J Psychological Disorders and Chronic Pain: Cause and Effect relationships 1996 In: Psychological Approaches to Pain Management. A Practitioners Handbook, Gatchel & Turk (eds) The Guildford Press, New York

Hawton K, Salkovskis P M, Kirk J, Clark D M 1989 Cognitive behaviour therapy for psychiatric problems. Oxford University Press, Oxford

Horowitz M J, Wilner N, Alvarez W 1979 Impact of events scale: a measure of subjective stress. Psychosomatic Medicine 41(3): 209-218

Jensen M P, Karoly P, Huger R 1987 The development and preliminary validation of an instrument to assess patients' attitudes towards pain. Journal of Psychosomatic Research, 31:393–400

Jensen M P, Turner J A, Romano J M, Karoly P 1991 Coping with chronic pain: a critical review of the literature. Pain 47:249–283

Jensen M P, Turner J A, Romano J M, Lawler B K 1994 Relationships of pain-specific beliefs to chronic pain adjustment. Pain 57:301–309

Jensen M P, Turner J A, Romano J M, Strom S E 1995 The Chronic Pain Coping Inventory; development and preliminary validation. Pain 60:203–216

Kori S H, Miller R P, Todd B D 1990 Kinisophobia: a new view of chronic pain behaviour. Pain Management Jan/Feb: 35-43

Landis J R, Koch G G 1977 The measurement of observer agreement for categorical data. Biometrics 33:159–174

Lorig K, Chastain R I, Ung F, Shoor S, Holman H R 1989 Development and evaluation of a scale to measure perceived self-efficacy in people with arthritis. Arthritis and Rheumatism 32:37–44

Main C J 1983 The Modified Somatic Perception Questionnaire. Journal of Psychosomatic Research 27:503–514

Main C J, Waddell G 1984 The detection of psychological abnormality in chronic low back pain using four simple scales. Current Concepts in Pain 2:10–15

Main C J, Waddell G 1991 A comparison of cognitive measures in low back pain: statistical structure and clinical validity at initial assessment. Pain 46:287–298

Main C J, Wood P L R, Hollis S, Spanswick C C, Waddell G 1992 The distress and risk assessment method. A simple classification to identify distress and evaluate the risk of poor outcome. Spine 17:42–52

McNair D M, Lorr M, Proppleman L F 1971 Manual for the profile of mood states (POMS). Educational and Industrial Testing Service, San Diego, CA

Parker H, Wood P L R, Main C J 1995 The use of the pain drawing as a screening measure to predict psychological distress in chronic low back pain. Spine 20:236–234

Ransford A O, Cairns O, Mooney V 1976 The pain drawing as an aid to the psychological evaluation of patients with low back pain. Pain 1:127–134

Riley J F, Ahern D K, Follick M J 1988 Chronic pain and functional impairment: assessing beliefs about their relationship. Archives of Physical Medicine and Rehabilitation 69:579–582

Rosenstiel A K, Keefe F J 1983 The use of coping strategies in chronic low back pain patients: relationship to patient characteristics and current adjustment. Pain 17:33–44

Snow-Turek A L, Norris M P, Tan G 1996 Active and passive coping strategies in chronic pain patients. Pain 64:455–462

Spielberger C D 1988 The State-Trait Anger Expression Inventory. Psychological Assessment Resources, Florida

Strong J, Ashton R, Chant D 1992 The measurement of attitudes towards and beliefs about pain. Pain 48:227–236

Tait R C, Chibnall J T 1997 Development of a brief version of the Survey of Pain Attitudes. Pain 70:229–235

Todd C, Bradley C 1996 Evaluating the design and development of psychological scales. In: Bradley C (ed) Handbook of psychology and diabetes. Harwood Academic, The Netherlands, ch 2, pp 15–42

Vakkari T 1990 cited in Harkapaa K, Jarvikoski A, Vakkari T 1996 Locus of control beliefs in back pain patients. British Journal of Health Psychology 1:51–64

Vitaliano P P, Russo J, Carr J E, Maiuro R D, Becker J 1985 The Ways of Coping Checklist: revision and psychometric properties. Multivariate Behavioral Research 20:3–26

Waddell G, Newton M, Henderson I, Somerville D, Main C 1993 A Fear-Avoidance Beliefs Questionnaire (FABQ) and the role of fear avoidance beliefs in chronic low back pain. Pain 52:157–168

Wallston K A, Wallston B S, DeVellis B 1978 Development of the Multidimensional Health Locus of Control (MHLC) scales. Health Education Monographs 6:160–170

Williams D A, Thorn B E 1989 An empirical assessment of pain beliefs. Pain 36:351–358

Williams R C 1988 Toward a set of reliable and valid measures for chronic pain assessment and outcome research. Pain 35:239–251

APPENDIX: THE ASSESSMENT OF PSYCHIATRIC DISORDER

It has been estimated that a significant proportion of chronic pain patients have identifiable psychiatric illness. In the majority of chronic pain patients there is evidence of emotional disturbance such as anxiety, depression or anger. Frequently the emotional intensity is not sufficient to indicate the need for formal psychiatric evaluation. Psychiatric disorder may antedate the development of pain, coexist with the presence of a pain syndrome or develop as a consequence of it. In patients in whom the reason for their distress is not associated with their pain, or in whom the severity of their distress is an obstacle to pain management, a formal assessment of the need for primary psychiatric treatment should be undertaken. (An example of an interview questionnaire used for this assessment is given at the end of this appendix.)

The most commonly used assessment systems are the International Classification of diseases and related health problems, now in its 10th edition (ICD-10), and the Diagnostic and Statistical Manual of Mental Disorders (DSM), now in its fourth edition (DSM-IV 1994). Currently the most commonly used system (certainly in the UK) appears to be the DSM-IV. Assessment of psychiatric disorder requires specialised training but for those not familiar with it a brief description of a number of the more commonly found diagnoses in pain patients is offered here. The actual diagnostic criteria from DSM-IV, together with their classification numbers, are also reproduced.

GENERALISED ANXIETY DISORDER

Generalised anxiety disorder is characterised by excessive anxiety and worry on more days than not for the previous 6 months; it is associated with a number of other symptoms such as restlessness, fatigue, difficulty concentrating, sleep disturbance and muscle tension, and the anxiety itself causes significant distress or impairment.

Pain patients are normally focused on *specific* concerns about pain, its effects and its significance. The major characteristics for generalised disorder are:

- excessive anxiety and worry occurring more days than not for at least 6 months, about a number of events and activities
- difficult in controlling the worry
- associated with three or more of the following symptoms:
  - restlessness or feeling keyed up or on edge
  - being easily fatigued
  - difficulty in concentrating or the mind going blank
  - irritability
  - muscle tension
  - sleep disturbance
- focus not confined to features of another axis I disorder
- anxiety, worry or physical symptoms causing clinically significant distress or impairment in functioning
- not due to direct physiological effects of a substance.

The full diagnostic criteria for generalised anxiety disorder (classified as 300.02 in the DSM-IV) are presented in Box 10A.1.

ANXIETY DUE TO A GENERAL MEDICAL CONDITION

Anxiety due to a general medical condition is clinically significant anxiety judged to be due to the *direct physiological effects* of a general medical condition. In a sense the physiological effects mimic primary psychological symptoms (such as tachycardia). Such features can usually be diagnosed only if a disorder other than a pain syndrome is present. The full diagnostic criteria for an anxiety disorder secondary to a medical condition (classified as 293.84 in the DSM-IV) are shown in Box 10A.2.

Box 10A.1 Diagnostic criteria for generalised anxiety disorder

A. Excessive anxiety and worry (apprehensive expectation), occurring more days than not for at least 6 months, about a number of events or activities (such as work or school performance)
B. The person finds it difficult to control the worry
C. The anxiety and worry are associated with three (or more) of the following six symptoms (with at least some symptoms present for more days than not for the past `6 months). **Note:** Only one item is required in children.

  (1) restlessness or feeling keyed up or on edge
  (2) being easily fatigued
  (3) difficulty concentrating or mind going blank
  (4) irritability
  (5) muscle tension
  (6) sleep disturbance (difficulty falling or staying asleep, or restless unsatisfying sleep)

D. The focus of the anxiety and worry is not confined to features of an axis I disorder, e.g., the anxiety or worry is not about having a panic attack (as in panic disorder), being embarrassed in public (as in social phobia), being contaminated (as in obsessive–compulsive disorder), being away from home or close relatives (as in separation anxiety disorder), gaining weight (as in anorexia nervosa), having multiple physical complaints (as in somatisation disorder), or having a serious illness (as in hypochondriasis), and the anxiety and worry do not occur exclusively during post-traumatic stress disorder
E. The anxiety, worry, or physical symptoms cause clinically significant distress or impairment in social, occupational, or other important areas of functioning
F. The disturbance is not due to the direct physiological effects of a substance (e.g. a drug of abuse, a medication) or a general medical condition (e.g. hyperthyroidism) and does not occur exclusively during a mood disorder, a psychotic disorder, or a pervasive developmental disorder

---

Box 10A.2 Diagnostic criteria for anxiety disorder due to … [indicate the general medical condition]

A. Prominent anxiety, panic attacks, or obsessions or compulsions predominate in the clinical picture
B. There is evidence from the history, physical examination, or laboratory findings that the disturbance is the direct physiological consequence of a general medical condition
C. The disturbance is not better accounted for by another mental disorder (e.g. adjustment disorder with anxiety in which the stressor is a serious general medical condition)
D. The disturbance does not occur exclusively during the course of a delirium
E. The disturbance causes clinically significant distress or impairment in social, occupational, or other important areas of functioning

Specify if:
  with generalized anxiety: if excessive anxiety or worry about a number of events or activities predominates in the clinical presentation
  with panic attacks: if panic attacks predominate in the clinical presentation
  with obsessive–compulsive symptoms: if obsessions or compulsions predominate in the clinical presentation

Coding note: Include the name of the general medical condition on axis I, e.g. 293.84 anxiety disorder due to pheochromocytoma, With generalized anxiety; also code the general medical condition on axis III.

DEPRESSION

The importance of depression has been discussed at length in Chapter 2. As previously discussed, although history of depression constitutes an increased risk for the development of chronic pain, pain is a stronger predictor of depression. The depression observed in many pain patients would not be sufficiently intense to constitute the basis for a diagnosable psychiatric illness. In fact pain management is arguably the preferred treatment option for depression secondary to pain-associated incapacity.

The principal features of clinical depression are shown below. Five of the following nine symptoms must be continuously present over a 2-week period:

• depressed mood
• loss of pleasure or interest in most activities
• weight or appetite changes
• increased or decreased sleep

Box 10A.3   Criteria for major depressive episode

A. Five (or more) of the following symptoms have been present during the same 2-week period and represent a change from previous functioning; at least one of the symptoms is either (1) depressed mood or (2) loss of interest or pleasure.

Note: Do not include symptoms that are clearly due to a general medical condition, or mood-incongruent delusions or hallucinations.

(1) depressed mood most of the day, nearly every day, as indicated by either subjective report (e.g. feels sad or empty) or observation made by others (e.g. appears tearful). **Note:** In children and adolescents, can be irritable mood
(2) markedly diminished interest or pleasure in all, or almost all, activities most of the day, nearly every day (as indicated by either subjective account or observation made by others)
(3) significant weight loss when not dieting or weight gain (e.g. a change of more than 5% of body weight in a month), or decrease or increase in appetite nearly every day. **Note:** In children, consider failure to make expected weight gains
(4) insomnia or hypersomnia nearly every day
(5) psychomotor agitation or retardation nearly every day (observable by others, not merely subjective feelings of restlessness or being slowed down)

(6) fatigue or loss of energy nearly every day
(7) feelings of worthlessness or excessive or inappropriate guilt (which may be delusional) nearly every day (not merely self-reproach or guilt about being sick)
(8) diminished ability to think or concentrate, or indecisiveness, nearly every day (either by subjective account or as observed by others)
(9) recurrent thoughts of death (not just fear of dying), recurrent suicidal ideation without a specific plan, or a suicide attempt or a specific plan for committing suicide

B. The symptoms do not meet criteria for a mixed episode
C. The symptoms cause clinically significant distress or impairment in social, occupational, or other important areas of functioning
D. The symptoms are not due to the direct physiological effects of a substance (e.g. a drug of abuse, a medication) or a general medical condition (e.g. hypothyroidism)
E. The symptoms are not better accounted for by bereavement, i.e., after the loss of a loved one, the symptoms persist for longer than 2 months or are characterised by marked functional impairment, morbid preoccupation with worthlessness, suicidal ideation, psychotic symptoms, or psychomotor retardation

---

- increased or decreased psychomotor activity
- fatigue
- feelings of guilt or worthlessness
- reduced ability to concentrate/make decisions
- recurrent thoughts of death or suicide.

Criteria for a major depressive episode are presented in Box 10A.3.

SOMATOFORM DISORDERS

The term 'somatiform disorder' is used to cover a variety of disorders in which physical symptoms suggesting a physical condition cause significant distress or impairment, but are not fully explained by a general medical condition. The major types are shown in Box 10A.4.

Recently, the term 'somatisation' has become popular. Somatisation disorders (formerly described as hysteria, or Briquet's syndrome) are characterised by multiple symptoms, beginning before the age of 30 years, extending over many

---

Box 10A.4   Types of somatiform disorder

- Somatisation disorder
- Undifferentiated somatiform disorder
- Conversion disorder
- Pain disorder
- Hypochondriasis
- Body dysmorphic disorder
- Somatiform disorder not otherwise specified

---

years and including a combination of pain, gastrointestinal, sexual and pseudoneurological symptoms. They differ from 'psychological factors affecting medical condition' in that there is no diagnosable general medical condition to account for the physical symptoms. A lesser variant (undifferentiated somatiform disorder) has been evoked to classify patients not quite fulfilling the criteria for a somatisation disorder. The major criteria for somatisation disorder (classified as 300.81 in the DSM-IV) are shown in Box 10A.5.

Box 10A.5 Diagnostic criteria for somatisation disorder

A. A history of many physical complaints beginning before age 30 years that occur over a period of several years and result in treatment being sought or significant impairment in social, occupational, or other important areas of functioning.

B. Each of the following criteria must have been met, with individual symptoms occurring at any time during the course of the disturbance:

(1) *four pain symptoms:* a history of pain related to at least four different sites or functions (e.g. head, abdomen, back, joints, extremities, chest, rectum, during menstruation, during sexual intercourse, or during urination)

(2) *two gastrointestinal symptoms:* a history of at least two gastrointestinal symptoms other than pain (e.g. nausea, bloating, vomiting other than during pregnancy, diarrhoea, or intolerance of several different foods)

(3) *one sexual symptom:* a history of at least one sexual or reproductive symptom other than pain (e.g. sexual indifference, erectile or ejaculatory dysfunction, irregular menses, excessive menstrual bleeding, vomiting throughout pregnancy)

(4) *one pseudoneurological symptom:* a history of at least one symptom or deficit suggesting a neurological condition not limited to pain (conversion symptoms such as impaired coordination or balance, paralysis or localised weakness, difficulty swallowing or lump in throat, aphonia, urinary retention, hallucinations, loss of touch or pain sensation, double vision, blindness, deafness, seizures; dissociative symptoms such as amnesia; or loss of consciousness other than fainting)

C. Either (1) or (2):

(1) after appropriate investigation, each of the symptoms in criterion B cannot be fully explained by a known general medical condition or the direct effects of a substance (e.g., a drug of abuse, a medication)

(2) when there is a related general medical condition, the physical complaints or resulting social or occupational impairment are in excess of what would be expected from the history, physical examination, or laboratory findings

D. The symptoms are not intentionally produced or feigned (as in factitious disorder or malingering).

Box 10A.6 Diagnostic criteria for conversion disorder

A. One or more symptoms or deficits affecting voluntary motor or sensory function that suggest a neurological or other general medical condition

B. Psychological factors are judged to be associated with the symptom or deficit because the initiation or exacerbation of the symptom or deficit is preceded by conflicts or other stressors

C. The symptom or deficit is not intentionally produced or feigned (as in factitious disorder or malingering)

D. The symptom or deficit cannot, after appropriate investigation, be fully explained by a general medical condition, or by the direct effects of a substance, or as a culturally sanctioned behaviour or experience

E. The symptom or deficit causes clinically significant distress or impairment in social, occupational, or other important areas of functioning or warrants medical evaluation

F. The symptom or deficit is not limited to pain or sexual dysfunction, does not occur exclusively during the course of somatisation disorder, and is not better accounted for by another mental disorder

Specify type of symptom or deficit:
with motor symptom or deficit
with sensory symptom or deficit
with seizures or convulsions
with mixed presentation

Conversion disorder

Conversion disorder is characterised by unexplained symptoms or deficits affecting voluntary motor or sensory function that suggest a neurological or other general medical condition. Psychological factors are judged to be associated with the symptoms or deficits. Such a diagnosis should be made with extreme caution, since it may lead to complacency in proper investigation of the physical basis of a complaint; and lead to the patient being labelled perjoratively and taken less than seriously. The diagnosis is usually unhelpful in the context of chronic pain since it is safe to assume (unless proved otherwise) that there *is* a physical basis for the complaint. Although less fashionable than formerly, patients will sometimes be given such a diagnosis. The full diagnostic criteria (classified as 300.11 in the DSM-IV) are shown in Box 10A.6.

Box 10A.7 *Diagnostic criteria for hypochondriasis*

A. Preoccupation with fears of having, or the idea that one has, a serious disease based on the person's misinterpretation of bodily symptoms
B. The preoccupation persists despite appropriate medical evaluation and reassurance
C. The belief in criterion A is not of delusional intensity (as in delusional disorder, somatic type) and is not restricted to a circumscribed concern about appearance (as in body dysmorphic disorder)
D. The preoccupation causes clinically significant distress or impairment in social, occupational, or other important areas of functioning

E. The duration of the disturbance is at least 6 months
F. The preoccupation is not better accounted for by generalised anxiety disorder, obsessive–compulsive disorder, panic disorder, a major depressive episode, separation anxiety, or another somatoform disorder

Specify if:
with poor insight: if, for most of the time during the current episode, the person does not recognise that the concern about having a serious illness is excessive or unreasonable

---

Hypochondriasis

The essential feature of hypochondriasis is preoccupation with the fear of having, or the idea that one has, a serious disease based on one's misinterpretation of bodily symptoms. In the context of chronic pain, a primary diagnosis of hypochondriasis (as with conversion hysteria) should be made only with considerable caution after a comprehensive cognitive and behavioural evaluation has been undertaken. Diagnostic criteria for hypochondriasis (classified as 300.7 in the DSM-IV) are shown in Box 10A.7.

ADJUSTMENT DISORDERS

An adjustment disorder is characterised by clinically significant emotional or behavioural symptoms in response to an identifiable psychosocial stress or stressor. The symptoms must develop within 3 months of the stressor and resolve within 6 months of its termination, although it may persist for a prolonged period (i.e. longer than 6 months) if occurring in response to a chronic stressor (e.g. a chronic disabling medical condition). Almost all patients could be considered to fall within this category, and therefore the diagnosis does appear to be particularly helpful. The diagnostic criteria for adjustment disorders (classified as 309.0 → 309.9 in the DSM-IV) are shown in Box 10A.8.

POST-TRAUMATIC STRESS DISORDER

The essential characteristics of post-traumatic stress disorder or PTSD are the development of a set of psychological and physiological symptoms following a traumatic event (such as a serious road traffic accident). Assuming the event can be considered of such an nature as potentially to fulfil criteria for the basis of such a disorder, the person must persistently re-experience the event in a number of ways, demonstrate persistent avoidance of stimuli associated with the trauma and experience persistent symptoms of increased arousal. If the individual demonstrates sufficient evidence of feaures in each of these categories, and if the duration of the symptoms is greater than 1 month, then the individual may be considered to be suffering from a diagnosable post-traumatic stress disorder. The specific criteria (classified as 309.81 in the DSM-IV) are shown in Box 10A.9.

PAIN DISORDER

The DSM-IV classification of pain disorder is unhelpful. It purports to distinguish three subtypes, depending on the relative importance of the psychological factors in comparison with the general medical condition. It is wise to assume that all significant pain problems have both a

---

Box 10A.8 Diagnostic criteria for adjustment disorders

A. The development of emotional or behavioural symptoms in response to an identifiable stressor(s) occurring within 3 months of the onset of the stressor(s)
B. These symptoms or behaviours are clinically significant as evidenced by either of the following:
   (1) marked distress that is in excess of what would be expected from exposure to the stressor
   (2) significant impairment in social or occupational (academic) functioning
C. The stress-related disturbance does not meet the criteria for another specific axis I disorder and is not merely an exacerbation of a pre-existing axis I or axis II disorder
D. The symptoms do not represent bereavement

E. Once the stressor (or its consequences) has terminated, the symptoms do not persist for more than an additional 6 months

Specify if:
   acute: if the disturbance lasts less than 6 months
   chronic: if the disturbance lasts for 6 months or longer

Adjustment disorders are coded based on the subtype, which is selected according to the predominant symptoms. The specific stressor(s) can be specified on axis IV.
   309.0 with depressed mood
   309.24 with anxiety
   309.28 with mixed anxiety and depressed mood
   309.3 with disturbance of conduct
   309.4 with mixed disturbance of emotions and conduct
   309.9 unspecified

Box 10A.9 Diagnostic criteria for post-traumatic stress disorder

A. The person has been exposed to a traumatic event in which both of the following were present:
   (1) the person experienced, witnessed, or was confronted with an event or events that involved actual or threatened death or serious injury, or a threat to the physical integrity of self or others
   (2) the person's response involved intense fear, helplessness, or horror. **Note:** In children, this may be expressed instead by disorganised or agitated behaviour
B. The traumatic event is persistently re-experienced in one (or more) of the following ways:
   (1) recurrent and intrusive distressing recollections of the event, including images, thoughts, or perceptions. **Note:** In young children, repetitive play may occur in which themes or aspects of the trauma are expressed
   (2) recurrent distressing dreams of the event. **Note:** In children, there may be frightening dreams without recognisable content
   (3) acting or feeling as if the traumatic event were recurring (includes a sense of reliving the experience, illusions, hallucinations, and dissociative flashback episodes, including those that occur on awakening or when intoxicated). **Note:** In young children, trauma-specific reenactment may occur
   (4) intense psychological distress at exposure to internal or external cues that symbolise or resemble an aspect of the traumatic event
   (5) physiological reactivity on exposure to internal or external cues that symbolise or resemble an aspect of the traumatic event
C. Persistent avoidance of stimuli associated with the trauma and numbing of general responsiveness (not

present before the trauma), as indicated by three (or more) of the following:
   (1) efforts to avoid thoughts, feelings, or conversations associated with the trauma
   (2) efforts to avoid activities, places, or people that arouse recollections of the trauma
   (3) inability to recall an important aspect of the trauma
   (4) markedly diminished interest or participation in significant activities
   (5) feeling of detachment or estrangement from others
   (6) restricted range of affect (e.g. unable to have loving feelings)
   (7) sense of a foreshortened future (e.g. does not expect to have a career, marriage, children, or a normal life span)

D. Persistent symptoms of increased arousal (not present before the trauma), as indicated by two (or more) of the following:
   (1) difficulty falling or staying asleep
   (2) irritability or outbursts of anger
   (3) difficulty concentrating
   (4) hypervigilance
   (5) exaggerated startle response

E. Duration of the disturbance (symptoms in criteria B, C, and D) is more than 1 month
F. The disturbance causes clinically significant distress or impairment in social, occupational, or other important areas of functioning

Specify if:
   acute: if duration of symptoms is less than 3 months
   chronic: if duration of symptoms is 3 months or more

Specify if:
   with delayed onset: if onset of symptoms is at least 6 months after the stressor

Box 10A.10 Diagnostic criteria for pain disorder

A. Pain in one or more anatomical sites is the predominant focus of the clinical presentation and is of sufficient severity to warrant clinical attention

B. The pain causes clinically significant distress or impairment in social, occupational, or other important areas of functioning

C. Psychological factors are judged to have an important role in the onset, severity, exacerbation, or maintenance of the pain

D. The symptom or deficit is not intentionally produced or feigned (as in factitious disorder or malingering)

E. The pain is not better accounted for by a mood, anxiety, or psychotic disorder and does not meet criteria for dyspareunia

Code as follows:

307.80 pain disorder associated with psychological factors: psychological factors are judged to have the major role in the onset, severity, exacerbation, or maintenance of the pain. (If a general medical condition is present, it does not have a major role in the onset, severity, exacerbation, or maintenance of the pain.) This type of pain disorder is not diagnosed if criteria are also met for somatisation disorder

Specify if:
acute: duration of less than 6 months
chronic: duration of 6 months or longer
307.89 pain disorder associated with both psychological factors and a general medical

condition: both psychological factors and a general medical condition are judged to have important roles in the onset, severity, exacerbation, or maintenance of the pain. The associated general medical condition or anatomical site of the pain (see below) is coded on axis III

Specify if:
acute: duration of less than 6 months
chronic: duration of 6 months or longer
Note: The following is not considered to be a mental disorder and is included here to facilitate differential diagnosis.

pain disorder associated with a general medical condition: a general medical condition has a major role in the onset, severity, exacerbation, or maintenance of the pain. (If psychological factors are present, they are not judged to have a major role in the onset, severity, exacerbation, or maintenance of the pain.) The diagnostic code for the pain is selected based on the associated general medical condition if one has been established or on the anatomical location of the pain if the underlying general medical condition is not yet clearly established—for example, low back (724.2), sciatic (724.3), pelvic (625.9), headache (784.0), facial (784.0), chest (786.50), joint (719.4), bone (733.90), abdominal (789.0), breast (611.71), renal (788.0), ear (388.70), eye (379.91), throat (784.1), tooth (525.9), and urinary (788.0)

---

physiological and a psychological component (Chs 1 and 2) unless there is overwhelming evidence to the contrary. The diagnostic criteria for pain disorder are shown in Box 10A.10.

PERSONALITY OR CHARACTER DISORDER

In addition to the identification of psychiatric disease, DSM-IV offers an appraisal of various types or personality disorder or character disor-

der, the identification of which is considered by clinicians to indicate a poor prognosis for outcome from pain management, or even be a contraindication to acceptance for treatment. The major types of personality disorder are illustrated in Box 10A.11.

In general clinical practice, however, such classifications are seldom helpful and, as Gatchel, Polatin & Kinney (1995) have indicated, the scientific evidence for such disorders being contraindications for treatment is not clearly established.

REFERENCES

DSM-IV 1994 Diagnostic and Statistical Manual of Mental Disorders, 4th edn. American Psychiatric Association, Washington DC

Gatchel R J, Polatin P B, Kinney R K 1995 Predicting outcome of chronic back pain using clinical predictors of psychopathology: a prospective analysis. Health Psychology 14:415–420

ICD-10 1994 International Statistical Classification of Diseases and related health problems, 10th edn. World Health Organisation, Geneva

---

Box 10A.11   Major types of personality disorder

- *Paranoid personality disorder* is a pattern of distrust and suspiciousness such that others' motives are interpreted as malevolent
- *Schizoid personality disorder* is a pattern of detachment from social relationships and a restricted range of emotional expression
- *Schizotypal personality disorder* is a pattern of acute discomfort in close relationships, cognitive or perceptual distortions, and eccentricities of behaviour
- *Antisocial personality disorder* is a pattern of disregard for, and violation of, the rights of others
- *Borderline personality disorder* is a pattern of instability in interpersonal relationships, self-image and affects, and marked impulsivity

- *Histrionic personality disorder* is a pattern of excessive emotionality and attention seeking
- *Narcissistic personality disorder* is a pattern of grandiosity, need for admiration and lack of empathy
- *Avoidant personality disorder* is a pattern of social inhibition, feelings of inadequacy and hypersensitivity to negative evaluation
- *Dependent personality disorder* is a pattern of submissive and clinging behaviour related to an excessive need to be taken care of
- *Obsessive–compulsive personality disorder* is a pattern of preoccupation with orderliness, perfectionism and control

---

AN EXAMPLE OF A STRUCTURED INTERVIEW FORM

Name:_____ D.O.B. _____ Date: _____

N.B. The ratings shown at the end of each category are not intended to represent literal descriptions of your clinical impression, they merely form a means of characterising an index of severity/intensity of response.

INTRODUCTION

Before I begin my assessment, allow me to explain why a clinical psychologist is involved in the management of chronic pain I would like to empha sis at the outset, that none of the staff at this centre believe that your pain is imagined, or all in the mind; we take your pain seriously. However, most people who suffer chronic pain tell us that it effects their work life, social life, family life and indeed sometimes how they view themselves; most people recognise that suffering for long periods of time can have such effects. My involvement therefore, is to determine what impact pain has had on your life and whether the programme can address some of your needs. Whilst I have certainly examined your medical notes, they obviously don't reflect your experiences, thoughts or feelings about what has happened to you. Finally, in order to help me put your present life circumstances into perspective, I would like to understand how you have coped with any other challenges that you have faced prior to the onset of your back pain.

HISTORY OF RECOVERY FROM PAIN ONSET/INJURY

1) When did you first experience back pain?   Month:_____   Year: _____

2) On that occasion how did your back pain start?
_____
_____

3) Did you see a specialist at that time? Did treatment help you to get over this first episode of pain?
_____
_____

4) How did your most recent episode of pain come about?
_____
_____

5) How many specialists have you consulted for your pain problem?
_____
_____

6) Considering your present level of pain, how long has it been like it is now?
_____

Optional question if patient had accident or injury:

7) Following your accident, were you troubled by frightening memories or dreams; (if yes) do they still bother you?
_____
_____

Rating: (Circle)
Insidious Onset/Traumatic Onset   Recurrent Episodes/Continuous Episode

CAUSAL BELIEFS

Obviously you have seen a number of doctors and specialists about your pain, what have they told you?

1)

a) Don't understand what was said: _____

b) Disc disease/collapse: _____

c) Bulging disc: _____

d) Nerve entrapment: _____

e) Nerve damage: _____

f) Arachnoiditis: _____

g) Rheumatoid/Osteo-Arthritis: _____

h) Unstable spine: _____

i) Muscle spasm: _____

j) Fibromyalgia: _____

k) Normal age-related wear & tear: _____

l) Other diagnosis: _____

2) Do you worry that the medical examinations may have missed something (eg. cancer)?

_____

_____

3) I obviously don't expect you to be a doctor, but what do you think is wrong?

_____

_____

4) Are there any treatments or examinations that you feel you should have had?

_____

_____

5) When activity increases the pain, do you think *actual* physical damage has occurred?

_____

_____

6) Do you expect your condition to change over the next 5 years?

_____

_____

7) If you do not get relief from your pain, how do you see the future?

_____

_____

Rating:

Firm conviction of ongoing pathology 3
Confused, has negative prognosis, will need convincing 2
Confused, open mind about prognosis, appreciate explanation 1
Reasonable understanding and appropriate view of future 0

IATROGENIC DISTRESS

1) Do you feel angry or aggrieved as a result of the way you have been treated by the health profession?

_____

_____

2) Has your partner been upset by the way you have been treated?

_____

_____

3) If you knew before your surgery/injections/physiotherapy what you know now, would you still agree that it was appropriate?

4) Have you been told that it is dangerous to do certain activities by health professionals?

5) To what extent do you feel that advice was appropriate?

6) In the course of your previous treatment was there ever a suggestion that you see a psychologist or psychiatrist? (patient's reaction; content, duration and place of treatment).

Rating:

Iatrogenic Distress

Overt hostility and alienation 3
Unresolved, situational anger, complacent 2
Resolved previous anger 1
No evidence of disaffection 0

Iatrogenic Dysfunction

Rigid compliance with inappropriate advice 3
Largely committed to maladaptive behaviour 2
Inconsistent compliance with inappropriate advice 1
Has maintained appropriate functioning 0

OCCUPATIONAL ISSUES

1) Have you been medically retired or laid-off because of your back pain? (How long?)

2) Do you feel that your employer was/is fair with you?

3) How have you coped with being out of work for ... months/years?

4) What aspects of that job did you like, and what things did you not enjoy?

5) If an employer was willing to employ someone with pain, do you think a future working life has something to offer you?

Rating: Occupational Ambition

Angry and frustrated in previous job, no occupational goals or incentives 3
Wants to work but overwhelmed by perceived obstacles 2
Wants to work but needs some help with confidence and sense of direction 1
Fully motivated, clear sense of direction, and actively seeking (or in) work 0

Analysis of Coping Behaviours

I'd like, if I may, to ask about how you manage your pain from day to day, and how changes in your lifestyle have affected those closest to you. May I ask first, with whom you share your home and what other people play an important part in your everyday life?

Home: Husband/Wife/Children Boys_____ (gender/age) Girls _____
Visitors: _____

Pain Management Stategies

1) What have you found to be the best way of managing your pain (*ask:* sitting/lying down; relaxation technique; distraction; activation; medication; massage; hot/cold pack)?

_____

_____

2) How much time during the day would you spend sitting/lying down? (good/bad day)

Good Day	Less than 1 hour	1–2 hours	2–4 hours	4+ hours
Bad Day	Less than 1 hour	1–2 hours	2–4 hours	4+ hours

3) On a bad day, how many tablets has the pain *made you take*?

_____

_____

4) Over the last month, how many bad days each week have you had, on average?

_____

5) Does alcohol help to ease your pain?

No/Moderately/Completely/Don't Drink

6) What would you drink on a weekday as opposed to a weekend?

_____

_____

6a) Have your drinking habits changed as a result of your pain?

_____

7) Apart from prescribed drugs, do you use other drugs (eg. cannibis) to manage your pain?

_____

8) Have you had to seek emergency pain treatment or GP call-out in the past year?

_____

9) When you have a good day, do you try to do as much as you can in order to make up for lost time? (explain)

_____

Rating: Pain Management Strategies

Passive, helpless, no good days, excessive drug (ab)use 3
Little evidence of active coping, mostly bad days, poor drug management 2
Active coping, reasonable drug regime, some inappropriate healthcare usage 1
Active coping, sensible use of drugs, non-reliance on primary care services 0

Family's Solicitous Behaviour

1) Has anyone in the family taken-over activities which used to be your responsibility? Ask about (circle):
Vacuuming: laundry: ironing: shopping: cooking: DIY: garden: childcare: parental care.
2) Who helps with these activities?

_____

3) What particular activities would they advise you against doing?

_____

4) When your family notice that you are suffering a lot, what do they do? Enquire (circle):
Console you; Advise remedial action; Take remedial action; Avoid you; Ignore you; Argue with you.

_____

Rating: Family's Solicitous Behaviour

Gross pain behaviour, completely dependent upon solicitous or disaffected care-givers . . .3
Obtrusive behavioural response to challenge, little independent function, solicitous carers 2
Partially obtrusive pain behaviour, capable of independent function, family challenged 1
Appropriate behaviour, independent functioning, role maintenance, family harmony 0

Famial & Social Adjustment

1) As far as your social and recreational life is concerned, what activities do you currently do? What have you stopped doing because of pain?

2) Does this cause difficulties with family life?

3) Has pain made you short-tempered or difficult to live with?

4) Has the way you cope with pain been the focus of family arguments?

5) *People have told me that living with back pain can often test a relationship, for eg., it can strain a close relationship but it can also bring a couple closer together.* Has there been a change in the way you and your partner relate to each other as time has passed?

(Optional) Security of Relationship

1) Is the security of your relationship threatened?

2) (If ambivalent about relationship) If your relationship were to end, how would this affect you?

Rating: Familial & Social Adjustment

Dysfunctional social withdrawal, major family conflict, relationship threatened 3
Goes out rarely, episodes of significant dysharmony, in otherwise stable relationship 2
Goes to external venues/visits people on good days, 'bad day' rows, stable relationship . . .1
Engages in full social and family activities, non-solicitous and harmonious relationship . . .0

Current Life Stress

During previous pain management programmes we have found that in addition to having to cope with the burden of pain, people were struggling with other problems of everyday life. In order to prevent us putting an over-whelming burden on you I'd like to check on a number of things which can cause difficulties in anyone's life.

1) *Financial:*

Do you find yourself pre-occupied with money worries? Are problems with debt getting on top of you?

2) *Welfare System:*

Have you had any difficulties getting or keeping your social security benefits?

3) *Medico-legal:*

Are you pursuing a claim for compensation? Is it progressing satisfactorily?

---

4) *Work Stress:*

Are you/your partner facing pressure from work?

---

5) *Dependent Relatives:*

Is the health of a close relative worrying you?

---

6) *Child Behavioural Problems:*

Sometimes children can be more of a handful when one parent is unwell; are you concerned about their behaviour or well-being?

---

7) *Post-Traumatic Stress:*

At some point in our lives we can witness or be involved in a tragic accident; has this happened to you? Do you continue to be troubled by memories or nightmares about this?

---

8) *Fears & Phobias:*

About half of the population experience a fear or phobia at some time during life, are you troubled by anxieties such as enclosed spaces; the feeling that things have to be perfect?

---

9) Is anyone close to you under-going a period of emotional distress?

---

10) Have you or any member of your family had any brushes with the law lately?

Rating: **Current Life Stress**

Chronic denial/over-whelmed by stressor(s), unable to fulfil minor responsibilities, ...3
Severely challenged but able to distract self and maintain core responsiblities 2
Situationally pre-occupied, but capable of fulfilling all responsibilities 1
No stressors or active problem-solving and effective stress management 0

Psychosocial History

You have helped me to gain a good understanding of your present situation. I would like now to put this into the context of how you managed to cope with the other major changes and challenges that can affect us during our life, from childhood onwards. For instance.

1) *Disruption during Childhood:*

Were you troubled by illness during the first ten years of life?

Were those years disrupted by any other unusual situations?

_____
_____
_____
_____

2) *Disruption during Adolescence:*

Between the age of 11 and 16 were you faced with any changes in lifestyle or family circumstances?

_____
_____
_____
_____

3) *Physical/Sexual Abuse:*

Nowadays society is more aware of the ways in which young people can be *maltreated* by adults, have you ever been subjected to anything which has left you feeling distressed? (Prompt if hesitant: *Something of an emotional, physical or sexual nature?*)

_____
_____
_____

4) *Adulthood:*

Employment and personal relationships provide the major sources of influence in our adult life; could you briefly describe these and the major changes, challenges or turning points in your life from the time you left secondary school to the onset of your back pain?

_____
_____
_____
_____
_____
_____

How did your life change at that time?

_____
_____

What jobs have you done and why did you change jobs?

_____
_____

Sometimes the onset of pain comes at a time when the family was dealing with challenging circumstances, did the start of your pain make any circumstances more difficult to deal with?

_____
_____

5) *Family Medical History:*

Has any member of your family suffered from chronic pain or any major medical or emotional difficulties?

_____
_____
_____

6) *Bereavement:*

One of the major events in anyone's life is the loss of a loved one – have you lost someone you cared for? Can you tell me when he/she died and how it happened?
Father: Mother: Brother: Sister: Partner: Child: Grandparent(s): Other family: Friend

_____
_____
_____
_____

Optional questions re: Unresolved grief.

6a) *Intrusive thoughts:*

Are you presently troubled by distressing images, thoughts, memories or dreams of X / someone you've lost?

6b) *Denial:*

Do you avoid, wherever possible, thinking or talking about X, or doing anything which reminds you of X? Have you found it difficult to accept his/her death?

6c) *Failure to adapt: (Beyond 13 months)*

Up to the present time, have you found it difficult to resume your social responsibilities or form new relationships.

7) *History of Psychological/Psychiatric Intervention:*

As a result of anything that has happened in the past, have you ever been referred to a Psychologist or Psychiatrist or Counsellor? How many times did you attend. What treatment did you receive?

How would you describe your mood over the last month or so?

Rating: Psychosocial History

Tragic life events/catastrophic response to events/unresolved/denial/impaired function. . . .3
Normal life events/extreme response to events/partially resolved/episodic active coping . .2
Normal life event recently/normal emotional reaction/? resolved/active coping 1
Functioning normally 0

Do you have any questions you would like the team to address during the feedback session?

Interview with Partner/Family member:

How do you think X copes with his/her situation?

How is the family coping with the present situation?

Is there anything that he/she presently finds distressing other than pain?

PLC

This is a questionnaire to find out how you see the causes and control of your pain. Just rate each statement by marking **X** in one of the boxes on the right which best shows how much you currently feel the statement applies to you.

CODES			
0	1	2	3

		Very true	True	Untrue	Very untrue
1	I need my medication to control my pain				
2	My pain will often go away if I let myself relax physically				
3	No matter what I do, I cannot seem to have an effect on my pain				
4	I can make my pain decrease if I concentrate on pain-free parts of my body				
5	I need the help of others to control my pain				
6	I can sometimes reduce pain by imagining the pain is really a pleasant stimulation				
7	Only I can help myself with the pain				
8	My pain level will go down if I remain passive and don't respond to it				
9	My pain professionals can help with my pain				
10	Sometimes I can reduce my pain by not paying attention to it				
11	I am responsible for how the pain affects me				
12	I can make pain go away by believing it will go away				
13	My pain just comes and goes, regardless of what I do or think				
14	My pain will decrease if I think of things going on around me				
15	Being in pain is never my choice				
16	I can reduce pain if I imagine a situation in which I have been pain free in the past				
17	Medication helps me control my pain				
18	My pain will get better if I think of pleasant thoughts				
19	My pain is out of control				
20	Just slowing down and regulating my breathing pattern often helps my pain				

CSQ

People who experience pain develop many ways of coping with it. Below is a list of common ways of dealing with pain. Actual activities and thoughts about pain are included.

For EACH question please indicate HOW OFTEN you do each of the activities by CIRCLING the number on the right which fits best. There are no right or wrong answers.

0 means you NEVER engage in the activity; 3 that you SOMETIMES engage in it; 6 that you ALWAYS do it—but remember you may choose any number from 0 to 6.

```
      0      1      2      3      4      5      6
   NEVER            SOMETIMES            ALWAYS
                                              N      S      A
```

1	I try to feel distant from the pain, almost as if the pain was in someone else's body	0 1 2 3 4 5 6
2	I leave the house and do something, such as going to the movies or shopping	0 1 2 3 4 5 6
3	I try to think of something pleasant	0 1 2 3 4 5 6
4	I don't think of it as pain but rather as a dull or warm feeling	0 1 2 3 4 5 6
5	It's terrible and I feel it's never going to get any better	0 1 2 3 4 5 6
6	I tell myself to be brave and carry on despite the pain	0 1 2 3 4 5 6
7	I read	0 1 2 3 4 5 6
8	I tell myself that I can overcome the pain	0 1 2 3 4 5 6
9	I take medication	0 1 2 3 4 5 6
10	I count numbers in my head or run a song through my mind	0 1 2 3 4 5 6
11	I just think of it as some other sensation such as numbness	0 1 2 3 4 5 6
12	It's awful and I feel that it overwhelms me	0 1 2 3 4 5 6
13	I play mental games with myself to keep my mind off the pain	0 1 2 3 4 5 6
14	I feel my life isn't worth living	0 1 2 3 4 5 6
15	I think someone will be here to help me, and it will go away for a while	0 1 2 3 4 5 6
16	I walk a lot	0 1 2 3 4 5 6
17	I pray to God it won't last long	0 1 2 3 4 5 6
18	I try not to think of it as my body, but rather as something separate from me	0 1 2 3 4 5 6
19	I relax	0 1 2 3 4 5 6
20	I don't think about the pain	0 1 2 3 4 5 6
21	I try to think of the years ahead, what everything will be like after I've got rid of the pain	0 1 2 3 4 5 6
22	I tell myself it doesn't hurt	0 1 2 3 4 5 6
23	I tell myself I can't let the pain stand in the way of what I want to do	0 1 2 3 4 5 6
24	I don't pay attention to the pain	0 1 2 3 4 5 6

	0	1	2	3	4	5	6
	NEVER			SOMETIMES			ALWAYS

		N	S	A
25	I have faith in medicine that someday there will be a cure for my pain	0 1 2 3 4 5 6		
26	No matter how bad it is I know I can handle it	0 1 2 3 4 5 6		
27	I pretend it's not there	0 1 2 3 4 5 6		
28	I worry all the time about whether it will end	0 1 2 3 4 5 6		
29	I lie down	0 1 2 3 4 5 6		
30	I replay in my mind pleasant experiences in the past	0 1 2 3 4 5 6		
31	I think of people I enjoy doing things with	0 1 2 3 4 5 6		
32	I pray for the pain to stop	0 1 2 3 4 5 6		
33	I take a shower or a bath	0 1 2 3 4 5 6		
34	I imagine that the pain is outside my body	0 1 2 3 4 5 6		
35	I just go on as if nothing happened	0 1 2 3 4 5 6		
36	I see it as a challenge and don't let it bother me	0 1 2 3 4 5 6		
37	Although it hurts, I just keep on going	0 1 2 3 4 5 6		
38	I feel I can't go on	0 1 2 3 4 5 6		
39	I try to be around other people	0 1 2 3 4 5 6		
40	I ignore it	0 1 2 3 4 5 6		
41	I rely on my faith in God	0 1 2 3 4 5 6		
42	I feel like I can't go on	0 1 2 3 4 5 6		
43	I think of things I enjoy doing	0 1 2 3 4 5 6		
44	I do anything to get my mind off the pain	0 1 2 3 4 5 6		
45	I do something I enjoy such as watching TV or listening to music	0 1 2 3 4 5 6		
46	I pretend it's not part of me	0 1 2 3 4 5 6		
47	I do something active like household chores or projects	0 1 2 3 4 5 6		
48	I use a heating pad	0 1 2 3 4 5 6		

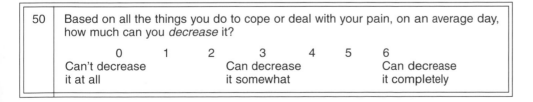

49	Based on all the things you do to cope or deal with your pain, on an average day, how much *control* do you feel you have over it?.
	0 1 2 3 4 5 6
	No Control Some Control Complete Control

50	Based on all the things you do to cope or deal with your pain, on an average day, how much can you *decrease* it?
	0 1 2 3 4 5 6
	Can't decrease it at all Can decrease it somewhat Can decrease it completely

11

Assessment of social, economic and occupational factors

Chris J. Main

INTRODUCTION

The purpose of a socioeconomic and occupational assessment in the context of pain management is to identify obstacles to recovery. Pain can have widespread and disabling effects. As discussed in earlier chapters, the effects of prolonged disability can be profound not only on individuals in terms of personal well-being but also on their family and ability to work. Relationships with family members, working colleagues and employers can change. Roles within families can change and 'overprotectiveness' may become a significant hindrance to recovery. With work loss of any significant extent, a degree of financial protection in terms of a variety of benefits or insurance-based wage replacement systems may come into place. In many societies, such assistance offers essential protection against significant hardship, but in the event of prolonged absence from work the person may become totally reliant on financial support, which is payable only with a certain level of certified incapacity. Partial recovery may threaten such financial benefits without guaranteeing the individual successful return to work or re-employment. This can leave individuals and their family in an exceedingly difficult dilemma. The problem is found in sharpest relief in circumstances in which litigation is involved. There may be little realistic hope of return to previous employment, there may be significant loss of earnings and individuals' only realistic hope of re-establishing their family's economic security may be to pursue litigation, the outcome of which is usually uncertain and the course of which may be prolonged. In consideration of suitability for pain management, it is important to recognise such factors as potential obstacles to rehabilitation and assess their significance in the context of clinical decision making. The nature and theoretical significance of these factors was discussed in Chapter 4. The purpose of this chapter is to offer some suggestions about how to assess their significance in the individual patient.

CULTURAL AND SUBCULTURAL FACTORS

The influences of cultural and subcultural factors on pain perception and disability were reviewed in Chapter 3. Cultural and subcultural factors are not in themselves obstacles to rehabilitation except in so far as they translate into difficulties in comprehension, mistaken beliefs about the nature of pain and disability, resistance to seek treatment, unwillingness to comply with treatment procedures or failure to accept a degree of personal responsibility for the outcome of rehabilitation. Each of these factors should be assessed as an obstacle in its own right (Box 11.1).

It can be seen that, with the exception of the first factor in Box 11.1, these potential obstacles are not culturally or subculturally specific. In appraisal of the influence of clinical history, however, it is important to consider whether such biases may have influenced the manner and content of treatment that has previously been offered to the patient.

The influence of gender and age

The influence of age and gender on perception of pain, and reaction to it, has already been discussed in Chapter 3. Although there is clearly a biological influence of both sex and age on health, a modern approach to assessment must take into account the socially determined influences of gender and age. A number of the key considerations are depicted in Box 11.2.

Box 11.1 Potential influence of cultural and subcultural factors

- Difficulties in language or comprehension
- Mistaken beliefs about pain and disability
- Resistance to treatment seeking
- Unwillingness to comply with treatment
- Failure to accept responsibility for treatment outcome

Box 11.2 Potential influence of gender and age

- Initial biases and assumptions
- Manner of assessment
- Whether to offer treatment and what treatment to offer
- Expectations of treatment outcome

Initial biases and assumptions

People are often unaware of the extent of their own biases in relation to matters of race, social class, gender and age. Racial and religious differences form the basis of cultural stereotyping ranging from (perhaps) relatively harmless humorous anecdotes and stories to family strife and divided communities. There is no point in pretending that such biases do not exist or that they can be eradicated from our consciousness. Clinicians, however, must try to become aware of, acknowledge and critically examine, the possible influence of such biases on their clinical decision making.

Manner of assessment

Patients often perceive doctors as patronising and dismissive. Previous experiences with health-care professionals may have led to a deep level of mistrust, distress and anger, which can adversely affect willingness to disclose information. (The role of iatrogenic distress and anger in the development of disability was discussed specifically in Ch. 5.) Such patients need to be listened to both carefully and sensitively. If individual members of the team are seen to be significantly influenced in the manner of their assessments by the age or gender of the patients, then the matter must be brought to their attention by other members of the team and appropriate steps made to rectify the problem. If patients have been made to feel uncomfortable by the manner of their assessments, they should be encouraged to bring this to the attention of one of the team.

Whether to offer treatment and what treatment to offer

Clinical decision making is complex (Ch. 12) and has many facets but the two overriding considerations in whether to offer treatment are, firstly, whether there is evidence that the treatment works and, secondly, whether the patient is suitable.

The most important consideration regarding treatment is the strength of evidence for its effectiveness. Flor and colleagues in a meta-analysis found evidence of effectiveness of pain management as a type of treatment (Flor, Friedrich & Turk 1992). In the field of pain management, however, there are very few well-designed clinical trials. In a more recent review, Morley, Eccleston & Williams (1999) concluded: 'Published randomised trials provide good evidence for the effectiveness of cognitive behavioural therapy, and behaviour therapy for chronic pain patients'. However, no trials have explicitly addressed the relationship between gender or age in response to treatment and there is no evidence therefore to indicate that pain management is not an appropriate type of treatment for particular gender or age subgroups.

In summary, although there is some evidence of age- and gender-related differences in outcome of treatment, at least some of the explanation may lie in selection biases. Gender per se should not be a factor in offering treatment and the patient's age should be considered only in so far as physical capacity or comorbidity may make the patient unsuitable for treatment.

The influence of the family

As mentioned in Chapters 3 and 4, the patient's family can have a significant influence on a patient's perception of pain and response to treatment.

Box 11.3 Assessment of family influences on decision to treat
• Corroboration of factual information • Psychological effects on family members • Family's perception of the nature of pain and disability • Family's role in treatment seeking • Acceptance of shared goals for intervention • Role of family in the rehabilitative process • Resistance to change

In assessment of the role and significance of family relationships, a number of factors need to be considered. They are shown in Box 11.3.

Corroboration of factual information

As part of the assessment of the patient, it is also desirable (and essential in the view of some) to interview members of the patient's family. It offers the opportunity to identify or clarify background details that the patient may be unable to recall, but also offers the opportunity to confirm the picture presented by the patient. The patient may be emotionally affected by the assessment and may unwittingly give a distorted picture of events, particularly if desperate for help. Not uncommonly, the patient's partner will have a clearer picture of what was said during previous consultations or of the medication regimen that has been prescribed. In a minority of cases, the team members may gain the impression that the patient is not being fully open with them. An independent interview with a family member may serve to allay anxieties or indeed confirm suspicions.

Psychological effects on family members

It is important to recognise that members of the patient's family may have significant emotional and practical problems as a direct result of the patient's pain-associated incapacity. This is seldom recognised. Research has shown that how a *partner* copes with a patient's pain has a significant effect on treatment outcome. What started as an individual's pain problem can develop into a shared relationship problem or even an entire family problem. As has already been stated, a clear-cut distinction between assessment and treatment is inappropriate if not impossible. Diagnostic clarification and installation of a degree of optimism can be therapeutically beneficial not only for the patient, but also for the patient's partner. Conversely, if patients partners are significantly distressed or angry about a patients' pain, the way they have been managed, the extent of their persisting incapacities or their prognosis then *their* reactions may be significant contributory factors in the patients' distress profiles. In cases of significant relationship disharmony, conjoint psychological therapy may be indicated. Sensitive attention to the partner's concerns will normally be sufficient and may reap rich rewards in assisting the patient's rehabilitation.

Family's perception of the nature of pain and disability

The patient's family may have a quite different perception of the nature of the patient's pain or pain-associated incapacities. It is important to identify what the partner thinks is wrong. The partner may have fears that they have not disclosed to the patient, or may feel that the patient has been reluctant to disclose the true extent of difficulties to the assessment team. The partner may feel that the patient has been too reluctant to seek clarification or treatment. As part of the investigation of the family's perception of the situation, the team can also gain an impression of the family coping strategies.

Family's role in treatment seeking

Perhaps surprisingly, it is not always immediately evident why patients have sought treatment. They themselves may have little expectation as far as further treatment is concerned. Other family members may have been the prime instigators of the seeking of treatment. Alternatively, they may have persuaded the patient to comply with the recommendation of other health-care professionals to attend for assessment for pain management. Many patients are initially suspicious that they have been 'fobbed off', are being offered a second-rate treatment, or are resistant to a treatment approach based on 'self-help' or cognitive–behavioural principles. Alternatively, the family may have a negative view of pain management and be dismissive or unsupportive of the referral for pain management.

Acceptance of shared goals for intervention. If the patient is accepted for pain management, it is important to capitalise on the potential assistance that can be offered by family members to the patient's rehabilitative efforts. Many pain management programmes include family members not only at the stage of initial assessment and consequent clinical decision making, but also during the pain management programme itself. It is usual practice in the Manchester and Salford Pain Centre, for example, to invite partners or significant others to attend, and indeed participate in, both the initial and the final session of the programme. In successfully 'selling' the programme to a patient's partner, the team may gain a valuable ally at times during the rehabilitation process when the patient begins to lose confidence or experience setbacks.

Role of family in the rehabilitative process

It should be clear from the above that involvement of the family, if not essential, is certainly highly desirable. Indeed in some of the North American programmes, active involvement of the family is a *prerequisite* of acceptance on to a treatment programme Unfortunately not all patients have supportive relationships, and indeed lack of appropriate sympathy, support and encouragement may be a major feature of patients' psychological difficulties in coping with their pain. While it is certainly desirable therefore to engage partners, it would seem somewhat harsh to reject patients because they do not have a supportive and appropriately concerned relationship. Problems of social isolation (and the lack of self-confidence that often underpins this) may be tackled during the treatment process itself. Training in anxiety reduction, confidence building and assertiveness within a problem-solving framework (Ch. 13) may also assist the reconstruction of emotionally damaged relationships.

Resistance to change

Finally it is important to assess resistance to change in the patient's family. A number of objectives will have been discussed with the patient, both at the time of preliminary assessment and at that of clinical decision making. The objectives almost inevitably will necessitate changes in the patient's daily life. Some of these changes may have a direct effect also on other family members. The role of the family in this specific matter can easily be overlooked. All stated difficulties and reasons for resisting change should be carefully examined and discussed. This can be done in a sympathetic manner. It is not uncommon to find, for example, that a partner has become the 'carer' of the patient. The partner may have a considerable emotional investment, and sometimes even a financial stake, in sustaining the role of carer. The importance of such 'dynamics' in consideration of suitability for pain management may become evident only when specific excuses are made or obstacles offered to implementation of the treatment plan. (Unfortunately these resistances are not always openly acknowledged and may emerge only as obstacles to change during the course of the treatment process itself.)

ECONOMIC CIRCUMSTANCES

The health-care system is not empowered to make significant differences to a patient's economic circumstances. As aforementioned, however, the financial consequences of being unable to work may be considerable. Economic factors may influence both a patient's presentation for treatment (willingness to consult) and their response to treatment. In terms of recovery and return to work, they can represent both enabling factors (in offering incentives to recovery) and positive disincentives (in terms of potential loss of sickness and invalidity benefits).

> **Box 11.4** Key economic considerations
>
> - Current financial circumstances
> - Comparison with status prior to injury
> - Degree of current financial stress
> - Impact on self-esteem and confidence
> - Impact on significant others
> - Litigation (status and anticipated outcome)

As discussed in Chapter 4, rules and regulations about benefit entitlement as a consequence of social policy have a direct bearing on the nature and extent of pain-associated incapacity. Assessment of entitlement to benefit is not properly, and should not be, a matter for the health-care team, whose primary concern should be clinical recovery or maximum restitution of function. The economic implications of change in function, however, can be considerable and therefore need to be assessed as potential obstacles to recovery. A number of the key features that should be investigated during an assessment for pain management are shown in Box 11.4.

Impact of financial adversity

Current financial circumstances

In the evaluation of current financial circumstances, it is important to consider the finances in terms of the whole family rather than just in those of the individual patient. There may be no short or long term financial effects of the patient's chronic pain. More often, however, particularly when the patient's pain is limiting function and ability to work, the effect may be considerable. Financial difficulties may represent a considerable and sometimes major component of the patient's level of distress. Disputes about benefit entitlement and associated allowances may consume a large proportion of the patient's emotional reserves. Patients may show reluctance to disclose details of their financial affairs. It should be explained that such enquiries by the health-care team are carried out solely with the purpose of investigating possible hindrances to rehabilitation. An assurance may have to be given about degree of confidentiality. It may be possible for the health-care team to assist with matters such as travelling expenses to enable attendance for treatment, but it is *never* a good idea to become actively involved in support of benefits, allowances or the pursuit of litigation. This should be explained at the outset to patients, otherwise misunderstandings may arise and the important clinical relationship with the patient may be fractured beyond repair. If patients' prime reason for attending is to obtain assistance in remaining disabled rather than increase function, they should not be accepted for treatment. Such issues can be heightened still further in the context of litigation (see below).

Comparison with situation prior to injury

Evaluation of the economic effects of patients' pain makes sense only in the context of a comparison with their financial status prior to onset of their incapacity. In making such a comparison, it is important to consider not only basic earnings, but also opportunity for payment augmentation through overtime and extra working. It may be best to ask patients to estimate the difference between what they would have been earning (in terms of net income) compared with their net income now (incorporating all their benefits and allowances). An adjustment may have to be made for changes in earning by other members of the family, whether by accident or design. It must be stressed, however, that such investigations by the health-care team should not be either intrusive or unnecessarily detailed.

Degree of current financial stress

Economic investigations should be undertaken only to identify a level of distress that would compromise the patient's ability to engage in the programme fully, or to satisfy the team that offer of pain management was appropriate *at the current time* rather than at a future date.

Impact on self-esteem and confidence

It should be recognised that financial adversity can have a profound effect on patients' self-esteem and confidence. If it appears from patients' socio-occupational history that they have always been the breadwinners (or main financial supporters) for their families, then significantly reduced income as a consequence of inability to work may not only put their styles of life, and even houses, in jeopardy, but also distress them to the point of clinical depression. If it appears from initial assessment that such a state of affairs seems likely, an attempt should be made to discuss the situation independently with a patient's partner or significant other. It may be important to stress to both the patient and their partner that significant demoralisation, if not frank depression, is a common consequence of persistent pain, pain-associated incapacity and inability to work. It should be viewed as a *normal* reaction to significant and prolonged adversity. It can be put to the patient that improved function through pain management may represent the patient's best option in the circumstances.

Impact on significant others

As aforementioned, chronic pain can become a family rather than an individual problem. If partners appear significantly distressed, and do not appear able to muster any enthusiasm for their partners' participation in pain management, they may require psychological counselling or treatment in their own right. Occasionally it appears that the patients and their partners are competing for attention. Sometimes, a course of marital therapy may be appropriate prior to re-evaluation for pain management. The prime purpose in evaluating the impact on significant others, however, is to evaluate the extent to which the reaction of the partner constitutes an obstacle to rehabilitation in its own right, or conversely can be used to assist the plan of rehabilitation.

The special case of litigation (status and anticipated outcome)

Litigation can perhaps be viewed as a special case of 'economic influences' although it sometimes becomes a process of major psychological

---

Box 11.5 Influences of litigation on clinical decision making

- Distrust of veracity of patient's complaint
- Dislike of patient
- Fear of future litigation in the event of unsuccessful treatment
- Concern that patient may not be able to 'focus fully' on rehabilitation

---

importance over and above the potential economic benefit. The influence of litigation on treatment outcome has already been discussed above in Chapter 4. Involvement in litigation, however, has a major impact on willingness to treat as well as acceptance of treatment. Clinicians (and treatment facilities) differ considerably in their willingness to accept for treatment patients who are currently involved in litigation. There appear to be a number of reasons for this. Justification is often given in terms of statistics demonstrating poorer outcome in patients involved in litigation, but there are other less clearly stated factors that appear to affect clinical decision making. They are shown in Box 11.5.

Distrust of veracity of patient's complaint

If a country does not have a 'no-fault' compensation system for individuals involved in accidents or personal injury, the patient may have little alternative to becoming involved in adversarial litigation. In such a system, there are both claimants and defendants. To be successful in the UK in personal injury litigation, the burden of proof, on the balance of probabilities, lies with the claimant. By the same token, defendants (frequently car insurance companies) have a right to defend themselves. In so doing they will hire experts to limit the value of the claim. In cases of putative whiplash injury following a road traffic accident, the process may involve challenging not only the nature of the injury and its relationship with the claimant's complaint, but also the legitimacy of the complaint, and by implication the genuineness or veracity of the claimant. Adverse comments about the patient (sometimes available to clinicians prior to assessment), and

stated disaffection for medical assessors by the patient, may bias clinicians (or teams) in their assessment of the patient's need for likelihood to benefit from pain management.

Dislike of patient

Some clinicians, particularly those with a lot of prior experience of personal injury litigation, appear to develop a dislike for patients involved in litigation. If such is evident, then the matter should be discussed openly with the pain management team.

Fear of future litigation in the event of unsuccessful treatment

Advances in medical technology, increasing expectations from treatment and need to find 'someone to blame' increases willingness in the population to pursue perceived medical negligence within a legal framework. This process has been stimulated at least in part by an apparent increase in lawyers offering assistance to potential claimants, sometime with the additional incentive of a 'no-win–no-fee' arrangement. Providers of health care have in response put increasing resources into 'risk management' within the framework of 'clinical governance' or peer audit. Such changes in the health-care system are still at a relatively early stage in the UK, but it is hard to imagine that such a process will not have an influence on clinical decision making in patients involved in litigation who present for treatment.

Concern that patient may not be able to 'focus fully' on rehabilitation

A final concern is that ongoing litigation may have an adverse influence on patients' willingness to undergo treatment or indeed benefit from it. There is no consistent scientific evidence either for or against this proposition. It is in our view important first and foremost to retain a clinical perspective in this matter. Ongoing litigation is undoubtedly a potential obstacle to rehabilitation. In our experience, it is best to be absolutely open with patients about the matter. Sometimes they will acknowledge the potential obstacle and suggest or agree to defer treatment until a later date. Some patients are so distressed at the persistence of their pain and the limitations it imposes on them that they are willing to forgo litigation completely. It is hard to develop any hard or fast rules. It should be recalled that it is not always the patient who has been the active pursuant of litigation. Perhaps each patient should be treated as an individual case and the fact of ongoing litigation assessed simply as one of a number of potential obstacles that need to be evaluated as part of the clinical decision-making process.

OCCUPATIONAL CONSIDERATIONS

In Chapter 4, a clear differentiation was made between different sorts of obstacles to recovery. It was considered important to differentiate clearly between risk factors for chronic incapacity and specific obstacles to rehabilitation. In this chapter, consideration will be given primarily to occupational factors as potential obstacles to rehabilitation, but it is important first to consider the relationship between occupational factors and objectives of pain management.

Linking assessment with purposes of treatment

Pain management programmes differ widely in their content, stated objectives and funding arrangements (Ch. 6). Some programmes are funded with the *specific objective* of returning patients to work. In many programmes, return to work is certainly considered a desirable if not the most important outcome of pain management. These differences in explicit objectives affect not only evaluation of outcome, but also specific occupationally focused content. In the more occupationally oriented programmes such as at PRIDE, the original functional restoration programme (Mayer & Gatchel 1988), the overriding emphasis is on the restoration of physical function, an essential part of which is a paced

programme of occupational rehabilitation incorporating muscle strength, exercise tolerance and restitution of a range of specific ergonomic tasks. Like every other treatment approach, functional restoration has its advocates and its critics. Some pain management programmes contain elements of specific occupational 'retuning' often delivered by occupational therapists with a particular enthusiasm for ergonomics. Some programmes have links with specific vocational retraining programmes to which patients 'graduate' on completion of the pain management programmes and indeed new developments in UK health-care policy have been recommending new links and partnerships across health and occupational agencies (Ch 18 and 19). These various approaches to the management of pain-associated muscular disorders in industrial settings (in terms of both work retention and return to work) are described more fully in Chapter 19.

Currently, however, although return to work is a specific objective for many patients entering pain management programmes, pain management is usually directed towards increasing exercise and postural tolerance, reducing stress and overcoming obstacles to rehabilitation rather than being focused primarily on occupational rehabilitation. There are many components of pain management none the less that may assist return to work by helping patients overcoming obstacles preventing specific engagement in occupational rehabilitation. Occupationally oriented pain management programmes are specifically discussed in Chapter 19.

A number of occupational considerations in accepting for management are presented in Box 11.6.

Box 11.6 Specific occupational considerations in selection for pain management programmes

---

• Clarity of objectives and expectations
• Job vulnerability and practical constraints in attendance
• Nature and severity of job stress
• Occupational 'blue flags'

Clarity of objectives and expectations

It is important to clarify specific objectives articulated by patients concerning their current work status, return to work or future occupational plans. It is important to be candid about what the programme has to offer. If it should be viewed realistically as a 'first step' to return to work, this should be openly admitted, without being unduly apologetic. If a patient is completely physically deconditioned, exhausted through impaired sleep, misunderstands the nature of hurting/harming and has lost all self-confidence, then pain management may be an essential prerequisite to occupational rehabilitation. The publicity materials for the programme should state clear treatment objectives and outcome measures. These will have to have been found acceptable to the funding agencies (Ch. 15) and a similar level of clarity is needed for patients.

Job vulnerability and practical constraints in attendance

Many chronic pain patients, if not already unemployed or medically retired, may be vulnerable in terms of continued employment. It is not uncommon, for example, for pain management programmes to be viewed as a final option with the outcome determining the patient's future employment.

There are also patients who are still at work, rather than on sick leave. They may have real difficulties in obtaining permission to attend for the treatment programme. Once again, each patient has to be assessed individually. There may be possibilities of running the programmes at different times of the day, or in assisting in other practical ways such as travel, but ultimately of course the patient has to take responsibility for making the necessary practical arrangements to attend. Sometimes, practical difficulties are a thinly veiled excuse for a more fundamental reluctance to participate in the pain management programme.

Nature and severity of job stress

As mentioned in Chapter 4, there are both real and perceived job stresses and it is not realistic to expect to have direct influence on a work setting from a health-care facility such as a hospital-based pain management programme. Many components in pain management, however, can be of relevance to how an individual understands and copes with the stress of work. Improved sleep decreases fatigue and improves tolerance for stresses of all sorts. A competent stress reduction programme will not only contain a set of approaches to physical and mental stress, but also incorporate careful analysis of stressors and their effects. If the patient's prime objectives are work oriented, relevance of these techniques to the management of work stress legitimately can be claimed.

Occupational 'blue flags'

In addition to the management of stress, other components of pain management may be relevant to perceived obstacles to return to work. Increase in fitness can improve tolerance for exercise and maintenance of fixed postures. The general 'problem-solving' approach may lead to a less impressionistic and more careful analysis of perceived work difficulties, and thereby offer opportunities for the development of new or more effective pain-coping strategies. Removal of mistaken beliefs about hurting and harming may have specific relevance to some of the physical aspects of work. Finally, improvement in mood and increase in confidence may improve tolerance for less than ideal working conditions (or indeed workmates). Identification of occupational concerns at the time of initial assessment therefore may turn out to be rehabilitative opportunities rather than obstacles to rehabilitation as such. When assessment is placed in the context of motivational interviewing it is possible to identify a range of ways in which pain management programmes can be of direct relevance to returning to work, even if some aspects of rehabilitation necessitate a sharper focus on occupational issues.

CONCLUSION: 'TALKING THE TALK' AND 'WALKING THE WALK'

Assessment of socioeconomic and occupational factors in consideration for pain management is therefore of fundamental importance. This chapter has attempted to offer a framework within which such factors can be evaluated. They can be viewed on the one hand as obstacles to rehabilitation or on the other hand as opportunities to broaden the relevance of pain management. There has been more research specifically in psychological assessment than in socioeconomic or occupational assessment (in terms of recovery and successful return to work). It is possible to use a range of checklists and disability measures to obtain a general impression about patients' levels of functioning (and incapacities). Although a number of new screening instruments are under development (Chs 18 and 19) they are not yet sufficiently sophisticated or well

developed to obviate the need for an individualised assessment of the socioeconomic and occupational context within which each patient exists. We are beginning to identify some of the key issues in this field. The conceptual shift from the fairly narrow theoretical models of 'work stress' to a broader understanding of socioeconomic and occupational obstacles to rehabilitation would seem to offer an exciting opportunity for pain management. It might be said that, in terms of engagement of patients, we have become moderately successful in assisting them to 'talk the talk'. Careful assessment is an essential part of this process. Our next compelling challenge is to enable and persuade them to 'walk the walk'.

KEY POINTS

- In consideration of socioeconomic and occupational factors within the context of pain management, the primary emphasis is likely to be on potential obstacles to recovery rather than the identification of treatment targets as such.
- Members of the family may have played a powerful role in shaping the patient's perception of pain, adjustment to disability and treatment seeking.
- Family influences may be either a benefit or a hindrance to recovery.
- Social aspects of previous consultations may have led to significant iatrogenic confusion or distress, which, if not addressed, may prove to be an insuperable barrier to engagement in treatment.
- Economic and occupational factors may serve as obstacles to recovery as well as positive treatment opportunities.
- Appraisal of such factors should be carried out on an individual basis with care and sensitivity.
- It should be remembered that appraisal of such factors may be therapeutic for patients and enable them to reappraise their priorities. As such, the assessment may be viewed as a potential first stage of engagement in treatment.

REFERENCES

Flor H, Friedrich T, Turk D C 1992 Efficacy of multidisciplinary pain treatment centers: a meta-analytic review. Pain 49:221–230

Mayer T G, Gatchel R J 1988 Functional restoration for spinal disorders: the sports medicine approach. Lea & Febiger, Philadelphia

Morley S, Eccleston C, Williams A 1999 Systematic review and meta-analysis of randomised controlled clinical trials of cognitive–behavioural therapy and behaviour therapy for chronic pain in adults, excluding headache. Pain 80:1–13

12

Clinical decision making

Chris C. Spanswick   Chris J. Main

INTRODUCTION

Literature review

It became clear on searching the published literature that there is a dearth of publications on 'clinical decision making in an interdisciplinary setting'. Much of the literature on clinical decision making relates to specific clinical problems, for example the management of femoral neck fracture (Bray 1997). Such references do not seem to shed any particular light on the complex problems of clinical decision making in a team setting.

There are a number of papers in the nursing literature regarding clinical decision making. These are mainly from maternity and accident and emergency fields. They are largely concerned with triage mechanisms and specific clinical areas.

Boney & Baker (1997) have pointed out the potential for bias in decision making, this has been reinforced by Clark, Potter & McKinlay (1991) who have shown the potential effect of the patient's gender, age, socioeconomic status and race as well as the professional's training and experience. It seems that even the order in which data are presented may influence clinical decisions (Cunnington et al 1997).

Jones (1995) in his review of clinical reasoning and pain outlines the importance of the therapist's organisation of clinical and biomedical knowledge. He emphasises the need to involve the patient in the decision-making process and to look beyond diagnosis alone as the key factor to treatment decisions. He suggests that clinicians should challenge their own beliefs and be aware of the potential of inappropriate allegiance to one approach.

A recent review of medical decision making (Lurie & Sox 1999) has pointed out the potential problems with reaching consistent decisions when they are complex or uncertain. In addition to examining sensitivity and specificity of tests the paper discusses mathematical models of decision making. Although quite complex the underlying concepts are important in putting the patient's response to tests and the weighting and interpretation of those tests into perspective.

Finally, the most relevant publications that shed some light on team decision making are to be found in the psychological and psychiatric literature. McCarthy, Dugger & Lazarus (1997) discuss the decision-making process in the management of a patient with psychiatric illness. They outline the need for a broad systems perspective. This includes the need to address medical and social needs, to differentiate between necessary and desirable treatment and realistic from ideal goals. This involves both the development of clinical pathways and organisational systems that serve the patient and the team.

Benbassat (1998), in his review of patient's preferences for participation in clinical decision making, points out that published surveys show that patients wish to be involved in the management of their illnesses. While much of the paper relates to the single doctor–patient relationship and not explicitly to team decision making many of the important factors are relevant to team working. He points out that patients who ask questions, elicit treatment options and express their preferences have better outcomes than those who do not. He concludes that most patients do wish to be involved in the decision-making process although up to 8% may prefer to remain passive. However, he emphasises that the only way of finding out patients' wishes is by direct enquiry.

Implications for conceptualising clinical decision making

Any sort of clinical decision making depends on a complex series of judgements involving a wide range of elements of information. Sound judgement requires both skill and objectivity. Skilled judgement relies on knowledge of the subject and adequate clinical competence in the evaluation of patients with pain. Adequate clinical training, with an introductory 'apprenticeship' during clinical induction (see below) should enable clinicians to reach the required degree of clinical competence (Ch. 16).

Systematic bias in judgement is more problematic. This can be particularly evident for example in the context of medicolegal assessments, during which experts may differ markedly in their estimation of the proportion of their clients who are exaggerating their symptoms or even deliberately faking. Distorted judgements may also arise in routine clinical assessment. These may result from prejudices of which clinicians are unaware. They may, for instance, have a mistaken belief that patients with red hair have significantly lower pain tolerance than others, and therefore offer them less treatment. The clinician may have a dislike of people who wear tinted glasses. Another member of the team may have a tendency to reject patients who show irritability or anger. Such emotional responses colour judgement. The individual may not be aware that this is happening, but it will become apparent to colleagues. If one member of the team is arriving at consistently different clinical judgements from those of colleagues, this must be resolved within a team meeting. Such factors can also affect the team decision and the team's ability to present a coherent view to the patient and influence the decision to attempt to change the patient's opinion. Ultimately, there is little point in further intervention unless the patient is convinced and trusts the judgement of the team. A decision has to be made regarding how much effort and time the team is prepared give to convince the patient otherwise. If the patient is discharged the reasons for this must be explicit and the referring agent must be informed. Such decisions need to be well founded and not distorted by poor clinical judgement.

THE PROCESS (GENERAL ISSUES)

The process of clinical decision making involves complex computation of the various sorts of data and information that have been gathered during assessment. It involves reaching agreement between the members of the team and negotiating with the patient. The decision rules should be explicit to allow audit, ensuring that a logical approach has been taken to address the important issues identified during assessment.

The stages of the decision-making process

There are a number of stages to the decision-making process (Fig. 12.1). Some are general issues and must be agreed prior to setting up the assessment system and pain management programme. Some are specific to individual patients and result in the decision to treat after agreement between team members and the patient at feedback.

Agreement must be reached on the following:

- philosophy
- professional competence of team members
- treatments to be offered
- workload capacity of the team
- assessment data including method of collection
- inclusion/exclusion criteria for the treatment options.

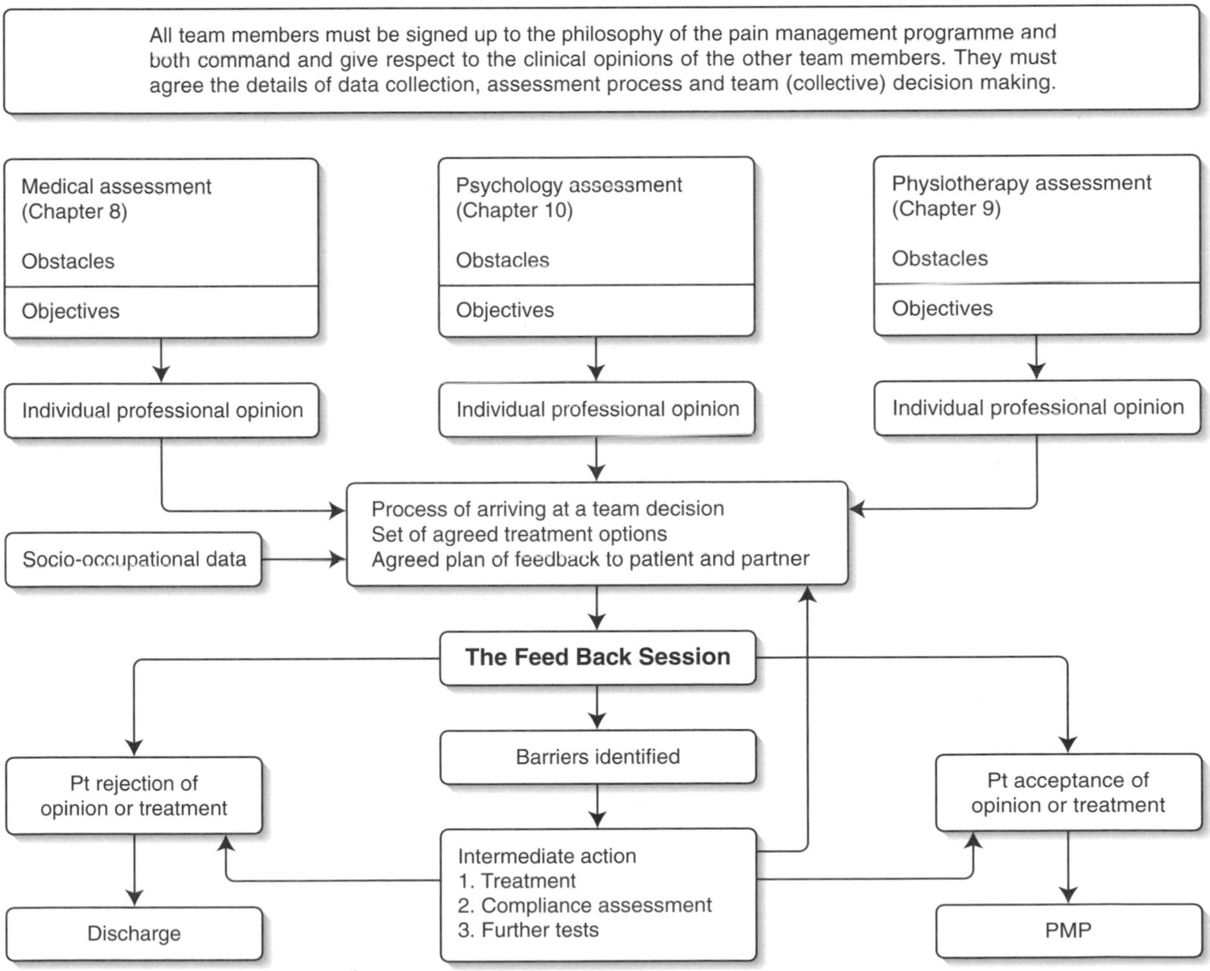

Figure 12.1   Stages of the decision-making process.

> **Box 12.1** Shared philosophy
>
> The philosophy of the 'pain management team' includes an understanding of the following:
> - The nature of pain and incapacity
> - The content and purpose of pain management programmes
> - Collective decision-making process
> - Techniques of communication (need for shared discussion with patients)

Rules of decision making and weighting of data

All of the team members must understand and be 'signed up to' a common philosophy (Box 12.1). They should have a good understanding of and agreement with the central aims, 'pain management' techniques and cognitive–behavioural therapy. Such an approach is a powerful tool in managing patients with difficult pain problems. Patients are adept at picking up discord and differences between team members. It is vital, therefore, that all team members contribute actively to a common aim.

It is important to plan a significant induction period for all new members of staff, no matter how senior. Specific skills in decision making (both individual and collective) need to be acquired. Such new members can inadvertently cause major problems both at assessment, feedback and treatment. It is strongly recommended, therefore, that all new members of a team (both senior and junior) should go through a period of induction and orientation before they are allowed to become clinically active independently. They should sit in on the clinics of all other members and the programme itself. In essence they will be serving a short but focused apprenticeship. The aim of this is to ensure that the new member explicitly understands the model of working and is able to adopt the different style of working. Although few problems are likely to occur with junior or trainee members some difficulties may be encountered with senior new members who may feel that they 'know it already'. It is vital, however, that all new

members feel able to work within the team framework and agree to the aims of the service.

The clinical team must discuss in detail all of the general issues relating to philosophy, team working, assessment and treatment options prior to setting up the service. Explicit rules and criteria for assessment and inclusion on a pain management programme must be agreed. It is unlikely that these rules will remain unchanged, but they should be made explicit and written down in order to allow the team to evaluate their effectiveness and if necessary change the rules in the light of experience. If this is not done, the team members will have no idea of the accuracy of their assessments; nor will they be able to monitor the effect on outcome of any changes to the decision rules.

Clinical competence

The individual team member must be able both to command and to give respect to the clinical opinions of the other team members. Members need also to be able to command respect from their peers within their own profession. This will require the members to be at a minimum level of seniority within their own profession (Ch. 16). There is no room for 'hidden agendas' or 'egos' within the team if it is to be successful. If such issues are not agreed prior to setting up the system, arguments and major disagreements are likely to occur during the 'case conference' or the 'feedback'. Mixed messages will be given by the different team members to patients, serving only to confuse them further. Patients are less likely to opt for pain management programmes if there is no agreement on treatment from their health carers.

Treatments offered

The team must resist at all costs the temptation to accept uncritically any patient referred with a chronic pain problem. Ideally the assessment process should allow the team to decide what is the most appropriate treatment for a particular patient and then institute that treatment. In many centres resources will limit treatment options.

The team must clarify precisely what treatment options are to be made available and what criteria will be used in the decision-making process. The treatment options may be restricted to a group pain management programme, or resources may allow a number of other options. These might include, for example: individual pain management, individual physiotherapy, medical management (e.g. including injections, drug management), individual psychological help or varying combinations of the above.

Few centres will be able to offer expertise in all available treatments for pain, but explicit plans should be made for those groups of patients who require treatments outside the resources of the team. The referral system should be set up to allow a smooth transfer of the patient with the least delay. The pain management team should speak directly with the providers of the other treatments to gain a full understanding of the provider's inclusion/exclusion criteria and the expected outcomes. For example, specific criteria for referring patients to spinal surgery should be agreed between the services to prevent inappropriate referrals. Only then can patients be counselled adequately and given realistic expectations for their assessments and treatments.

If patients are to be referred elsewhere for intermediate treatments (see below) careful discussions with the clinical team providing such treatments must take place. The provider of the intermediate treatment must have a good understanding of what the pain management team requires of them (this will need to be reiterated in the referring letter). The system of referral should be put in place to reduce delays and prevent the patient being lost in the system, being inappropriately reinvestigated and perhaps being offered completely different treatment from that originally intended.

Work-load capacity

It is very important that the team assesses realistically and agrees on the maximum capacity of work load and the type of work that they are willing and able to undertake (Ch. 15). Pressure will be brought to bear on the team to see ever-increasing numbers of patients. Failure to assess patients adequately both in depth and in breadth will lead to important findings being missed and inappropriate or unhelpful treatments being given (Box 12.2). The costs, therefore, of *not* assessing patients adequately may be considerable and will put patients at significant risk (e.g. missed pathology/problems leading to inadequate or inappropriate treatment). Experience has repeatedly shown that teams who are skilled in the identification of patients' needs may unwisely agree to offer treatments for which they simply do not have the time or resources. This leads to either a long waiting time for the treatment offered and/or rushed and poor quality treatment. Perhaps the most important serious negative effect is the potential to produce rapid 'burn out' amongst the team members. In addition, poor quality treatment may leave the patient worse off than prior to treatment and potentially sensitised against further attempts at 'pain management'. An example is given in Case study 12.1.

One of the commonest problems is identifying the need for individual psychological help but without adequate sessional commitments from a suitably trained psychologist being available. Individual psychological work with patients is not only time consuming but also taxing and should not be offered unless there are enough resources to provide this in addition to the assessment clinics and group programmes.

Box 12.2 Costs of inadequate assessment

- Missed organic pathology
- Failure to identify important factors that influence pain and disability
- Failure to identify important factors that should influence which treatment is offered
- Wrong treatment given
- Failure to respond to treatment (e.g. difficulties on pain management programme)
- Unnecessary reinvestigation
- Iatrogenically induced increase in disability
- Demoralised, disenfranchised patient
- Poor reputation for service

Case study 12.1

Mr W. is a 28-year-old social worker with a 5-year history of unremitting back pain. He has not worked for 12 months. He has been assessed by a spinal surgeon and has been told that surgery will not help his problem. He was referred for 'the pain management programme'. He was assessed briefly and enlisted for a programme. Because of the brevity of his assessment a number of important factors were missed and he did not feel able to disclose a number of problems that worried him. These are listed below:

• he had not been convinced that there was not something seriously wrong with his back

• he was worried that he might have a severe arthritis as his father had had a similar problem when he was younger
• he had resorted to using high doses of medication and illicit substances to 'distance himself' from the pain
• he found his job very stressful, did not want to return to it under any circumstances and began to ask for help in convincing his employers to 'medically retire' him.

These problems became evident only whilst attending the programme. It caused significant disruption to the running of the programme and the morale of the rest of the group as he dropped out after some acrimony. He took his own discharge and his GP referred him to another spinal surgeon for a further opinion.

If no resources for individual psychological help are available what should be done with the distressed patients? Skill in communication is of prime importance. The following points should be born in mind when explaining the nature of the problem and proposed treatment to the patients:

• stress the reality of their pain
• emphasise that distress and psychological effects of pain are 'normal'
• explain the interaction between feelings, pain and activity
• encourage patients to address all of the factors making life difficult for them
• list areas that need further assessment, treatment, or both
• agree the treatments that are to be offered
• explain the need to use outside help if necessary
• offer empathy and moral support.

It is important for the team to establish good links with other clinical services. This is particularly important with regard to providing individual psychological help for patients who might otherwise be enlisted for a group pain management programme. Patients often feel they have been passed from pillar to post in the health-care system. If local resources are not available for individual psychological treatment, then patients should be referred to colleagues outwith the pain management service. It must be made clear to patients, however, that this is simply to enable

further treatment to proceed later when they are ready for pain management and that they are not being discharged or fobbed off.

If such resources are not available within the same hospital then referral to another hospital will be necessary. Formal links with other services should be developed with explicit decision rules for referral and shared care. This should involve setting up joint meetings and agreement on assessment criteria. The members of the other team should be treated much as new members of staff within the pain management team (see above) if the system is to work well.

The assessment procedure

The collection of assessment data is discussed elsewhere (Ch. 7). The team must agree on the nature and method of collection of such data. All members must be clear about their responsibility for the collection, recording and presentation of specific data. This will enable the team to identify missing data and ensure that clinical decisions are made on the basis of the agreed and explicit data rather than the 'gut feelings' of the clinicians involved. The team must decide what action should be taken in the event of missing data. It may require the postponing of the decision or it may allow provisional decisions to be made. For example, an X-ray may have been reported as normal, but the patient is convinced that the problem is a crumbling spine. The X-ray must, therefore, be shown to convince the person otherwise. It is a matter of judgement for the team 'at the time' as to whether the decision for treatment has to be postponed until the X-ray has been shown to the patient, or whether the treatment can be planned 'subject to' the X-ray being shown. Ultimately the team must assess patients' understanding of their own problems. If the team members feel they have gained patients' confidence and are convinced that showing patients their X-rays is simply a formality then treatment can be planned. If the team has *not* convinced the patients, then the decision should be postponed until the X-rays have been located and shown to the patients. Only then can patients' beliefs be challenged and decisions made.

Inclusion/exclusion criteria for the pain management programme

The team must agree the specific inclusion and exclusion criteria for 'pain management' or any of the alternative treatments that may be offered. These are discussed at greater length later (Ch. 13 part 1). There are within these inclusion/exclusion criteria some 'absolute' and some 'relative' exclusions (Box 12.3). These need to be made explicit to give the assessing team confidence in decision making. It is difficult to decide how 'relative' exclusions are and how much of a risk the team is prepared to take in offering treatment to any given patient. There are no hard and fast rules and the team will become more proficient in this skill over a period of time. It is for this reason that continuous audit of clinical decision making and outcome of treatment should be done.

It may not be possible at a single visit to judge the relative importance of a particular barrier to progress in any individual patient. The system must therefore allow for some form of assessment of whether the barriers are significant or not. This may be done by setting the patient specific tasks related to the barrier identified. The decision for treatment can then be based on documented evidence rather than inference. This might be, for example, asking patients to increase gradually the time they spend up and out of bed each day. They would have to document this and their partner would have to monitor progress. This would enable the patient to demonstrate willingness to address the barrier and improved physical fitness, which is necessary for inclusion on a programme.

Summary

Having established the treatment options that are to be made available, the team must agree on the following:

Box 12.3   Criteria for 'pain management'

Absolute criteria
- The patient should have been adequately investigated to exclude treatable pathology (clinical red flags)
- There should be no other treatment option that will substantially change the patient's pain
- There should be no further outstanding treatments or consultations with others for the same problem
- The patient must have agreed to stop other consultations
- There must be recoverable loss of physical function
- The patient must demonstrate evidence of psychological distress
- There should be no major psychiatric illness or personality disorders suggestive that patients will sabotage treatment for themself or others

Relative criteria
- The patient must be physically fit enough to take part in the exercise part of the programme
- There should be no major medical barriers to participating in the programme (e.g. severe angina or asthma)
- There should be no major drug or substance abuse
- There should be no other independent psychological problems (e.g. unresolved bereavement reaction) that are likely to interfere with patients addressing their pain and disability
- There should be no physical barriers to pain management (e.g. severe osteoarthritis of knees)
- The patient must be prepared to risk social and other disability benefits and litigation
- The patient's partner should be prepared to support the patient actively in rehabilitation

1. the basic ground rules regarding what information is to be used in the decision-making process
2. the relative importance or weighting of various data
3. willingness to negotiate and change the rules in the light of auditing the team's decision making
4. the important barriers to change including relative and absolute inclusion and exclusion criteria for pain management
5. liaison with other services if necessary to provide individual psychological help
6. options in the event of the patient being unwilling to consider pain management.

CLINICAL DECISION MAKING FOR THE INDIVIDUAL PATIENT

Forming an individual professional opinion

During the assessment process all the relevant professionals are responsible for the collection of relevant data to enable them to form a clinical opinion and identify specific barriers to rehabilitation. Although the data collected by the various team members will differ, the integration will enable the team to come to a decision concerning the suitability of a pain management programme or alternative treatment for the patient. All team members should be able to form a clinical opinion from their own standpoint (Box 12.4). They must be able to justify that opinion (if necessary to their peers) and demonstrate the logic of their own process of diagnosis. In addition they

---

Box 12.4 Individual professional opinion
• Provide a diagnostic formulation from the individual professional's standpoint • Identify specific barriers to rehabilitation • Formulate plan to address barriers (if not absolute) • Identify alternative treatment if appropriate • Identify any concurrent treatment for other problems

---

must be able to: identify for the team any specific obstacles to pain management, weigh the obstacles (i.e. are they absolute or relative exclusions to pain management?), present a plan to address the obstacles or identify appropriate alternative treatment.

Arriving at a team decision

Each of the different professions will have its own perspective on some of the common issues. For example, the level of reported and observed disability may justifiably have slightly differing explanations from the different professions. The physician to the team may emphasise degenerative changes in the spine, the mechanical effects of previous surgery and residual nerve irritation. The physiotherapist may feel that significant paraspinal muscle spasm and deconditioning of muscles may be of prime importance. The clinical psychologist may emphasise the patients' fears of damaging themselves because of their previous experiences. Each of these explanations may be valid but offer only a partial explanation of the overall level of disability. The team may arrive at a consensus only after discussion. It is important none the less to respect individual opinion. It should be remembered that, even if genuine differences of opinion remain, a consensus must be presented to the patients.

Treatment during assessment

The most important reason for the explicit nature of the ground rules for assessment, and criteria for the treatment options, is that some of the 'management' of the patient will need to begin during the gathering of information and prior to team members discussing the problems together at the end of the case conference. Team members must, therefore, have a first-hand working knowledge of how each other works. This is to ensure that mixed messages are not given to the patient during the assessment. For example each team member must 'know' how each other might deal with certain misconceptions that the patient might have, so that these may be dealt with

---

Case study 12.2 Example of major misattributions

Mr A. is a 32-year-old ex-manual worker. He has worked since the age of 16 in horticulture. He has had back pain for several years. He was told by one of his previous medical specialists that he had 'arthritis of the spine'. This has frightened him into very protective and avoidant behaviours. He has given up his job as a gardener and now rests most of the time for fear of damaging his spine further. He has noticed he now gets pain on very little activity, which he feels proves he has a major problem with arthritis in his spine. He is 'convinced' that exercise will damage his back further and he is very apprehensive throughout the assessment process.

Box 12.5 Purposes of team meeting (case conference)

To produce a clear description and assessment of:
1. The nature of the patient's pain
2. The patient's disability and associated problems
3. The patient's understanding of the problem
4. Any potential or further treatments
5. The completeness of the assessment information
6. Any barriers to progress

---

immediately rather than necessarily waiting until the very end of the assessment process. (An example is given in Case study 12.2.) This can be vital in some cases as erroneous beliefs may actually hinder collection of accurate data and willingness to disclose information, upon which the team will be reliant to make decisions regarding treatment.

The correction of misconceptions is often, however, left to the 'feedback' session with the patient, partner and the whole team at the end. Certainly any correction should be reinforced at the feedback session even if it has already been dealt with during assessment. Simply explaining to the patient that the particular issue in question will be discussed in more detail later may be all that is necessary during the gathering of data.

In order to gain the confidence of such patients it is necessary to address their misconceptions directly during the assessment process. This may be best done by the doctor in the first instance and reinforced by the rest of the members of the team. Such a flexible method of working is not possible unless all of the team members have a working knowledge of how each will deal with such patients.

The team meeting (case conference)

After all team members collect their data set and formulate their own assessment of the patient there follows a team meeting or case conference,

the purposes of which are listed in Box 12.5. This is to enable team members to present their evaluation of the patient's problems to the team. All of the team members may have to modify their opinion in the light of additional information gained from the other members of the team.

The negotiations in the case conference must produce a clear description of the nature of the patient's pain, disability and associated problems, the patient's understanding of the problem, any potential or further treatments and the completeness of the assessment information. There should be enough information for the team to judge whether pain management is an option and identify and specify any barriers to progress.

All team members should present their assessments of the patient from their own standpoints. They should not attempt to anticipate what the other team members might feel or modify their opinions until all of the evidence has been presented and discussed. There is a tendency for those involved in pain management to concentrate on the common ground in the biopsychosocial model. Team members must be reminded that their responsibility to the group is to be meticulous and focused in their data collection and to offer their particular professional opinion.

It is frequently only following the team discussion that individual opinions can then be put into context and appropriate weighting given to their findings. Although the team will have some general guidelines, the group should decide the weighting of each member's assessment at the time of discussion as this may vary from case to case. Ultimately the final view must be that of the team.

In addition to the objective assessment of the patient's pain and associated problems, the team must actively investigate a patient's understanding of the problem. This may be wide of the mark. Educating the patient therefore may be an integral part of the proposed treatment. This process usually starts during the feedback process although occasionally some correction of misconceptions may have been given during the assessment process. Indeed, further treatment, investigations or pain management may not be possible until patients' misunderstandings have been specifically addressed. It may even be necessary to institute further investigations or 'show' patients the results of previous investigations in order to convince them that further or specific treatment is not indicated.

Negotiations within the team

Following the presentation of the data and opinions of the individual team members, the team must agree the next course of action. Providing there is enough data available to make a decision then the team should discuss the following two major questions:

1. Is this patient suitable for a pain management programme?
2. Is this the right time to be offering a pain management programme, or are there currently barriers to progress?

Potential barriers to progress

The identification of 'barriers' to pain management (Box 12.6) is the most important aspect of the case conference and indeed the whole assessment process. The list above is not exhaustive or absolute, nor should it be regarded as anything other than an aide mémoire to focus the team's discussion. The team must not only identify the barriers, but also decide what action is necessary in order to overcome these barriers.

The team may feel that the patient is not suitable for pain management. A decision must be made as to whether this decision is 'absolute' (i.e. that the patient is *never* likely to benefit from a pain management programme), or 'relative' in which case the team must identify the specific barriers that must be addressed. In the event that the patient is to be turned down, the manner in which this is communicated needs to be agreed by the team prior to the feedback. Alternative guidance about future management, both to patients and to their referring agent and GP, should then be given as in Box 12.7.

Box 12.7 Advice to referring agent and GP

- Encourage patient to keep as active as possible despite pain
- Avoid repeated referrals for the same problem
- Monitor medication use and effects
- Encourage pacing of activities
- Encourage patient to take a realistic view of future
- Do not reinforce belief in 'cure' for problem
- Support the patient and family in 'managing' pain and associated disability.

Box 12.6 Potential barriers to progress

Biomedical
- Inadequate previous investigation of the patient's pain
- Inadequate previous treatment of the patient's pain
- Concurrent major medical or surgical problems
- Major drug and/or substance abuse
- The patient is currently being offered alternative treatment

Functional
- Inadequate fitness to cope with the demands of the programme
- Unable to look after personal care (e.g. wash, dress)

- Major concurrent musculoskeletal problems (e.g. awaiting hip or knee replacement surgery)
- Unable to remain up and active from 9 to 5

Psychosocial
- Concurrent major psychiatric illness.
- Concurrent major psychological problems
- Major misattribution (patient or partner)
- Financial (benefits and litigation)
- Family (e.g. solicitous spouse)
- Apparent lack of distress
- Anger (previous treatment, accident)
- Willingness to change

The management of barriers to pain management

Biomedical

Inadequate previous investigation of the patient's pain. The physician to the team has specific responsibilities to ensure that the patient's pain has been adequately investigated. This should not only be to the physician's satisfaction but also to the patient's and even the patient's partner's satisfaction. It may be that further investigation is clinically indicated, but more commonly the results of previous investigations have not been interpreted into layman's terms for the patient. However, safety is of prime importance. Patients with tumours have been known to slip through the net.

If further investigations are required the reasons must be explained to the patient and the antic-ipated results should be outlined. This is of particular importance if these are being done for the sake of completeness and negative results are anticipated. The patient will otherwise be further convinced that there is something wrong and therefore be even less willing to consider rehabilitation.

Inadequate previous treatment of the patient's pain. An assessment of the completeness and efficacy of previous treatments should be made. This should include not only ensuring that all appropriate treatments have been tried, but that they have been performed properly. It is easy for example to blame a patient or the pain for the failure of an epidural to help, but there must be some evidence that the epidural was correctly placed (i.e. produced numbness in the area required) in the first place.

It can be difficult to know when to discontinue further attempts at pain reduction. Many treatments for chronic pain do not have a high likelihood of producing long term improvements in pain. Patients with high levels of distress do not respond well to treatment. Continuous 'failed' treatment is demoralising to both patient and doctor and will contribute to further distress. If no further pain-relieving treatment is to be offered this should be explained with the reasons carefully to patients and their partners. Pain management will not be possible until both patients and their partners are convinced that further attempts at pain reduction will not be helpful.

Concurrent major medical or surgical problems. Concurrent medical or surgical problems should not be regarded as absolute exclusions to pain management. There may be some that obviously totally preclude taking part in the physical rehabilitation aspect of the pain programme (such as awaiting investigation of severe angina), but many can be 'managed' on a programme providing all the team members are aware of the problems (patients awaiting elective surgery for a non-related problem, for example, may simply require the timing of attending the programme to be arranged around the surgery).

If there is any doubt regarding the physical fitness of a patient to take part in the programme, then specialist advice must be sought (see below). This is particularly important with a patient with angina, for the protection not only of the patient, but also that of other members of staff.

Major drug and/or substance abuse. Many patients with chronic pain problems end up taking more medication than is helpful. Some have major problems with medication and substantial alcohol or substance abuse. Part of the pain management programme is aimed at helping patients to reduce their dependency on drugs and other substances. Patients in whom the level of medication and other substance use is such that their cognitive functions are impaired should not be put straight on to a pain management programme. They will require a specific drug reduction programme prior to attending the programme. Indeed, successfully reducing medication should be a condition of attending the programme.

The patient is being offered further treatment. On occasions patients are referred to a number of different clinics at the same time. They may also be consulting practitioners in the private sector for both conventional and complementary treatments. This is usually a function of the sense of helplessness and desperation in the referring agent. Patients cannot be put into a pain management programme if they are currently being offered treatment elsewhere, since it will compromise their compliance with the pain management programme.

Patients may be left in something of a dilemma. They may not know whether they should accept other pain reduction treatment or proceed with pain management. The team cannot make decisions on behalf of patients. They may advise patients about which questions might be asked of the other specialist. Patients should also be appraised of realistic outcomes of other treatments. Advice should be based, wherever possible, on published data rather than speculative opinion. Care should be taken in doing this. Patients themselves should be encouraged to ask appropriate questions of the specialist, consider the situation and then report their decision to the pain management team.

This problem of possible alternative treatment can be difficult to resolve satisfactorily, especially if none of the members of the assessment team is, for example a spinal surgeon, and the patient is being offered surgery. It is therefore very important for the team to have established good clinical links with other specialists in order to seek appropriate advice as necessary. The other specialists must also have an understanding of the aims and objectives of pain management.

Functional

Lack of physical fitness Some patients are so disabled that they are unable to sit for more than a few minutes at a time. They may not be able to walk more than a few yards. Such patients will need to spend some time prior to the programme working on sitting, standing and walking tolerance in order to become fit enough to take part in the programme.

Such patients are often very fearful of increasing levels of physical activity. It may be necessary to spend some time with them on a number of occasions to help them overcome their fear and to chart their activities. This will enable an assessment of motivation and allow time for them to gain a better understanding of the aims and expectations of the programme. The patients in turn will be able to clarify their own goals and thus be more focused in their attempts to improve their quality of life.

Unable to look after personal care. Inclusion in a group pain management programme is simply not possible if patients' levels of physical functioning are such that they are not self-caring. The inability to look after personal care is indicative of substantial levels of disability. Most pain programmes are run as either 'day' programmes (the patients attend each day and return home each night) or with hostel-type accommodation only. The latter requires patients to be able to care for their own needs (including, washing, dressing and feeding). In such circumstances both patients and their partners must decide what they wish to do. The team should outline the level of physical activity necessary for a patient to be included on the programme and the reasons why. The patients and partners then have to decide whether they wish to attempt to improve activities enough to gain a place. If they express a wish to try then the team should offer practical help and advice as to how they may achieve their goal.

Individual appointments may be required to monitor progress. During these it is important to help patients move towards realistic goals and to understand that the inclusion on a programme is but the beginning of a long term change in lifestyle.

Major concurrent musculoskeletal problems. Concurrent musculoskeletal problems normally should not be a reason for not including patients in a pain management programme. Concurrent musculoskeletal problems must be of a very major degree (e.g. awaiting surgical treatment for large joint problems) to prevent inclusion. There are programmes for patients with osteoarthritis and other musculoskeletal problems. Patients should be excluded only if there are other pain-reducing treatments that have not been given, or if the patient is awaiting treatment.

Unable to remain up and active from 9 to 5. Patients should be able to tolerate activities for a full day (9 a.m. to 5 p.m.). Many patients will have become very inactive and may not be used to being up and active throughout the day. They commonly will rest or lie down at some time during the day. It is important to inform patients what is required of them so that they can begin to increase their tolerance of being active during the day.

Psychosocial

Concurrent major psychiatric illness or personality disorder. Major psychiatric illness requires treatment in its own right. This is almost without exception an absolute exclusion criterion for pain management. The patient must be able to comprehend the teaching and cope with being in a group. Patients with major personality disorders will not only not benefit from a programme, but can be very destructive in the group (Chs 2 and 10).

Concurrent major psychological problems. Only through a thorough and careful psychological interview do some of the hidden issues become apparent. A number of patients have other psychological issues, which will interfere with their ability to benefit from a programme. Unresolved grief and previous physical or sexual abuse, for example, are not uncommon. The psychologist on the team will need to ensure that the relevance of any problems is highlighted. This may require specific intervention before pain management. It may even preclude pain management altogether.

Major misattributions (or misunderstandings) by patients. Many patients have significant misunderstandings regarding the cause of their pain. They are often convinced that there is 'something serious wrong'. They usually equate increases in their pain with further damage. The mechanical nature of chronic low back pain, for example, tends to reinforce the patient's model (i.e. more movement equals more damage equals more pain). The patient's previous medical advisors may have reinforced this by pointing out 'arthritic' or 'degenerative' changes on X-rays. Some of the explanations given by health-care professionals may well reflect their own bias rather than be based on objective evidence.

Major misunderstandings may be addressed during the assessment process. Specific enquiry about the patient's beliefs will have been made. This should be checked again during the feedback process to allow further explanation if necessary. It should be done in a positive manner. Denigrating other professionals' opinions is not helpful. An explanation of why certain terms (e.g. spinal arthritis) have been used and what was actually meant is more appropriate. Occasionally patients are not reassured by the explanations given, or clarification of the nature of their problems is required. It may require, therefore, a specialist opinion (e.g. that of a spinal surgeon) to reassure the patient finally that is it safe to rehabilitate and that further 'treatment' is not appropriate or required.

Pain management programmes are not common. Most patients and many health-care professionals know little about them. Therefore, both patients and their referring doctors may have a number of misunderstandings about the nature and purpose of a pain management programme. Enquiry should be made as to what the patient may have been told about the programme and any misconceptions corrected. Specific reassurance regarding the psychological content as well as the exercise content should be given. It is often helpful to give written information about the nature, purpose and content of the programme.

Financial (benefits and litigation). The team must have an understanding of the financial and other consequences of patients improving their level of physical function. It is important to be non-judgmental and open in discussions with the patient. Neither litigation nor the receipt of substantial state or other benefits should be regarded as absolute exclusions to pain management.

There may be substantial financial risks to patients if they undergo rehabilitation. Rehabilitation may lead to improved physical functioning, but not sufficiently to enable return to employment. Patients may therefore not be prepared to jeopardise their family's welfare.

Many patients none the less are anxious to get back to work or training for work and are willing to risk their benefits and medicolegal claims in order to improve their quality of life. Provided patients have convinced the team of this then they should be offered a place on the programme. Conversely if patients feels they cannot afford to take such a risk then there is little point in proceeding.

Family. Continuous seeking for cures may be driven as much by patients' partners or families as by patients themselves. Their close relatives often feel helpless, as they are unable to do anything specifically to help the patient. Partners may be convinced that there is either something specifically wrong or that somewhere there must be someone who can stop the pain. They can be very protective of patients and may be anxious to prevent them doing anything which might worsen their condition.

The team must be convinced that the patient's partner and family are not going to undermine, either actively or unwittingly, a patient's participation in a programme by being overprotective. Although efforts can be made to persuade the partners, and if possible include them in the introductory part of the programme, the team will have to decide as to whether the family's behaviour is such as to constitute a barrier to inclusion.

Apparent lack of distress. Some patients are 'comfortable' in the sick role. Such patients display an absence of distress and indicate they have become resigned to their way of life. (This role may have been reinforced by the partner or other relatives.) Indeed in some cases, the patient's level of incapacity may have prevented the family from breaking up. Changing this family dynamic may be extremely hazardous since it can represent a major threat to the relationships and roles within the family. In such circumstances the team must come to a judgment as to the likely benefit of rehabilitation, taking into account both likely costs as well as potential benefits. If there is substantial resistance by both patient and the family, then the team may decide not to invest time and effort in a patient who is

---

> **Box 12.8** The potential sources of anger
>
> *The pain*
> * The limitations that the pain imposes
> * Patient's inability to 'cope' with the pain
>
> *Misunderstandings*
> * Communication style of health-care professionals
> * Failure to find cause
> * Failure to respond to treatment
>
> *Socioeconomic and occupational implications*
> * The benefit system
> * Litigation system
> * Occupational circumstances

unwilling to address the necessary changes in lifestyle.

Anger. The patient may be angry for a number of reasons (Box 12.8) and this may vary in intensity from mild irritation through passive–aggressive non-compliance to open hostility. Some of the major aspects of anger have been discussed previously (Ch. 2). In the context of clinical decision making for pain management, the three commonest sources of anger and distress are:

* the pain itself (with its disabling effects)
* failure of or misunderstandings about previous treatment
* the socioeconomic and occupational implications of the pain-associated incapacity.

The cause of the anger must be clarified during the case conference and plans set for tackling it during the feedback process. In teams that are used to working together, this may have already happened during the assessment process by any one of the members. Commonly the physician will have begun to defuse any anger aimed specifically at the medical profession. There will still be a need to complete this process during the feedback session. It may be necessary to exclude patients from a programme if it is impossible to defuse their anger sufficiently to allow them to set it behind them and thus concentrate on the future.

Patients often feel a sense of anger and frustration at their pain and the limitation it places on their physical activities. This may not necessarily be overtly expressed, but is often disclosed by the patient when inquiries are made. Anger and frustration are not helpful and commonly lead to progressive demoralisation and depression. It is helpful to assist patients to recognise this even at the time of initial assessment.

Many patients express anger with the way other health-care professionals have treated them. They often feel they have been treated dismissively or that judgements have been made about the veracity of their pain. Patients whose pain has been caused by the negligence of others often remain angry with that person and are anxious for some from of censure. This frequently leads them into litigation, which partly due to its adversarial nature unfortunately reinforces this. Such litigation rarely adequately 'compensates' people for their loss and is in itself a stressful process.

Pain that leads to loss of physical capacity may be compensable by the state in the form of financial benefits. The benefits are designed to cover the increased costs of the patient's disability and frequently require medical examination. Disputes between patients and the benefits agency are commonly seen amongst patients with chronic pain. This often leads patients to feel they are being treated unfairly and subsequently develop anger at the system and the doctors employed by the benefits agency.

Further resentment may be evident at the occupational implications of their incapacity. (The role of economic and occupational influences on responses to rehabilitation are discussed more fully in Ch. 4.)

Unless the anger is dealt with early on in the assessment/treatment process the patient will not make much in the way of progress on a pain management programme. There is also a significant danger that unless the cause of the anger is identified and dealt with the patient may become disruptive on the programme.

Willingness to change. Willingness to change is one of the most important issues and potential barriers to progress. Clearly some patients have never contemplated stopping seeking cures and managing their pain instead. Most patients attend pain centres in the expectation of a cure or at least pain reduction. They may expect this even when referred to a pain management programme. This expectation may have been enhanced by the referring agent. Providing there is no evidence that there is any curative treatment, patients must therefore be introduced to the notion that there is no cure and that pain reduction techniques will not be of any help. They will have to learn to 'manage' their pain.

An assessment of the patient's willingness to change must be made. The team will have to come to a judgement as to whether this patient is prepared to put in the effort into making substantial changes in activity in the face of unchanging and perhaps short term increase in pain. Some information will have been gathered during the assessment process. This may need to be explored further during the feedback session. Patients ultimately have to convince the team that they want to be given the chance on a programme (Box 12.9). If doubt is raised during the case conference then the team members may press the point more during the feedback in order to convince themselves.

Finally the team must have a clear plan for discussing its recommendations to patients and

---

Box 12.9 Specific answers needed to assess 'willingness to change'

- Has the patient understood that no curative or palliative treatment is available?
- Does the patient understand the benefits of pain management?
- Does the patient understand that continuing to seek cures is not a successful long term strategy?
- Is the patient prepared to focus on rehabilitation in spite of pain?
- Is the patient prepared to put in the considerable physical and mental effort required?
- Is the patient prepared to suspend judgement and take the risk of failure?
- Does the patient have specific identifiable goals and targets?
- Is the patient prepared to 'plan' and 'institute' the necessary changes?

their partners (Box 12.10). It must decide who will lead the discussion and how the other team members will support, what information will be given and how 'pain management' will be 'sold' to the patient if necessary.

Selling the proposed management to the patient (the feedback session)

The assessment process and in particular the proposed treatment plan may be very different to what the patient had expected. The team must therefore formulate precisely how the results of their assessment and the proposed treatment will be explained and if necessary 'sold' to the patient and their partner. Prior to the 'feed back' to the patient and their partner,

the team must have a clear plan of what information is to be fed back, how this is to be done and by whom. The team must also agree on what it will do if the patient takes a different stance from the expected one. The more the team members work together the better they will be at handling unexpected responses from patients. An example is given in Case study 12.3 of an unexpected response from a patient. In this particular case the team members changed the direction of the feedback session mid discussion without the need for further discussion among themselves.

The nature of the patient's problems

The first part of the feedback process should be to give patients a clear and careful description of their problems. Each member of the team should do this and patients should be asked specifically if they understand everything that has been said to them. The team must also be explicit in inviting questions and queries about the assessment and the conclusions that have been reached. If the patients simply do not understand some aspects they must made to feel comfortable in asking for further explanation and they must feel able to express fears or doubts about what has been said. The team should take care not to overload patients with too much information, otherwise they will not remember much of what was said.

Clinicians should be wary of making judgements about the severity of patients' pain. If it is implied that their pain isn't really as bad as they

---

Box 12.10 Summary of case conference

By the end of the discussion the team should have a clear plan of action covering the following points:

1. Is pain management an appropriate treatment for this patient?
2. Can this patient be listed for a pain management programme now?
3. What are the specific barriers to pain management?
4. What are the plans to address these barriers?
5. How will 'pain management' be 'sold' to the patient and their partner?
6. What other treatments are appropriate if pain management is not appropriate?
7. What advice should be given to the patient, the referring agent and the general practitioner if pain management is not appropriate?

Case study 12.3 Example of changing tack during the feedback process

During the case conference all of the team members were convinced that Mrs X. was 'comfortable' in the sick role and would not be interested in managing her pain more successfully. The team members were not convinced of her willingness to sustain the necessary effort to benefit from a rehabilitation programme. They agreed simply to offer some advice on exercise and discharge her after feeding back the details of the assessment to her.

In the feedback session Mrs X. became more communicative and animated. She understood the model of hurt not necessarily meaning harm and expressed interest in learning not only to manage her pain better but also to improve her level of activities. This was totally unexpected. The team, without further consultation, immediately changed tack and began to 'sell' the pain management programme positively to Mrs X. She responded and, on checking with her, she had clearly understood the aims and objectives. She was given more written information and invited to contact the team again with her decision following reading more about the programme.

She was subsequently listed and did very well on the programme.

claim, then the communication link will almost certainly be lost irretrievably and immediately. Instead one should attempt to offer a logical understanding of how and why pain has persisted, why incapacity may have developed and why treatment has not restored them. The emphasis should finally be that there may be room for recovery of some of the patient's lost activities. It is important to use non-threatening and non-judgemental terms. Explaining that the team has seen many similar patients with similar problems will help give credence to the team's assessment and proposed plan of treatment.

It is important to appreciate two major points. First, this assessment probably will have been very different from previous assessments that patients are likely to have undergone. They may be quite mystified about the necessity for such an in-depth assessment. Secondly, they will be faced with a large amount of new information in a short time, which may serve only to confuse them rather than help them make decisions about their future. It is often helpful to explain to patients that the team is aware of these issues so that they are put more at ease and feel able to ask questions. Clinicians should not move on to the proposed treatment or further investigations unless the team is convinced the patient under-stands the points that have been raised in the assessment. Patients should also be given time to reach their own decisions. It is far better to emphasise a few important points and to ask patients to return on a further occasion. This will allow them time to think through the conse-quences of what they have been told. If necessary patients can be given written advice about pain management and its relevance to their particular problem.

The proposed plan (following feedback from the patient)

Options for further treatment

There are a number of options that should be considered (Fig. 12.2). The team will have consid-ered these prior to the feedback, but often the decision as to which is ultimately appropriate for 'this' patient cannot be taken until the team has had feedback directly from the patient during this session.

If the patient accepts the team's opinion then matters can proceed. Management may involve further investigations or may include some inter-mediate treatment to help address any barriers. If the plan includes further investigations or other specific interventions prior to pain management,

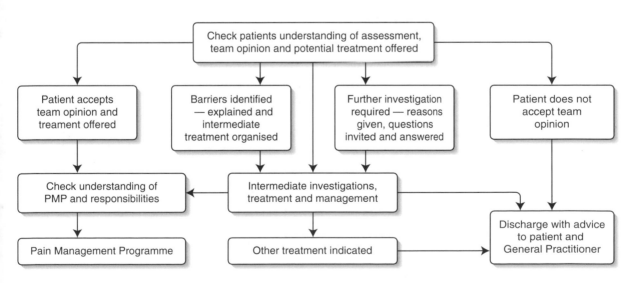

Figure 12.2 Options for further treatment.

the team members must explain their reasons carefully. The team should check whether patients understand what they have been told and invite questions from them or their partners. Patient then can be listed for a pain management programme.

Some patients will not accept the team's opinion or need a lot of convincing to undertake a rehabilitation programme. The team should try to be aware of any potential biases in its own assessment of how much effort is likely to be required to try to engage the patient appropriately. It must, however, arrive at a realistic assessment of whether a satisfactory result can be achieved within the resources available. If the patient is to be discharged the team should offer advice regarding the patient's future management of the pain. This should be consistent with the advice sent to the referring agent and GP.

Intermediate treatment. During the feedback process the team may consider that further interventional treatment is indicated. It is important to ensure that all appropriate treatments have been completed before the patient is listed or offered a pain management programme. The team should be explicit about the expected outcome of such treatment and should encourage the patient to think of it as a means to achieving maximum benefit from the pain management programme.

Some treatments may be necessary to enable patients to become fit enough for the programme, having identified specific barriers. For example, if patients have severely limited sitting tolerance, they may not be able to participate in the programme without some preparatory therapy specifically aimed at overcoming this obstacle to participation.

Such patients will need to be reviewed prior to inclusion on the programme.

Determination of likely compliance

The team may not be convinced of patients' willingness to address all of the necessary issues concerning their pain. Patients may state willingness, but they need to actually demonstrate compliance. Setting specific physical goals can be helpful in identifying patients who are willing to put effort into the programme. Failure to achieve targets (set well within patients' capabilities) is an indication that they are unlikely to do well when pressed hard on a programme. This technique of setting preliminary targets may be applied to problems with medication use as well as physical function. If patients are misusing medicines to the extent they cannot concentrate, setting a simple target of medication reduction is not only necessary, but will give an indication of motivation.

Listing for a programme

Before patients are listed for a pain management programme, time should be taken to confirm the aims and purposes of such programmes. The team will need to be explicit about the expected outcome, if necessary emphasising that a cure or reduction in pain is not expected. Emphasis should be placed on the positive outcomes of improved activities, confidence, fitness, mood, etc. The team, the patient and partner must share the same goals, otherwise the treatment process is doomed to failure.

Having explained the nature of the programme the team must check with patients their understanding of what is being offered. The responsibilities of the team and the patient must be made clear, together with any risks that may be involved. This is particularly important for those involved in litigation. Although completing a programme may help patients' cases in demonstrating motivation, dropping out may be detrimental to their cases. Patients must be made aware of this.

The timing of the programme should be confirmed so that patients can make appropriate arrangements to attend all of the sessions. Should there be any anticipated problems these should be highlighted at the time of listing rather than at the beginning of the programme.

Finally, to reiterate, the team must appreciate that patients will have been given a lot of totally new information in a very short time. Many patients recall being very confused at the end of the assessment process and feedback session. Patients should be given simple written summary covering all of the points discussed in the feedback session, details of the programme and if necessary details of further reading. If it is not possible to arrange this immediately following the feedback session, it should be arranged as soon as possible thereafter.

Summary

At the end of the feedback session patients and their partners should have a clear understanding of the following:

* the nature of their pain, its cause (if known) and prognosis
* the meaning of all the investigations, including any further investigations that may need to be done
* the likelihood of cure or substantial reduction of their pain
* the treatment options available including the pain management programme
* the specific barriers to rehabilitation that the team has identified and how they may be overcome
* if listed, the philosophy and practical details of the programme together with their necessary commitment.

The team should have a clear plan of the following:

* the nature of the patient's pain (diagnosis)
* safety of rehabilitation (does this patient's pain mean damage?)
* concurrent important medical, physical and psychological problems

* a list of the specific barriers to pain management together with action plans
* either a date for inclusion on a pain management programme, a review following specific investigation, further opinion or individual treatment or discharge with advice to the patient and referring agent.

In addition to imparting the plan of treatment based on thorough clinical assessment, much of the feedback process is aimed at merging opinions of the team members, the patients and their partners. At the end of the process all must have a common understanding of the nature of the patient's pain, disability and associated problems, goals for treatment and expectations of outcome with an agreed course of action.

CONCLUSION

It is clear that clinical decision making is a complex task in which a wide variety of information is used to clarify clinical issues, goals and barriers to progress. The final decision is probabilistic. Not all patients will do well. Some patients whom the team feels are unlikely to do well surprise everyone and make major positive changes in their lifestyle. Others who are expected to do well sometimes fail.

An understanding of the clinical decision-making process, following structured assessment, will give a clearer picture of the individual's problems, which in turn can inform and shape future clinical decision making. Ensuring an appropriate treatment plan will increase the likelihood of a worthwhile outcome of treatment.

KEY POINTS

- The process of clinical decision making should follow explicit rules and be subject to audit.
- Clinical decision making within the interdisciplinary context requires all members to subscribe to a shared philosophy.
- The shape of the clinical service must be defined and agreed in detail.
- Good and consistent team decision making requires constant practice as a team.
- Team members must perform to the highest standard within their own professional field in order to advise the team.
- The assessment of all patients for pain management must be complete in both breadth and depth.
- Agreement of an appropriate treatment plan between the team and the patient is essential.
- Audit and review of team working should be performed regularly.
- The identification and management of barriers to progress are an essential part of team-based assessment.

REFERENCES

Benbassat J, Pipel D, Tidhar M 1998 Patient's preferences for participation in clinical decision making: a review of published surveys. Behavioural Medicine 24(2):81–88

Boney J, Baker J D 1997 Strategies for teaching clinical decision making. Nurse Education Today 17(1):16–21

Bray T J 1997 Femoral neck fracture fixation. Clinical decision making. Clinical Orthopaedics and Related Research 339:20–31

Clark J A, Potter D A, McKinlay J B 1991 Bringing social structure back into clinical decision making. Social Science and Medicine 32(8):853–866

Cunnington J P W, Turnbull J M, Regehr G, Marriott M, Norman G R 1997 The effect of presentation order in clinical decision making. Academic Medicine 72(10):S40–S42

Jones M 1995 Clinical reasoning and pain. Manual Therapy 1:17–24

Lurie J D, Sox H C 1999 Principles of medical decision making. Spine 24(5):493–498

McCarthy P R, Dugger D E, Lazarus A 1997 Case management and clinical decision making. In: Schreter R K, Sharfstein S S (eds) Managing care not dollars: the continuum of mental health services. American Psychiatric Press, Washington DC, ch 15, pp 229–243

The pain management programme

SECTION CONTENTS

Although it is recognised that clinics may vary considerably in the programme delivery, content and staffing, a number of common features characterise pain management. The successful programme blends specific uniprofessional skills into an integrated package that is consistent in terms of its overall philosophy of care and balance of emphasis. In a mature programme, there will have developed a degree of commonality across the professionals involved. *What* is delivered is more important than *who* delivers it. Most of the programmes would acknowledge primarily a cognitive–behavioural emphasis, although other psychotherapeutic perspectives may be incorporated. The primary focus is on improvement of function rather than cure of pain and the development of personal responsibility and self-help skills appear to be fundamental to success. Until relatively recently, the specific importance of addressing maintenance of change and the management of 'flare-ups' has perhaps been insufficiently recognised. These issues are addressed in Chapter 14.

13

Clinical content of interdisciplinary pain management programmes

---

PART 1 CONTENT OF THE GROUP PROGRAMME

Chris C. Spanswick   Helen Parker

INTRODUCTION

This section of the book outlines the specific content of interdisciplinary pain management programmes. It is best to consider the goals and expected outcome of pain management and then to detail the content, which is designed to help the patients make the necessary changes.

The aims of pain management programmes (Box 13.1.1) are well known and have been documented in other texts (Main & Parker 1989). How these aims are addressed and delivered will vary

---

> **Box 13.1.1**   Aims of interdisciplinary pain management programmes
>
> ---
>
> - To improve patients' management of their pain and related problems
> - To help patients improve their level of physical functioning
> - To help patients reduce their use of medication
> - To help patients become less dependent upon the health-care system
> - To reduce patients' use of the health-care system
> - To reduce patients' level of depressive/anxiety symptoms
> - To improve patients' level of self-confidence and self-efficacy
> - To address patients' fear and avoidance of activity that may be painful
> - To help patients return to useful and gainful activities

between programmes. This may be dependent more upon local resources, rather than philosophy. Nevertheless, there is a minimum amount of input that is required to produce change. Most, if not all, programmes should include three main components of delivery. These include education, skill acquisition and practice/implementation. All of the professionals involved in the running of the programme will take part in most, if not all, of the above.

Commonly much of the medical input will be almost exclusively educational although this should be as interactive as possible and not simply a number of didactic lectures. The professionals involved in the psychological and physical activity sessions will use all three techniques (i.e. education, skill acquisition, practice and implementation). The types of technique used are listed in Box 13.1.2.

At the time of writing the group programme at Salford is run from 9 a.m. to 5 p.m. 5 days a week for three consecutive weeks (see timetable in Table 13.1.1). Patients attend a pre-programme session the week before the programme to allow collection of data (psychometric questionnaires and measurement of physical function) to be used for outcome measurement. Patients also attend follow-up sessions at 1 month, 3 months and 6 months following the programme. These are regarded as an integral part of the programme requiring patients and their partners to commit to 7 months.

There will be a small number of sessions at which all of the team members will need to be present. The first session is the most important. Most sessions, however, will be conducted by one team member at a time. The reader will notice that there are a number of topics that will be covered

by more than one professional (e.g. pacing of activity and management of flare-ups). Although the topic may be the same, individual professionals will cover that topic from their own standpoint at the same time as pointing out the links with other team members' sessions. This will provide a consistent message from the different team members and add weight to its importance.

For the sake of clarity this chapter of the book has been divided into a number of parts, each addressing a specific aspect of the programme. This part deals with the initial programme session, at which all team members must be present. Subsequent parts deal with the sessions relating to physical exercise, psychology and medical education. These are likely to be led by a single team member, although all team members should have worked in sessions jointly to ensure consistency of approach. The final part outlines the general principles of the group programme and how to prepare the patients for managing their pain at home.

PREPARATION

Before the programme commences the team involved in the delivery of the programme must meet to discuss the timetabling and the content of the programme. Adequate time for this must be set aside. All team members must be aware of their responsibilities. The team should discuss each of the patients on the programme specifically to identify individual barriers to progress. It is worth going over the assessment data again at this stage. The team members may not have been involved in the assessment of every patient so it is important that they become familiar with the details of each patient prior to starting the programme. This will enable the team to plan the specific content of the programme more efficiently. It should allow the team to anticipate problems rather than simply reacting to events on the programme. In addition the team will be able to agree a common strategy with any of the anticipated problems that may arise on the programme thereby presenting a common message to the patients.

The group programme by its nature will address general issues that may or may not be

---

Box 13.1.2 Techniques of pain management

- Didactic teaching (e.g. pain pathways, anatomy)
- Interactive teaching (e.g. drugs, problem solving)
- Skill training (e.g. stretches, exercises, relaxation, pacing)
- Practice (e.g. problem solving, exercises)
- Evaluation and check on progress

Table 13.1.1   Manchester and Salford Pain Centre 30-session pain management programme

		Monday	Tuesday	Wednesday	Thursday	Friday
Week 1						
a.m.		10.00 Pre-programme assessments in-patients (physiotherapist)	9.00 Pain pathways (doctor) 10.30 Communication and working principles (psychologist)	9.00 Brain, body, beliefs Imaging and rehearsal of stress Group discussion Relaxation (psychologist)	9.00 Problem solving 1 (psychologist) 11.15 Practical, group discussion, relaxation (psychologist)	9.00 Individual feedback for patients (whole team)
p.m.		1.30 Introductory sessions (whole team)	1.30 Introduction to exercise Pain and activity (physiotherapist) 3.30 Speed walk (physiotherapist) 4.00 Relaxation (psychologist)	1.30 Intro to pacing Exercise Speed walk (physiotherapist) 4.00 Drugs I (doctor)	1.30 Exercise Pacing/introduction to goal setting Speed walk (physiotherapist)	1.30 Exercise Pacing/goal setting (physiotherapist) Staff info: Doctor available for medical issues
Week 2						
a.m.		9.00 Basic anatomy Exercise Speed walk (physiotherapist)	9.00 ABC of stress 1 Practical Group discussion Relaxation (psychologist)	9.00 ABC of stress 2 Practical Group discussion Relaxation (psychologist)	9.00 Dr/patient (doctor and psychologist) 10.00 Coping with change at home Relaxation (psychologist)	9.00 Group feedback for patients (physiotherapist and psychologist) Presentation of task assignment (psychologist)
p.m.		1.30 Problem solving 2 Practical Group discussion Relaxation (psychologist)	1.30 Posture Exercise Speed walk (physiotherapist)	1.30 Exercise Aerobic exercise Speed walk (psychologist) 4.00 Drugs II (doctor)	1.30 Exercise (physiotherapist) 3.00 Exercise in water (local swimming baths, physiotherapist) Speed walk (physiotherapist)	1.30 Partner info session (whole team)
Week 3						
a.m.		9.00 Assert yourself 1 Practical Group discussion Relaxation (psychologist)	9.00 Exercise Aerobic exercise Speed walk (physiotherapist) 11.30 Emergency card (doctor)	9.00 Task assignment (physiotherapist and psychologist)	9.00 Feedback task assignment (physiotherapist and psychologist) Postprogramme assessment (psychologist) Relaxation (psychologist)	9.00 Postprogramme assessment Questionnaires (physiotherapist and psychologist)
p.m.		1.30 Exercise Posture/body mechanics Speed walk (physiotherapist)	1.30 Task preparation (psychologist) 2.00 Assert yourself 2 Relaxation and guided imagery (psychologist) 4.00 Task (psychologist)	1.30 Exercise 3.00 Exercise in water (local swimming pool) Speed walk physiotherapist	1.30 Video assessments Video feedback (physiotherapist) 4.00 Maintaining home exercise (physiotherapist)	1.30 Staff info. Programme discharge letters (whole team)

There will be a 30 minute break each morning and afternoon session.

relevant to any particular patient. In practice most of the issues covered will apply to most of the participants but the programme must allow for some individualisation in order to address any specific problems that individual patients may have. Some time must therefore be allocated to individual sessions. The remaining patients can quite reasonably be set other tasks that they can be doing during such sessions.

THE INITIAL SESSIONS(S) OF THE PROGRAMME

The first session of the first day is probably the most important session (Keefe, Beapre & Gill 1996). All team members *must* be present. The patients should attend with their partners or 'significant others'. The fundamental purpose of this session is to explain again (this should have already been done before the patients were listed for a programme) the reasons why the patients have been invited to attend the programme. The patients and their partners will need reassurance that the patients' pain is real and is taken seriously by the team. The patients should have been convinced that no further treatment or investigation is indicated and that focusing on activity rather than pain is the only option. The patients' partners must be similarly convinced.

The session should outline the details of the programme and the expectations of outcome. The house rules regarding behaviour, attendance and the disclosure of sensitive information should be explained (see Appendix to this chapter, p. 267). Patients (and partners) who are not comfortable with continuing on the programme following this session must either be convinced or removed from the programme. It is important that every effort is made to elucidate the patients' and partners' feelings about starting on a rehabilitation programme. Only then can any specific worries or fears be tackled. These may be addressed either in the group setting or on an individual basis. It cannot be emphasised enough that major barriers to progress must be addressed early on in the programme and preferably before the end of the first session.

The patients and partners will need some time to get to know each other. Time should be made for patients and partners to introduce themselves and express their expectations of the programme. In addition to general issues and making introductions it is worth ensuring that there are short presentations from each of the team members. This gives an opportunity for team members to introduce themselves and to explain their role in the programme. This should cover reassuring patients' fears about activity and 'psychology' and giving them realistic expectations of outcome.

Both patients and partners are often confused and faced with a large amount of information on the first day. Therefore try not to overload them with too much information. The prime aim is to sell the programme to them and identify specific barriers that will need addressing as early as possible. Box 13.1.3 lists general points to be covered in the initial session.

The medical introduction

One of the functions of the doctor in pain management programmes is to give credence to the programme and techniques used. Unfortunately patients do still take more notice of what doctors say than other professions. It is for this reason it is worth letting the doctor start the introductory session. The introduction should be pitched at a very simple level and a number of points emphasise that will

---

Box 13.1.3 Points for the initial session

- Check patient's (and partner's) understanding of the purpose of the programme
- Explain again the purpose and specific aims of the programme
- Reassure the patient (and partner) of the reality of the pain
- Allow the patient (and partner) to raise questions concerning treatment and investigations
- Outline and explain the reasons for 'house rules'
- Short introductions from each team member outlining the future sessions
- Sell the programme
- Allow time for patients to get to know each other
- Try not to overload the patient (and partner)

Box 13.1.4 Medical points in the introduction

- The patients' pain is real
- Chronic pain is different from acute pain
- Explain the relationship (and lack of it) between pain and injury
- Explain the reasons for previous investigations
- Patients have been 'selected' for pain management because there are no other options
- It is 'safe' to participate in a rehabilitation programme
- Hurt does not mean harm
- Very briefly mention other topics the clinician will cover in future sessions

---

be repeated by colleagues in the team later (Box 13.1.4).

Limitations of the medical model

The reliance of numerous professions on the medical model in the management of chronic pain has been reproached throughout this book and the reader will be under no illusions about the limitations of this model. Such a model has use in the management of acute pain problems and diseases of an identified pathology. Until the commencement of their current chronic problem patients may have been successfully treated by the medical model for different problems and have always held out hope that it would triumph in the end. To this end they may have subjected themselves to many interventions most of which will have failed totally and some of which may have offered only temporary relief. The ability to produce temporary relief may well have reinforced their view that cure may be ultimately possible. This has to be challenged.

Being told that one's pain is unlikely to go away, that the actual cause (such as in musculoskeletal pain) may not be clearly identifiable and that the results of scans and X-rays are not helpful in explaining the current situation is very upsetting for the patient (van Tulder et al 1997). This in turn may lead to a degree of hostility or anger. Doctors must be prepared to be the 'Aunt Sally' and accept that patients' anger with their previous medical and other advisors may be directed at them. It is not helpful simply to blame

other doctors or health-care professionals for the patient's predicament (Loeser and Sullivan 1998).

Great care must be taken to emphasise that the absence of obvious or treatable pathology does not imply the pain is imaginary or 'psychological'. It is helpful to explain the complexity of the pain system in a lay person's terms. This should reinforce the reality of the pain experience in the absence of ongoing tissue injury or damage. A number of models may be used. Most patients have heard of amputees feeling pain in an absent limb and understand sports players may not experience pain from an injury until the game is finished.

The complexity of the pain system. The complexity of pain transmission, and the multiple factors that affect pain perception, is one of the early topics of education because it is fundamental to achieving the belief in patients that they can gain control over the intrusive nature of the pain. Most patients have rudimentary understanding of pain via nerve conduction and that the pain is 'felt' in their brain. Unfortunately most are likely to have had reinforced the misconception that persistent pain can be explained only by persistent nociception. In addition they also believe, again erroneously, that the intensity of pain is determined solely by the severity of the tissue injury or damage (Ch. 1).

It is best to use examples of (acute) painful experiences that the patients may have had in the past to explain the variable pain experience from any given injury. Individual experiences can be recalled to suggest the important role of attention, anticipation, fatigue, stress and emotion in the perception of pain. This will allow the introduction of the 'gating mechanism'. It is important that the participants are made aware of the difference between increased perception of pain and increased nociceptive transmission. The role of descending inhibitory influences on 'shutting the gate' or modulating the pain gate can then be used as a reason for the teaching of pain-modulating techniques such as relaxation, distraction and mobilisation.

The value of diagnoses and tests. Many patients, like many clinicians, have a 'fixation' about identifying a structural component or cause of their pain problem. They require a cause that can be clearly identified. Introducing them to the concept that pain may result from changes in the sensitivity of nerves and the 'mis-transmission' of previously non-painful stimuli can be very useful in offering an alternative explanation of their pain that does not require identification of a 'source' by scans, blood tests or other investigations. This, of course, is the basis of much current thinking on the role of neuroplastic change in the generation and maintenance of chronic pain (Ch. 1).

Doctors should emphasise that the patients have been carefully assessed and every effort has been made to check that there is no ongoing tissue injury or damage. They should explain this in a way that will allow any patients to challenge this if they feel that they have *not* been investigated adequately. This may need to then be dealt with on an individual basis if necessary. Often an explanation about the interpretation of investigations is enough to defuse such a problem. Despite careful assessment and counselling prior to listing a patient for a programme there will still be occasions when patients raise questions for the first time on the programme. Box 13.1.5 lists the major educational points to be covered in the first session.

Given that both patients and partners will be faced with an enormous amount of new information the doctor must finish with only one important message. This should be that 'hurt does not mean harm' in the case of chronic pain and it is 'safe' for the patients to exercise in spite of their pain. The team is happy that following a full assessment the patients will not damage themselves.

Physiological effects of pain and inactivity

At Salford this part of the introduction is given by the physiotherapist. It has to be said that many patients have had 'physiotherapy' and possibly 'exercises' to no avail. They therefore may view this part of the programme with some scepticism, suspicion and even fear. The physiotherapist must therefore gain the patients' confidence and explain how this programme will differ from their past experiences.

It is important to explain the differences between conventional physiotherapy, which the patient is likely to have had, and the physiotherapy on the pain management programme. Commonly the physiotherapist will outline the sorts of conventional treatment that the patient may have had (Box 13.1.6) and then encourage the patients to comment.

Most of the comments from the patients regarding previous physiotherapy are negative.

Box 13.1.6   Traditional physiotherapy treatments

- Types of treatment:
  — symptomatic pain relief e.g. electrotherapy
  — manipulation/mobilisation
  — other 'hands on' treatments
  — education/advice
- Aims of traditional physiotherapy:
  — seek cause for painful symptoms
  — directed towards alleviating and curing symptoms

Note: The physiotherapist is generally 'in charge' of the treatment and the patient is the 'passive recipient' of the treatment.

For chronic pain physiotherapy is likely to be of short term benefit only.

Box 13.1.5   Major educational points in the first session

- Simple explanation of the pain system:
  — injury does not *always* produce pain (e.g. sports injury)
  — pain can occur in the absence of injury (e.g. postamputation)
  — other factors influence pain perception
- Reasons for investigations:
  — limitations of investigations
  — interpreting the results
  — why doctors give differing answers

- Conclusions:
  — the patients have been carefully assessed to look for continuing damage
  — it is safe for the patients to exercise in the presence of their chronic pain
  — hurt does not equal harm
  — the programme aims to help patients improve physical functioning in spite of pain
  — the programme is designed to help the patients learn skills to manage their pain more successfully

At this point the physiotherapist should outline the problems with repeated or prolonged physiotherapy (Box 13.1.7). However, some patients may have had relief from some passive forms of therapy; in these cases it is important to get the patient to identify the difference between short term symptomatic relief and the gradual downward spiral of loss of function. From this the patient should be helped to discriminate between therapies that have short term benefit but have not addressed the problem of increased incapacity.

Most patients identify with the problems outlined in Box 13.1.7. This allows for discussion and reassurance from the physiotherapist that past experiences will not be repeated on the programme.

Most patients are very aware of the effects of inactivity (Bortz 1984). Through group discussion, the physiotherapist can get the patients to identify the changes that they have experienced since they have had chronic pain. Most will relate reduced strength and fitness, increased fatigue, weight gain and depressed mood.

Having explained about the effects of inactivity the physiotherapist should now outline the major benefits of exercise. The beneficial effects of exercise in the management of pain need to be understood early on in the programme if compliance with exercise is to be achieved (these are discussed later). Box 13.1.8 lists the goals of physiotherapy in pain management.

It is important to warn patients that they may expect discomfort and an increase in their pain following exercise. It should be explained that this is a normal concomitant of exercising muscles and joints that have not been used for some time. This is also critical if compliance with exercise is to be achieved.

A frequent charge made by patients is that the discomfort they feel following exercise in the muscles and joints away from the 'injured' area is not of the same quality or intensity of that coming from the 'injured' area. In this situation it may be useful to reinforce the points made by the doctor about the increased sensitivity of the pain system (neuroplastic changes). It is important to explain in understandable laymen's terms that non-painful stimuli (e.g. stretch) may be misrouted up the pain system in patients with chronic pain. Using the metaphor of an 'oversensitive burglar alarm system' may be helpful in conveying this difficult concept.

Finally the physiotherapist should outline briefly the approach to be taken in subsequent sessions, and the responsibilities of each party (Box 13.1.9). It should be explained that the focus will be on activity not pain, and emphasised that the physiotherapist is not being unkind. The

---

Box 13.1.8 The goals of the physiotherapy component of the pain management programme

- To learn about the effects of inactivity
- To learn about the importance and benefits of exercise
- To increase flexibility, strength, cardiovascular and respiratory fitness i.e. to recondition the body
- To increase levels of general activity and function despite the pain
- To manage daily activities more effectively (managing the over/under activity cycle)
- To learn about the benefits of goal setting and pacing
- To learn about posture and biomechanics and apply these skills in everyday activities
- To learn how best to manage acute flare-ups

Box 13.1.7 The adverse effects of repeated or prolonged episodes of physiotherapy for chronic pain

- Reliance on the physiotherapist for treatment
- The physiotherapist takes control of managing the pain problem
- The physiotherapist may actively discourage patients' attempts to manage their own problem
- Conflicting diagnoses/opinions
- Demoralisation as a result of repeated failed treatments

Box 13.1.9 Responsibilities of physiotherapist and patient

- Skills combined with other team members
- Aims to help the patient improve function and quality of life despite the pain
- Pain/symptoms are not the focus of attention
- Therapists are responsible for teaching pain management skills
- The patient is responsible for applying the skills

reality of patients' pain is not in question. There is little that can be done to change patients' pain in itself and there is therefore little point in the therapist responding to complaints of pain or pain behaviour. The physiotherapist should reinforce that the purpose of the programme is to help the patients manage their pain more successfully. Choosing simply to ignore the patient when they demonstrate pain behaviour without explanation can result in some people becoming angry (both patients and spouses). This is why it is essential to give this explanation of the staff action, or lack of it, right at the start of the programme.

The psychological effects of chronic pain

Almost all patients with chronic pain are suspicious of psychological issues and psychologists. They usually interpret any attempt to look at psychological issues as meaning that their pain is, in effect, imaginary. Past experience with health-care professionals has sensitised many against considering any of the psychological influences or consequences of pain. Many have had previous consultations in which the patient's pain has either implicitly or occasionally explicitly been said to be psychological. Psychologists in teams therefore have a difficult task ahead of them before they even speak. Many of these potential barriers will have been addressed at the assessment, but that may have been several weeks or months ago. Patients (and their partners) will require further reassurance that their pain is taken seriously.

Perhaps the best way to begin to gain the patients' confidence is to outline simply the normal consequences of chronic pain (Gatchel 1996). Presenting the details of a number of traps that patients find themselves falling into demonstrates that there are a number of profound and serious consequences to chronic pain. Individual patients will realise that they are no different from many other patients treated on the programme. The psychologist can then explain that not only is the pain a problem, but there are now a number of new other problems. These

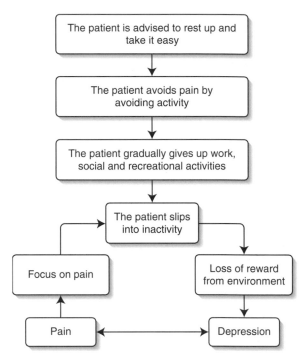

Figure 13.1.1 The 'take it easy' trap.
Adapted from Peck C, Love A 1986 Chronic pain

may well have occurred as a consequence of the pain, but nevertheless will need addressing.

Figure 13.1.1 shows how patients can slip almost insidiously into decreasing levels of activity following well-meaning advice to 'take it easy'. This ultimately can lead to withdrawal from all rewarding activities. a slide into depression and a subsequent focusing on and decreasing tolerance of pain. The pain alone is perceived as the barrier to any activity, when in fact many other barriers now exist. The use of such a simple model to outline the natural consequences of chronic pain and decreased activity enables patients to identify with it. They can begin to understand how they have become so disabled without blame being implied. By avoiding blame the patients are more likely to address the issues rather than become angry or resistant.

Figure 13.1.2 demonstrates the chronic treatment trap into which many patients fall. In the beginning both patient and doctor expect a resolution of the problem. In the case of the patient

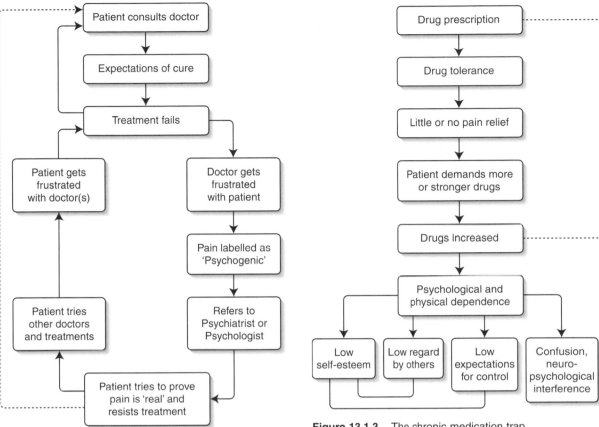

Figure 13.1.2 The chronic treatment trap.
Adapted from Peck C, Love A 1986 Chronic pain

Figure 13.1.3 The chronic medication trap.
Adapted from Peck C, Love A 1986 Chronic pain

with chronic pain, treatment fails to provide a cure. Other treatments will be tried and they too fail. The doctor becomes progressively frustrated with the patient. The failure to respond to treatment must be because the pain is not 'organic' and the patient is then sent for 'psychological' treatment. The patient, who knows the pain is real, resents such inferences and tries to prove the pain is real by not participating in psychological treatment and searching for more physical treatments. Unfortunately this is not only unsuccessful and leads to more and more failed treatment, which confirms to the doctor that the pain is mainly psychological or has a major psychological component.

Patients identify well with this model. They often feel they have been 'labelled' and treated dismissively. Giving an understanding of the

very different nature of chronic pain enables them to understand why treatment has failed and why doctors (and other health-care professionals) are frustrated as well. No blame should be aimed at either the doctors or patients. The purpose of demonstrating these models is to explain that what has happened to the patient is common and that the consequences of chronic pain are profound.

Figure 13.1.3 outlines the chronic medication trap. This is perhaps the commonest trap that ensnares patients. This occurs largely out of the helplessness of the doctor as well as the patient. The figure charts the development of tolerance leading to the patient asking for something stronger. Invariably psychological dependence occurs and in some cases physical dependence as well. Patients' reliance upon tablets makes them feel bad about their predicament and others will often point out they are becoming addicted, which only makes them feel worse. Patients do indeed become reliant on tablets as the only way to control or manage their pain and therefore do not attempt any other strategies. A number of patients suffer subtle neuropsychological changes as a consequence of either toxic doses of medicines or drug interactions. Most patients are not aware of this effect until they eventually withdraw from medication.

Some patients may have stopped analgesic medication because it does not help. Most patients, however, continue to take analgesics even when these are not helpful. All patients identify with the 'medication trap'. Many do not understand why this has occurred. The psychologist should not blame the doctor or the patient, but simply point out that this is simply what happens, that it is not helpful and will need to be addressed.

Figure 13.1.4 shows the effects of chronic pain upon relationships. Very few relationships emerge unscathed from the effects of the chronic pain and the associated incapacity. As can been seen from the figure the consequent incapacity leads to changes in the ability of the couple to enjoy activities together. This in turn leads to a less rewarding relationship and commonly to problems with communication. Ultimately the couple focus on the pain as the cause of all of their problems and its cure as the only solution. This topic is often the most important theme to emerge during the partner session later in the programme.

Some patients may be in the middle of one of the traps, or have been through some of the problems outlined. Most patients identify with most if not all of the 'traps' described above. No blame is attributed. The 'traps' are simply a description of what happens to people. On the basis of these 'ripples' from the pain and associated incapacity, the psychological issues can be addressed more openly and with little resistance or hostility from most patients. Such an explanation allows the psychologist to lay the ground for subsequent sessions and allay the fears of the patients.

The psychologist now moves on to begin to link mind and body in very simple terms. It should be explained that pain will have an effect

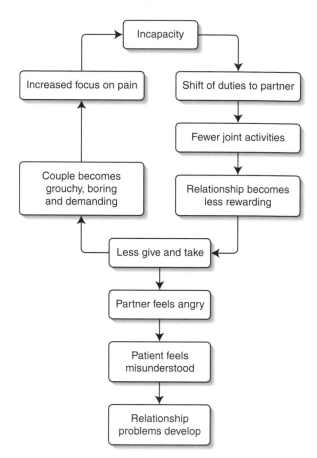

Figure 13.1.4 The chronic resentment trap. Adapted from Peck C, Love A 1986 Chronic pain

emotionally as well as physically and these in turn can affect each other. Patients will, therefore, have to address all of the effects of and the issues surrounding the pain if they are to take control and master it.

The psychologist will give a very brief outline of the sorts of things that the group will be doing during the sessions later in the programme. Finally questions are invited from patients and partners.

CONCLUSION

The whole process of the first day is carried out with as little didactic and as much interactive teaching as possible. The patients and partners are encouraged to interrupt if they do not understand anything. The patients are encouraged to stand up if sitting for any length becomes uncomfortable. This is the beginning of the patients taking more responsibility for their own condition.

KEY POINTS

At the end of the first day the patients should have an understanding of the following:

- their pain is real and taken seriously.
- they have been assessed to ensure that it is safe to exercise in the face of pain (hurt does not equal harm).
- The consequences of their chronic pain (physical and psychological)

are common and can be regarded as normal.
- The programme is designed to help them learn to improve their quality of life despite their pain.
- The philosophy of the programme is 'self-help' and they are responsible for their own management.

REFERENCES

Bortz W M 1984 The disuse syndrome. Western Journal of Medicine 141:691–694

Gatchel J G 1996 Psychological disorders and chronic pain: cause-and-effect relationships. In: Gatchel R J, Turk D C (eds) Psychological approaches to pain management: a practitioner's handbook. Guilford, New York, ch 2.

Keefe J K, Beapre P M, Gill K M 1996 Group therapy for patients with chronic pain. In: Gatchel R J, Turk D C (eds) Psychological approaches to pain management: a practitioner's handbook. Guilford, New York, ch 10

Loeser J D, Sullivan M 1995 Disability in the chronic low back pain patient may be iatrogenic. Pain Forum 4:114–121

Main C J, Parker H 1989 The evaluation and outcome of pain management programmes for chronic low back pain. In: Roland M, Jenner J R (eds) Back pain: new approaches to rehabilitation and education. Manchester University Press, Manchester.

Peck C, Love A 1986 Chronic Pain, In: Healthcare: A Behavioural Approach King NJ, Remengi A (eds) or 14. Grune & Stratton, Sydney

van Tulder M W, Assendelft W J J, Koes B W, Bouter L M 1997 Spinal radiographic findings and non-specific low back pain. Spine 22:427–434

APPENDIX: HOUSE RULES—MANCHESTER AND SALFORD PAIN CENTRE HOPE HOSPITAL

We wish to ensure that your stay here runs as smoothly and pleasantly as possible and that you have the best chance of benefiting from what the programme has to offer. Adherence to the following rules is expected both by group members and by staff.

The hostel is within a hospital setting with patients on the ward below. The facilities you use also serve as an assessment clinic during the day. You are obliged to respect others and to contribute to looking after the hostel during your stay.

1. Common room
   Please keep this room clean and tidy. You are sharing these facilities with other patients.
2. Other group members
   Group members both male and female share these facilities. You should respect each other's right to privacy and personal space.
   The group relies on honesty and confidentiality both within the group sessions and 'after hours'.
3. Going out
   It is reasonable for you to leave the premises in the evening. A booklet of local amenities compiled by a previous group is available. However, you must return quietly before 10.00 p.m. and must be able to participate actively in the programme the next day.
4. Visitors
   Family and friends may visit the hostel but must leave the premises by 10.00 p.m.
5. Alcohol, cigarettes and illicit drugs
   No alcohol or illicit drugs may be consumed on the hospital premises. This building operates a no-smoking policy. You cannot smoke inside this building.

If you, or other members of the group, are having difficulty in adhering to these rules, please contact a member of staff.

PART 2 MEDICAL COMPONENT OF THE PROGRAMME

Chris C. Spanswick

PAIN PATHWAYS

The patient's simplistic and inaccurate model of pain will have been challenged at the introductory session. It is important to expand on this later to give the patient a better understanding of the pain system and the reasons behind the variability in pain experience following injury. The patient should understand that the complexity of the pain system has only recently been understood and indeed we still have much to discover. It is important that emphasis is laid on the fact that our knowledge of the pain system is based on good scientific evidence and is not simply theory or pseudoscientific ramblings. Figure 13.2.1 is a simple model of the pain pathway.

It is not necessary to go into immense detail, but it is important to explain enough to give the patient an understanding of the reasons behind the various treatments that are used and why some treatments do not work (e.g. cutting nerves). The doctor should not be tempted to use only a didactic lecturing style. Because of the complexity of the pain system and the difficulty that we as professionals have in understanding it, the doctor should constantly check patients' understanding. It is best to use models and examples that patients may have experienced or know about already. For example, simply asking the patients about their experience of twisting an ankle in detail will bring out the detail of first and second pain. This then enables the doctor to show the patients that a single event (the injury

269

Pain Pathway

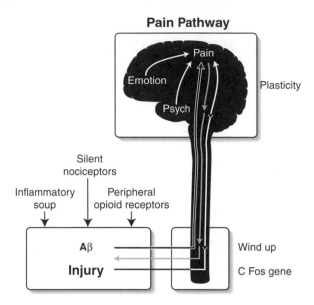

Figure 13.2.1 The pain pathway

to the ankle) produces two entirely different pains. The system therefore must be more complicated than a simple stimulus–response system.

It is often useful to explain that the nervous system modulates all incoming information from the peripheral nerves and will filter out unimportant information almost to the extent that the person may not be aware of it—for example, the selective deafness of children called to meal times, or the sensation of the wristwatch, which does not normally enter consciousness. Similarly the nervous system will enhance and pay much more attention to information that is deemed important, threatening or annoying—for example, the squeak in the car, the whimper of a newborn baby or the sound of footsteps behind one when walking in the dark.

Most patients can identify with examples of this. It should be explained that pain signals are treated in much the same way. They are, of course, regarded as important signals and may well be enhanced, especially if the patient is fearful of their meaning (Box 13.2.1 and Ch. 1).

At the end of the session(s) on pain pathways patients should be confident that their usual chronic pain does not signify further damage or harm and when it increases it does not signify a new injury. They should also understand that a new pain in an area they have not had pain in before *may* indicate damage and it may require attention. Patients should therefore become more confident of increasing activities in spite of their pain and become less fearful of movement. Unless patients understand the model of pain and are able to be confident that they will not deteriorate physically as a consequence of increasing their physical activities they will not participate in the programme or make any progress.

DIAGNOSES AND INVESTIGATIONS

This session has the potential to stir up a significant amount of anger that patients may have with the medical and other professions. The doctor entrusted with this session must be prepared to take the brunt of patients' anger with the medical profession in general. Patients' experiences are very variable. Most patients have had a lot of previous investigations and (unsuccessful) treatment. They often feel they have been passed from pillar to post with little explanation of their condition. They may have been given to

---

Box 13.2.2 Investigations, tests and diagnosis: the points patients should understand after the session on investigations, tests and diagnoses

- The reasons why certain investigations are performed
- The limitations of particular types of investigations
- The interpretation of the results of investigations
- What do people without pain show on investigations?
- What are the known causes of chronic pain?
- What treatments are available?
- Just how effective are the treatments?
- Why can't pain be stopped?
- What is the future likely to be for a patient with chronic pain?

Box 13.2.3 Medication use education

1. *1st session*
- Introduction to drugs
- Types of medicines
- Benefits, uses, side-effects and problems
2. *2nd session*
- Tolerance
- Addiction and dependence
- Physical and psychological dependence
- Withdrawal: problems and benefits
- Monitoring medicines
- When to use painkillers

---

understand that they have 'spinal arthritis' when the X-rays simply show degenerative change. It may have even been implied they are imagining their pain or it is not real pain.

It is sometimes helpful to invite a specialist from outside the team (e.g. a spinal surgeon). Care should be taken in choosing whom to invite. The relevant person should have a good understanding of pain management programmes and the specific reason for their session. They should be warned that patients on such programmes can often become very angry during this session. Patients often feel that investigation, tests and diagnoses have not been explained fully (Box 13.2.2). They frequently feel they have been treated dismissively. As a consequence they may become quite hostile to the doctor in this session. It is worth ensuring that another regular team member is at this session not only to provide some support for the doctor but also to gain first-hand knowledge of what was said.

Despite the risks it is often very much more powerful, however, if the message that surgery is not the answer to the patients' pain comes from a surgeon rather than a member of the team. Surgeons may be able to explain much more convincingly the limitations of tests and surgery. They will be able to put surgery into context and explain why certain investigations are performed and how they should be interpreted. Finally they may be able to give the patients an understanding that as yet some problems do not have a medical solution.

At the end of this session any residual fears of the patients should have been addressed. This may require time to be spent with individuals to either reassure particular patients or institute further investigations in order to reassure them. It must be said that investigating such patients further at this late stage should be very rare and will probably exclude them from the programme until the issues have been clarified. Most issues, however, can be more than adequately addressed in the group setting. The team should feel able to draw a line under these issues and feel comfortable that no further discussions should be held unless an entirely new problem occurs.

MEDICINES: HOW TO GET THE BEST OUT OF THEM

There is quite a lot of information to impart concerning medications, their use and the problems associated with them (Box 13.2.3). It is best to tackle these at two sittings, avoid didactic teaching (remember how boring pharmacology lectures were!) and get the patients to do most of the work.

A significant proportion of patients with chronic pain problems persist in using medication of various types despite little in the way of prolonged or sustained benefit. Many have been prescribed medication, which is normally designed to help with short term problems during the initial phase of the pain. There is evidence in the literature that the level of medication usage, and in particular misuse, correlates with the level of psychological distress (Spanswick & Main 1989). In other words the more distressed patients are the more likely it is that they will use analgesics and/or tranquillisers and also the more likely that they will use them in doses above the recommended maximum. It is for this reason that some education regarding medication usage is important. It cannot be assumed that medication usage will automatically change following a pain management programme unless it is specifically addressed.

Patients should be warned in one of the first sessions by the doctor that they may well experience more pain in the first few days or weeks of the programme. This is usually because they are using muscles they have not used for some time. They should be asked specifically *not* to increase their medication usage, but to begin to take it on a time-contingent basis rather than a PRN (pro re nata) or pain-contingent basis (Fordyce 1976). They should complete a drug usage form (see Appendix to this chapter, p. 283) and to fill this in each day recording *all* pain-related and psychotropic medication they use. This will enable the team to establish the patient's baseline use of medication.

Introduction to medicines

Many patients have no understanding of the medicines they are taking or the rationale for their prescription. The medications are often taken in a haphazard way. Frequently patients gain little benefit despite high doses.

It is important, therefore, to offer some education addressing the points above. It is useful to allow patients to do much of the work in finding out about the various types of drugs and to get them to report back the detail of what they have learned. However, it is important to give a basic structure into which they can hang the detail.

The patients should, therefore, have been set 'homework' in one of the sessions prior to this first session on medicines. They should be given copies of the British National Formulary (BNF) and asked to look up a number of drugs including the medicines they are likely to either be taking or have taken in the past. The group is asked to divide themselves into subgroups and to allocate to each subgroup a specific type of medicine to look up. At this session each subgroup is asked to tell the rest of the group what they have learned about the various medicines they were asked to investigate. In order to help the patients make sense of the information they will discover they should be directed to searching out the benefits, the side-effects and the major problems with each type of medication they look up.

The patients may be quite daunted by this task and will need some guidance. The doctor's task is to act as interpreter, as the BNF is not designed for the layperson. The doctor should guide the patients through the meaning of the medical terms and translate the information in terms that the patients can understand. Patients may be frightened by the description of side-effects and complications. The doctor should take care to reassure patients about the safety of the medicines they have read about and put the side-effects into context.

At the end of the presentations and the subsequent discussions within the whole group and with the doctor the patients should have an understanding of the various types of medication outlined in Box 13.2.4. They should understand the basic mode of action of NSAIDs, opioids, tranquillisers and night sedatives. They should understand why such medications are prescribed. It is important to reiterate what has been said in the introductory session. No blame

---

Box 13.2.4 Medication

- NSAIDs
- Opioids and opioid-containing medicines including Co-compounds
- Paracetamol
- Tranquillisers (benzodiazepines)
- Antidepressants (tricyclic antidepressants, newer antidepressants, SSRIs)
- Anticonvulsants
- Others

> **Box 13.2.5** NSAIDs: main teaching points
>
> - Act by inhibiting enzymes that normally enhance pain
> - A peripherally acting painkiller
> - Not addictive
> - Some potential problems with gastric side-effects
> - Some central side-effects

> **Box 13.2.6** Opioids
>
> - Related to morphine
> - Work at morphine receptors
> - Key-and-lock mechanism
> - Physical dependence
> - Psychological dependence
> - Development of tolerance
> - Withdrawal effects
> - Long term use effects (possibly enhancing pain)
> - Interaction with benzodiazepines (central effect)
> - Why use them
> - The body's own morphine

of either the patient or their doctor should be implied. The patients may become angry at realising they have been prescribed medication that has not been helpful and may have caused significant problems. The doctor must emphasise that most of the medications discussed are very useful in the early phase of a pain problem or during the acute episode.

The opportunity should also be taken to answer any questions, doubts or worries about any other medication that the patients may be taking.

NSAIDs

Box 13.2.5 shows a simple outline of the important points to be made with regard to NSAIDs. Explaining how the NSAIDs came to be discovered and used originally and why they have been so successful is important. The message should not be entirely negative about drugs, but rather putting their use into the context of other conditions and diseases (e.g. osteoarthritis). The emphasis should be made, as with all medication, that often patients do not necessarily find them helpful if taken all of the time, although they may be helpful during acute episodes of pain (McQuay & Moore 1998a).

Opioids

Many patients are horrified to discover that they are taking medication that includes an opioid, a drug related to morphine (Box 13.2.6). Some become quite angry, especially if they have become physically dependent on them. It is therefore important to explain the rationale for using opioids in acute pain and exactly how effective they can be. Their use in chronic pain,

however, is not associated with quite so much success (Jamison 1996, Molloy, Nicholas & Cousins 1997). Of course all episodes of chronic pain began with an acute episode and therefore it is quite reasonable to use opioids in the acute phase (McQuay & Moore 1998b). It is important to reinforce that no blame should be attached to either the prescriber or the patient.

Paracetamol

It is surprising how many patients do not know that the 'co-' compounds like co-proxamol or co-codamol contain paracetamol. It is, fortunately, becoming less common, but considering the potential danger of inadvertent overdose of paracetamol it is very important. Indeed it is the paracetamol rather than the opioid content that is dangerous in the taking of such 'co-' compounds in excessive doses. There are records of patients consuming as many as 28 co-dydradamol per day!

Emphasis should be made that in therapeutic doses paracetamol is safe and sometimes helpful even for chronic pain. More importantly it is not addictive and relatively free from side-effects such as gastric irritation.

Tranquillisers and night sedatives

Most patients with chronic unrelieved pain develop sleep problems if they did not have them before. In addition a proportion become increasingly anxious and worried about their

---

Box 13.2.7   Tranquillisers

- Sedatives
- May help sleep in short term
- Originally thought not to be addictive
- Now known to produce 'physical' dependence within 3 weeks
- Psychomotor effects
- Enhanced effect on cognition with concurrent opioid
- Withdrawal effects
- Psychological dependence, 'habit'

Box 13.2.8   Antidepressants

- Tricyclic antidepressants often prescribed as analgesics
- Analgesic effect separate from antidepressant effect
- Well-documented dose-response curve
- Useful non-addictive night sedation
- Significant side-effects can limit use
- More recent SSRIs less sedating; no known analgesic effect

---

pain and increasing disability. A significant number are prescribed night sedatives, which usually means a benzodiazepine. Fortunately there is a trend for fewer patients to be prescribed diazepam for pain even if some muscle spasm is associated with it. Such treatment almost invariably does not help the pain and simply sedates the patient, who subsequently finds it more difficult to cope. Some pointers about tranquillisers are given in Box 13.2.7.

Having already explained the mechanisms of the actions of opioids, it is a simple matter to use that basis for the teaching of the effects of benzodiazepines. It is worth putting benzodiazepines into context. It should not be implied that drugs themselves are bad, but rather that they need to be used appropriately in appropriate circumstances to reap the best benefit. The patients should have noted that they are not recommended for more than 6 weeks from their reading of the BNF.

Antidepressants

Depression as a part of the clinical picture with chronic pain is neither uncommon nor unsurprising (Ch. 2). A number of patients end up taking antidepressants of one type or another. Many, if they have already been to a pain clinic, will have been prescribed a tricyclic antidepressant for the analgesic effect rather than the antidepressant effect (Box 13.2.8). It is important to emphasise that the analgesic effect seems to be entirely separate from the antidepressant effect. Patients often need some reassurance that

antidepressants are not tranquillisers or addictive. The are frequently not aware of the reason for their prescription. It is therefore important to spend some time explaining their use. Mention should be made of the more recent SSRI (selective serotonin reuptake inhibitor) antidepressants. Some patients may have been prescribed these. Although their effectiveness in depression is not challenged, they do not appear to have a specific analgesic effect.

Anticonvulsants and other membrane stabilisers

A small number of patients will have been prescribed anticonvulsants (or other membrane stabilisers) for their pain problem (Bull et al 1969, Loeser 1994, Monks 1994). There is some evidence in the literature that they can be helpful, particularly in neurogenic pain of a shooting nature. Patients, pharmacists and some doctors become confused as to the rationale for their prescription. It is not possible to educate the whole of the medical and pharmacy staff. Therefore, educating patients is the most efficient way of ensuring these drugs are used in the appropriate way by them.

It is important that patients understand why they have been prescribed, how they work and how they should take them (Box 13.2.9). Many patients will take them 'as required', which is probably the least effective way of using them.

Other medication

During the medication education part of the programme it is often a good time for patients to ask the questions they always wanted to ask

---

Box 13.2.9 Anticonvulsants and other membrane stabilisers

- Useful in pain of a 'shooting' or paroxysmal nature
- Often used in pain of a neurogenic origin
- Needs to be taken regularly 'by the clock'
- May cause sedation, tremor, gastric irritation and other side-effects
- Long term use requires blood monitoring
- Not addictive

Box 13.2.10 Definitions in patients' language

Tolerance
- The ability of the body to 'get used to' a medicine
- Often leads to a decreasing effect from the drug and the need either to increase the dose or to move on to a 'stronger' medicine
- Does not happen with all medicines
- Most common with opioids, tranquillisers and night sedatives
- Can happen in a short time (less than 6 weeks)

Psychological dependence
- A habit
- Commonly results from repeated actions in association with a trigger
- Inability to perform the habit makes people feel anxious and focus on the original symptoms
- Easily reinforced

Physical dependence
- Involves the development of tolerance
- 'Physical symptoms', usually unpleasant, develop following sudden cessation of medication
- The physical symptoms may include some that are similar to those for which the medicine was taken
- All withdrawal symptoms stop eventually, even without treatment
- Withdrawal symptom profile varies according to the medicine and between individuals

---

about their other medicines. This should be actively encouraged, although it is obviously not the main thrust of the education. It is important to emphasise to patients that although they will be encouraged to make less use of analgesics and tranquillisers they should continue on all their other medicines that they take for other purposes (e.g. blood pressure tablets).

Patients should be set a homework task at the end of this session. It is worth indicating the topics to be covered in the next session and ask the patients to prepare some questions they may wish to ask and to put some thoughts down on paper. Given that the next session will be on addiction and tolerance, the group should be asked to prepare any questions they have and write down their thoughts about addiction and getting use to medicines.

Tolerance, addiction and how to get the best out of medicines

Although this second session on medication could be given in entirely a didactic way, it is best to use techniques that involve as much activity from the patients as possible. The doctor should check that patients understood the content of the previous session on medicines and that there are no further outstanding worries or questions. It may be worth reassuring the audience by explaining that many patients find these sessions difficult and often raise questions about tablets and medicines.

It is best to use the term 'dependence' rather than 'addiction'. The word addiction is often used in a judgmental way and is best avoided. The discussion should identify the difference between physical dependence and psychological dependence.

The doctor should then ask the group members to give their own understanding of dependence and tolerance. At the end of the discussion with the group it should be possible to write down definitions of physical and psychological dependence and tolerance (O'Brien 1996, Reisine & Pasternak 1996). The discussion can then move on to what the patient can do to avoid these problems.

Box 13.2.10 outlines the main teaching points of this part of the session. No blame should be attached to either patients or their prescribing doctor. This session should emphasise that this is simply what happens. It does not happen to everyone, nor does it represent a problem in everyone, even though they may have noticed some of the physical effects. The ultimate aim of this session is to point out that continuous use of some pain medicines is often not helpful and can be counterproductive.

Box 13.2.11 Reasons for reducing and withdrawing from medication

- Significant improvement in cognitive functioning (especially with opioid/benzodiazepine combination)
- Loss of potentially significant side-effects (e.g. constipation, gastric problems)
- Feel more 'in control'
- Improvement in self-esteem
- Analgesics often make little or no change to long term pain anyway
- Return of positive short term response for acute episodes (see tolerance above)

Box 13.2.12 Common reasons for failing to stop medicines

- Abrupt withdrawal leads to a much greater chance of profound withdrawal symptoms
- Stretching out the time interval between tablets produces withdrawal symptoms
- An increase in pain is a common withdrawal symptom, reinforcing the 'need' for tablets
- The patient has no other strategies to manage the pain to replace the tablets
- General practitioner may inadvertently reinforce regular medication

---

Box 13.2.13 Principles of drug withdrawal

- Choose to reduce or withdraw from one drug at a time
- Choose the easiest one first (probably the opioid)
- Start by stabilising level of medication usage
- Change from pain-contingent to time-contingent medication
- Keep timing of medication the same (do not extend time between medications)
- Reduce the amount taken by a small amount (half a tablet) at a time
- Reward success

Patients must be given some positive reasons for medication reduction and withdrawal (Box 13.2.11). These should be outlined before going on to techniques of how to withdraw from tablets.

Some patients become overenthusiastic and will wish to stop everything immediately. Some may become quite angry at any implication they are to blame as they have tried to stop medicines but have been unsuccessful because the pain becomes intolerable. Time should be taken to address these feelings and explain why many patients are unsuccessful in their attempts to stop tablets (Box 13.2.12). For example, simply stopping tablets or stretching out the time in between tablets is more likely to provoke withdrawal symptoms. This, however, is the commonest strategy that patients adopt.

At this point the principles of drug withdrawal should be outlined and the patients then set the task of working out for themselves precisely how they propose to come off all or some of their medication. However, before any attempt is made to withdraw patients should learn to change their habit of taking medicines. Patients must start to take their medicines on a 'time-contingent' basis or 'by the clock' rather that contingent upon their pain. This will help break the 'pain–pill' habit and must be in place before any attempt at withdrawal is made.

At this point, if not before, the patients are asked to keep a drug diary (see pain diary in Appendix to Ch. 7, p. 134) to help them monitor their own medication usage. This will give them an insight as to how much they actually are taking and may well change their behaviour just by the fact that they are monitoring the situation. Having established baseline patients should follow the guidelines outlined in Box 13.2.13 while continuing to monitor their tablet consumption.

The patient plan should first establish taking medicine on a time-contingent basis and not only as response to pain. Having established regular medication patients should concentrate on reducing the amount of drug/medication by a small amount every few days or weeks. This should be done with the aim of coming off the chosen medication within a specific period of time. This will vary according to which type of medication is being withdrawn. In general opioids may be withdrawn much quicker than benzodiazepines, which might take several months (Hobbs, Rall & Verdoon 1996). It may be necessary to change the patient's medication in order to facilitate withdrawal. For example, some compound analgesics that contain an opioid and paracetamol are best prescribed separately so that the opioid component can be withdrawn separately from the paracetamol or more slowly if necessary.

It is important to stress that if the patients do get any withdrawal symptoms these will eventually disappear. The negative aspects of withdrawal should not be overemphasised; many patients get none at all. Patients should be encouraged to plan the withdrawal and use the medication-monitoring forms to assess their progress and identify any problems. This allows patients to monitor their reduction of tablets and enables the staff to reinforce the changes the patient has achieved. Some patients may have difficulty in completing such forms so it is important to go through it with them individually if necessary. Patients should be encouraged to ask questions about their medication if they are not sure, and to check with the doctor on the programme that they are managing their medication correctly. Be sure to keep the patient's GP informed.

The patients must understand that medication reduction and withdrawal is a long term plan and should not be instituted in haste. They should not be expected to make major changes in a few weeks, particularly if they are increasing their level of exercise at the same time.

Much of the teaching about medication will have necessarily dwelt on the negative effects of continuous use. It is important to point out that medicines can be of significant help, particularly during acute episodes of pain. It is worth revisiting the 'mission statement'. This emphasises that continuous use of medicines for reducing pain is usually not helpful in the long term. Analgesic use for short periods during acute episodes has been shown to be helpful (McQuay & Moore 1998a–c). If patients are able to reduce their medication to the lowest level possible (preferably zero) then they are likely to gain some help during acute flare-ups without having to exceed the maximum recommended dose. In addition, patients will have been taught other techniques to help them manage acute episodes more effectively. This prepares the way for the last session with the doctor. An example is given in Case study 13.2.1.

THE MANAGEMENT OF FLARE-UPS

During the last week there is a session with the doctor that is entitled 'the emergency card'. An important part of this session is devoted to the 'sensible use' of medication. During the course of the programme the patients will have learned to use a range of skills in managing their pain. They are taught to recognise the difference between their usual pain, which may simply be increased

---

Case study 13.2.1   Chronic back pain

Mrs J. has had a chronic back pain problem for some 8 years. She has tried most medications but has found them not helpful and has become desperate to find something that works. Over a prolonged period she has ultimately ended up taking a significant number of different medicines. These include anti-inflammatory drugs (diclofenac), an opioid (dihydrocodeine), up to 16 tablets a day, a night sedative (temazepam) and an antidepressant (amitriptyline).

Despite the use of all of this medication her pain is still severe. It appears to get much worse if she tries to stop any of the tablets. She doesn't like taking all of this medication and tries to stretch out the time in between her ordinary painkillers (dihydrocodeine). This simply seems to make her pain much worse and reinforces her feeling that she needs to continue taking the tablets in spite of the fact they do not help very much. Mrs J.'s use of painkillers had become very haphazard and on

occasions she would take four or five at a time to try to get on top of the pain.

Towards the end of the pain programme Mrs J. had managed to organise her medication use so that she was taking her tablets on a regular time-contingent basis (even though still at a higher dose than the recommended maximum). She picked one medication (dihydrocodeine) and decided to reduce this slowly by reducing her consumption from four tablets every 6 hours to three and a half every 6 hours. When she had got used to the new level (after several days) she reduced this further to three tablets every 6 hours. She continued with this technique for several weeks until she was not taking any dihydrocodeine. She noticed by reducing her medication this way that there was very little change in her pain. She then planned to tackle her use of other tablets one at a time until she was on a minimal level of medication.

in intensity, perhaps as a response to unpaced exercise, and a new pain, which they have never had before. Patients are encouraged to pay little attention to their 'old' pain, and in particular not to continue to seek further curative treatment or to manage it solely with medication. With a new pain they are encouraged to seek appropriate advice if it does not settle in due course.

The session centres around the patients making their own plans for what they are going to do when they get an acute flare-up of their pain. The doctor poses the questions and the patients as a group have to come up with the answers. Thus the patients have an investment in the resulting plans. It is often useful to give an explanation of the 'emergency card' system that exists in many hospitals to make sure the hospital's response to a 'red alert' is not chaotic but well ordered and thought out. It should be pointed out that hospitals often 'practise' and then make changes in the light of experience. The patients should be encouraged to produce their own 'emergency card', and practise what they will do and make changes in the light of experience.

The group members should be taken through, step by step, exactly how they will feel when they have an acute flare-up and what they have learned that will help them to manage it more successfully than they have in the past. They should understand that they will need to plan what they are going to do during an acute episode as they are unlikely to think rationally at the time. The doctor's role in this session is simply to guide the discussion and make sure all the relevant points are made. Box 13.2.14 shows the points that should have been made by the group by the end of the session.

In the past tablets were the first and in some cases the only way many patients had of trying to cope with and manage their old pain and flare-ups of their old pain, even if it did not help much. The patients are encouraged to continue to use *all* the skills they have learned and not to resort to medication in the first instance.

The doctor should give specific recommendations for what types of medicines may be used and how they should be used during acute

---

> **Box 13.2.14**   Major points for the emergency card
>
> - Don't panic; this will get better
> - Assess 'is this a new pain or my old pain?'
> - Physical and mental relaxation
> - Possibly stretching exercise
> - May need to rest up (max. 2 days bed rest)
> - Keep active; potter if possible
> - Cut back on exercises
> - Begin to pace exercises up slowly again
> - May need some painkillers to help restore function
> - Visit general practitioner only for prescription for painkillers
> - Retain control; don't allow oneself to be referred again
> - Work out why this happened (lack of pacing, etc.)
> - Congratulate self for managing it well

> **Box 13.2.15**   Guidelines for the use of medicines during acute episodes of your usual pain
>
> - Keep on the lowest level of painkillers (preferably none) when not in the midst of a flare-up
> - Use all of the other techniques you have learned to 'manage' this episode
> - Medicines can be useful as a tool to help you institute the other techniques
> - NSAIDs (if they do not give you significant side-effects) can be used on a regular basis for a short time (4 weeks maximum) if helpful
> - Combination analgesics (e.g. co-codamol) may be added or used alone. These should be taken 'by the clock' (not on a pain-contingent basis) for a maximum of 3 or 4 weeks. The dose should then be reduced and stopped
> - The medicines should be used as a 'tool' to help in restoring activity

episodes. These guidelines are outlined in Box 13.2.15. They are not absolute, but should give an indication of how to get the best out of medicines. The doctor should inform the patients that these guidelines will also be sent to their GP, so that medicines are not inappropriately withheld during acute episodes and that the patients are supported in their efforts to keep medication to a minimum at other times.

The doctor should not, however, concentrate on medicines at this stage but rather encourage the group to come up with the solutions on the basis of what has been learned on the programme. It is often best to use a case example to focus the discussions. The patients should be set homework to make their own 'emergency card', which should detail what they are going to do when they have an acute flare-up. They should be encouraged to get the help of their partners (if appropriate) to help in the plan of action. This will give the partner a specific supportive role rather than overprotective role in helping patients to manage their own pain.

Finally the patients must be directed to practising their emergency system. Just as novices practise the routine *before* making a parachute jump, so the patients must practise their emergency plan when they are in a good phase so that their response to an acute episode becomes almost a habit.

A PATIENT'S GUIDE TO HOW TO SURVIVE THE HEALTH-CARE SYSTEM

It has been said that the health-care system itself should have a health warning! Many of the patients on pain programmes have been on a circuitous route before ending up on a pain management programme. They have little understanding as to why they have apparently been passed from pillar to post with no answers or helpful treatment (Loeser & Sullivan 1995).

Basing this session on the experiences of the patients in the group will make it more relevant to them. This is best done by briefly going through the referral pathway of one or two of the patients. Rather than simply giving answers as to why, for example, referral between a number of specialists occurred, the doctor should encourage the group to come up with some of the potential reasons. This should promote discussion on a number of topics ranging from 'why did I see a different doctor in the same clinic each visit?' to 'why didn't I get an MRI scan at my first visit?' Of course it is not possible to know the precise reasons in any given case, but the doctor should give the patients an idea of the thoughts that may have been going through the treating doctor's mind and a better understanding of how the health-care system works.

Patients have no understanding of differential diagnoses, what diseases different specialists see or the specificity and sensitivity of various tests. They do not usually have an understanding that test results are not necessarily absolute and that ultimately a judgement has to be made with regard to diagnosis and treatment.

One of the most important points to be made is the fact that doctors, be they GPs or specialists, are no less human than the patients they see and are subject to bias and other human frailties. If the doctor is pressurised by the patient to 'do something' at any cost, the patient should understand that the doctor may respond emotionally rather than intellectually. In other words, upon seeing a very distressed patient pleading for help, the doctor may be tempted to offer treatment to the patient even though the likelihood of major help is very small. This may be offered to help doctors cope with their sense of helplessness rather than being based on their knowledge and experience. The doctor and the patient usually regret this decision later. Patients frequently do not have an understanding of the effect of the pressures that they put upon their doctors. They tend to feel they are being denied treatment when the doctor is appropriately resistant to the patient's imploring that something must be done.

The group should be invited to come up with the solutions and answers as to how to get the best out of consultations with their doctors. This may be approached by asking the group to come up with ideas of how to make life as difficult as possible for the doctor. Having identified these behaviours the group could then be asked how they could modify their behaviour to put the doctor at ease and thus get the most out of the consultation.

It is impossible to anticipate all of the points that may be covered in this session. There are, however, a number of important learning points. These include the importance of the patients' behaviour in determining how the doctor reacts. The specific learning points are outlined in Box 13.2.16.

CONCLUSION

It is important not to overmedicalise the programme. The doctor's role in the programme

---

Box 13.2.16 Learning points for surviving the health-care system

- When consulting your general practitioner or specialist be explicit about what you want (e.g. 'I only need some pain killers for a short time').
- Put the doctor at ease
- Explain you are taking responsibility for managing your old pain
- Do *not* get angry or aggressive
- Do *not* pressurise the doctor if there is nothing that can cure your problem
- If you have a new pain, explain it is not your usual pain but a new one you have not had before
- If you are anxious take someone with you. The other person will remember what is said better than you
- Write down the questions you want to ask, so you don't forget anything
- If you are to undergo investigations ask what is being sought
- If you are offered treatment, ask what is the expected outcome and the risks
- Avoid being reinvestigated or treated for your old pain

---

should be supportive of the psychologist and physiotherapist. There are a small number of sessions in which the doctor may participate with other team members present. These include the initial session (see above) and the session with the partners. The reason for both is essentially the same: to reinforce the 'hurt does not equal harm' message and act as a resource to answer any remaining medical questions that may arise.

Finally the doctor may be required at any time during the programme to evaluate any new problems that may arise. There has been at least one patient on the programme at Salford who had a new episode of pain that was discovered to be due to another disc prolapse. The patient was assessed by the doctor on the programme and immediately referred for spinal surgery, which was successful.

KEY POINTS

- The medical component of the programme should integrate with and facilitate the sessions led by other team members.
- The following topics should be covered:
  —pain pathways
  —special tests, investigations and diagnosis
  —medication use and misuse
  —tolerance, physical and psychological dependence
  —the management of flare-ups
  —how to make the best of the health care system.
- Time should be set aside to answer patients' specific queries.

REFERENCES

British National Formulary 2000 British Medical Association, London and Royal Pharmaceutical Society of Great Britain, London

Bull J, Quinbrera R, Gonzalz-Millan H, Lozano C O 1969 Symptomatic treatment of peripheral diabetic neuropathy with carbamazepine: double-blind crossover study. Diabetologia 5:215–220

Fordyce W E 1976 Behavioural methods for chronic pain and illness. C V Mosby, St Louis

Hobbs W R, Rall T W, Verdoon T A 1996 Hypnotics and sedatives. In: Hardman J G, Gilman A G, Limbird L E (eds) Goodman and Gillman's the pharmacological basis of therapeutics, 9th edn. McGraw-Hill, New York, ch 17, pp 362–373

Jamison R N 1996 Comprehensive pretreatment and outcome assessment for chronic opioid therapy in nonmalignant pain. Journal of Pain and Symptom Management 11(4):231–241

Loeser J D 1994 Tic douloureux and atypical facial pain. In: Wall P D, Melzack R (eds) Textbook of pain. Churchill Livingstone, New York, pp 699–710

Loeser J D, Sullivan M 1995 Disability in the chronic low back pain patient may be iatrogenic. Pain Forum 4:114–121

McQuay H J, Moore R A 1998a Oral ibuprofen and diclofenac in post operative pain. In: An evidence based resource for pain relief. Oxford University Press, Oxford, ch 10, pp 78–83

McQuay H J, Moore R A 1998b Injected morphine in post operative pain. In: An evidence based resource for pain relief. Oxford University Press, Oxford, ch 13, pp 118–126

McQuay H J, Moore R A 1998c Paracetamol with and without codeine in acute pain. In: An evidence based resource for pain relief. Oxford University Press, Oxford, ch 19, pp 58–63

Molloy A R, Nicholas M K, Cousins M J 1997 Role of opioids in chronic non-cancer pain (editorial). Medical Journal of Australia 167:9–10

Monks R 1994 Psychotropic drugs. In: Wall P D, Melzack R (eds) Textbook of pain. Churchill Livingstone, New York, pp 963–989

O'Brien C P 1996 Drug addiction and drug abuse. In: Hardman J G, Gilman A G, Limbird L E (eds) Goodman and Gillman's the pharmacological basis of therapeutics, 9th edn. McGraw-Hill, New York, ch 24, pp 557–577

Reisine T, Pasternak G 1996 Opioid analgesics and antagonists. In: Hardman J G, Gilman A G, Limbird L E (eds) Goodman and Gillman's the pharmacological basis of therapeutics, 9th edn. McGraw-Hill, New York, ch 23, pp 521–555

Spanswick C C, Main C J 1989 The role of the anaesthetist in the management of chronic low back pain in back pain. In: Roland M, Jenner J R (eds) New approaches to rehabilitation and education. Manchester University Press, Manchester.

Appendix: Manchester and Salford Pain Centre medication chart

Name _____

Please list **all** the tablets and medicines that you take (including over-the-counter medicines). List the ones you take for pain in the first box and any others not for your pain in the second box.

Pain medicines	
Non-pain medicines	

Name:

Manchester and Salford Pain Centre
PAIN MEDICATION CHART

This chart is to help you record all the tablets and medicines you take FOR YOUR PAIN. Please record only drugs you have to take because of your pain. This may include pain killers, muscle relaxants, anti-inflammatory drugs, sleeping tablets and anti-depressants. It is designed to help you monitor how much you take and how often you have to take your tablets or medicines. Please use a new sheet for each week. If you are unsure how to record your medicine use please ask one of the staff.

Please write the name of the tablet or medicine in the left hand box. Write in the number of tablets that you take each day in the boxes on the right. There is a column with suggested times (e.g. breakfast) please write in the next column (Approximate time) when you actually took your tablet. It may be that you do not take your medicines at breakfast, lunch, teatime and bed time. In which case simply record when you take them in the 'Approximate time' column. The row 'Extras' is for you to record any extras you have to take during that 24 hour period. It may be you take 2 extra tablets in the afternoon and 2 extra tablets in the middle of the night. You would then record 4 in the 'extras' row. There is an example below to give you some idea of how you should complete your forms.

IMPORTANT
When you have completed the form please could you give it to either the Doctor or Karen in the Office

Use this for ONE drug for ONE week

EXAMPLE

Name of drug		Approximate time	Mon	Tue	Wed	Thurs	Fri	Sat	Sun
Co-proxamol	Breakfast	7 am	2	2	2	2	2	2	2
	Lunch	12 pm	2	2	2	2	2	1	0
	Tea time	3.30 pm	2	2	2	1	2	0	1
	Bed time	10.30 pm	0	2	2	2	2	2	2
	Extras		2 at 3am!			2 at 3am & 2 at 6pm			

PART 3 PHYSICAL ACTIVITIES PROGRAMME CONTENT

Paul Watson

INTRODUCTION

Physical activity is perhaps the most powerful component in pain management programmes. Increasing fitness is important not only in reversing the disuse syndrome, but in giving a powerful signal to patients that they are beginning to regain a degree of control over their musculoskeletal system. It is therefore extremely important from both the physical and the psychological point of view.

Effect of chronicity

Over time chronic pain patients will have reduced their levels of physical activity. The physiological effects of this are a gradual physical deconditioning of the patient (through the avoidance of exercise) characterised by reduced strength and flexibility and reduced aerobic capacity (Bengtsson et al 1994, Bennett et al 1989, Jacobsen, Wildshiodtz & Danneskiold-Samsoe 1991). Because of the reduced level of activity chronic pain patients are also more likely to be overweight than the normal population.

Effects of increase in physical activity level

Influence on mood

Increases in physical activity levels have been associated with an improvement in mood evidenced by reduction in depressive symptoms and anxiety. This does not, however, necessarily imply a cause–effect relationship. People who are depressed tend to be less active than those who are not depressed. Improvement in mood may be a result of improved self-efficacy or achievement and engagement in group activity rather than a direct result of the physical conditioning. Many of the studies that have identified a relationship between improvement in mood following exercise have been conducted on depressed or anxious populations rather than people with chronic pain (North, McCullagh & Tran 1990). Despite these reservations most research into the area does seem to indicate that exercise does improve mood.

Evidence of an analgesic effect

Data on an analgesic effect of exercise has been equivocal. Observations of endurance runners led some to infer that increased fitness was related to increased pain tolerance. Initial research into the area suggested that beta endorphins were produced during physical exercise and that this may occur at low levels of exercise intensity. However, the work of Gurevich, Kohn & Davies (1994) and Donovan & Andrew (1987) suggest that it occurs only at high levels of exercise intensity. To confuse the issue further Droste et al (1991) found that the *perceived* level of intensity was related to the biggest changes in pain thresholds and that this was independent of endorphin levels. Changes in pain report associated with participation in exercise has been widely reported (see below) although the mechanism still remains unclear.

Initial effect of increased exercise

Once patients attempt to restart exercise they will experience an increase in pain or post-exertional soreness, which most of us feel after unaccustomed exercise. This may reinforce their perception that they have re-injured themselves. Increased pain engendered by post-exertional pain in an unfit individual with chronic pain can also serve to increase excitation of pain receptors in an already sensitive pain system,

presumably through secondary central sensitisation (Corderre et al 1993, Henriksson & Mense 1994, Mense 1994).

Physical capacity as an outcome measure

Some authors have suggested that an increase in physical capacity leads to an improved outcome as measured by reduced disability and reduced pain report, a reduction of recurrence of symptoms and reduced work absence. These studies usually refer to programmes that rely on physical and psychological interventions. There is a wide variation in the improvements on each of the different physical measures within subjects (e.g. muscle strength, cardiovascular fitness and range of motion). It is extremely difficult to establish the influence of specific improvements on disability, recurrence and maintenance of change. Physical exercise sessions are a valuable tool to de-sensitise fearful patients by allowing them to approach physical exercise in a carefully regulated and safe way, thus overcoming their fear of activity.

PHYSICAL ACTIVITIES

The key aims of the physical activity component of the programme are summarised in Box 13.3.1.

Box 13.3.1 Aims of physical activity programme

- Overcome the effects of physical deconditioning
- Challenge and reduce patients' fears of engaging in physical activity
- Reduce physical impairment and capitalise on recoverable function
- Provide a safe and graded approach to the re-engagement in physical activity
- Help patients accept responsibility for increasing their functional capacity
- Promote a positive view of physical activity
- Introduce physically challenging, functional activities to rehabilitation

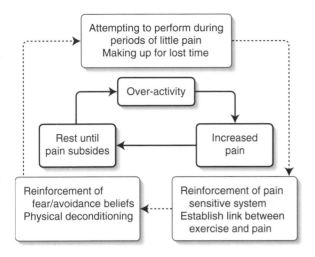

Figure 13.3.1 The over/under-activity cycle. From Keefe, Group Therapy for Patients. In Psychological Approaches to Pain Management 1996 edited by Gatchel RJ & Turk DC. Reproduced with permission of The Guildford Press, New York, USA.

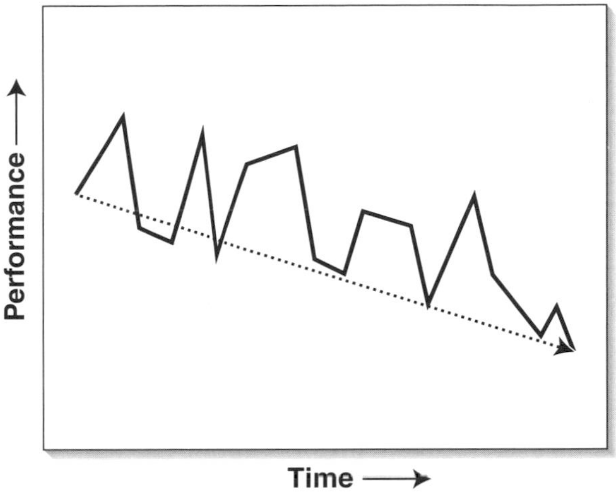

Figure 13.3.2 A graphic representation of poor pacing leading to a gradual reduction in performance.

TECHNIQUES FOR THE INCREASE OF PHYSICAL ACTIVITY

Goal setting and pacing

Limited physical capacity and lowered pain tolerance restrict function in chronic pain patients. As has been mentioned above, engaging in activity may exacerbate the pain immediately or some time after the activity has finished. Although patients are educated to remain active despite the pain it is essential that they do not precipitate the pain to such an extent that they have to limit their activity. Conversely some patients avoid activity to such an extent that they do not progress and do not achieve improvement.

Pacing exercise has been described by Gil, Ross & Keefe (1988) as moderate activity–rest cycling. It is a strategy to enable patients to control exacerbations of pain by learning to regulate activity and, once a regimen of paced activity is established, gradually to increase their activity level. The converse of this is the 'over-activity–pain–rest' cycle, illustrated in Figure 13.3.1.

Chronic pain patients often report levels of activity that fluctuate dramatically over time. On questioning at initial assessment they report that they frequently persist at activities until they are

prevented from carrying on by the ensuing level of pain. This leads them to rest until the pain subsides or until frustration moves them to action whereupon they then try again until defeated once again by the increase in pain. Over time the periods of activity become shorter and those of rest lengthen. Achievements become smaller and disability increases, as the individual becomes more anxious and fearful of activity and progressively demoralised. A typical pattern of activity can be seen in Figure 13.3.2.

The purpose of pacing and goal setting is to regulate daily activities and to structure an increase in activity through the gradual pacing up of activity. Activity is paced up by timing activity or by the introduction of quotas of exercise interspersed by periods of rest or change in activity (Fordyce 1976, Gil, Ross & Keefe 1988, Keefe, Beaupre & Gil 1996). Pacing activity requires the patients to break down activities into both activity and rest periods and to subdivide tasks into sections that enable rests to be taken. The patients must learn also to identify activities that they find stressful and pain provoking (often, but not always, the most strenuous). These activities are assigned longer rest periods and shorter activity periods. Gradually the length of the activity times can be increased and the rest periods reduced.

In summary, although patients are encouraged to remain active despite the pain, it is necessary not to precipitate pain to such an extent that they have to limit their activity. The important principle is that they remain active rather than descend into periods of prolonged rest. What may appear to be a relatively easy task in fact often requires a lot of discipline on the part of the patient. Once engaged in a task it is often easier to continue until it is completed rather than take time out to rest. Some individuals find the use of clocks or kitchen timers useful to remind them to change between activity and rest periods.

Goal setting

Goals should be set in three separate domains:

1. *physical*, which relates to the exercise programme the patient follows and sets the number of exercises to be performed or the duration of the exercise and the level of difficulty
2. *functional/task*, which relates to the achievement of functional tasks of everyday living such as housework or hobbies and tasks learned on the programme
3. *social*, where the patient is encouraged to set goals relating to the performance of activities in the wider social environment. It is important that goals are personally relevant, interesting, measurable and achievable.

THE INFLUENCE OF PSYCHOLOGICAL FACTORS ON PERFORMANCE

It is important to distinguish physical *capacity* from physical *performance*. Physical capacity is determined by physiological constraints. Thus, no matter how hard I try, I cannot touch the ceiling if my arm is not long enough. Physical performance on the other hand is influenced by many different psychological factors (as outlined in Ch. 2). Among the most important of the psychological factors is self-efficacy (or belief that one can actually carry out the task in question). In setting

goals therefore it is important to consider the patient's expectations.

Self-efficacy

The concept of setting goals in pain management is supported by two influential pieces of psychological theory. Locke in 1967 suggested that increased task performance was facilitated by the setting of specific but challenging and attainable goals. Demotivation and a sense of failure occur if the goals set are unattainable. According to Bandura (1977) two forms of expectation may lead to increased performance (Ch. 2). These are *efficacy expectations* (or the belief that one has the personal ability to perform actions that will lead to specific outcomes) and *outcome expectations* (or the belief that specific outcomes can be achieved as the result of specific behaviours). Of these efficacy expectations may be the most potent determinants of change in pain management. Previous research has demonstrated a close link between increased self-efficacy and good outcome from rehabilitation and pain management with respect to increased activity, increased positive coping and reduced pain behaviour (Bucklew et al 1994, Burkhardt et al 1994).

In the initial stages of the rehabilitation programme patients may suffer from low self-efficacy. Failure to perform a task (total inability to perform an exercise) or incompetent performance of the task (failure to reach the required level of performance, e.g. required number of repetitions) leads to a fall in perceived self-efficacy. Continued goal attainment will reinforce self-efficacy and lead to a perception of mastery over the task or problem (managing to exercise despite the pain). Increases in self-efficacy can be brought about in a number of ways or strategies (Box 13.3.2).

Box 13.3.2 Methods of increasing self-efficacy

- By information from others including professionals
- Vicarious learning from others
- Personal experience and practice
- Generating physiological arousal and 'psyching' oneself up to do things

From Bandura 1977, reproduced with permission.

In pain management programmes, many patients demonstrate lack of self-confidence. Being part of a group is often particularly helpful in facilitating progress. It is most important therefore that goals are set that encourage successes but are sufficiently challenging to ensure progress.

THE ESTABLISHMENT OF APPROPRIATE GOALS

The setting of goals should be a matter of negotiation between the patient and the therapist. The use of goal-setting charts is essential. An example of one such chart is shown in the Appendix to this part of the chapter (p. 297).

Patients set a target for activities each week and record their achievements on the charts. Through this process they not only monitor their progress but also become more accurate in setting attainable goals. Goal setting can also be used as a problem-solving exercise. Patients are asked to set specific goals (e.g. travelling to visit relatives). They then have to identify the physical goals (e.g. increase sitting tolerance) that will help them to be successful. The specific barriers to achieving those goals are also identified (e.g. increased stiffness/discomfort on a long journey). Strategies are developed to overcome these (e.g. taking breaks, performing stretches). It is also useful for patients to discuss the consequences of the goal, both positive (visiting friends, re-establishing contacts) and negative (possible increased pain the next day). They should plan how they are going to deal with the negative consequences (alteration in medication, stretching exercises and change in activity levels).

Involvement of relatives and family

As was illustrated in Chapter 3 it is usually desirable, and sometimes essential, to involve family members in the rehabilitation process. Introducing pacing may have a significant effect on the routines of the rest of the family. Patients may have to develop strategies that assist them in overcoming barriers presented by relatives and friends in a non-confrontational way. Care should be taken to explain the concepts of pacing and goal setting clearly to them also. They too can often be a barrier to the achievement of goals through their desire to protect the patient from injury. They should be advised not take upon themselves any task during the patients' rest period or complete tasks for them because patients are taking a long time to complete it. The way in which everyday work within the house is performed may need addressing. It may be usual for patients or their families to complete work around the house during the day and leave the evening for 'relaxing'. This usually results in a drive to complete tasks quickly rather than spread them throughout the day. It is sometimes difficult to facilitate such changes in family patterns of behaviour. Suggestions of change to family members may meet with resistance. Group tasks during pain management programmes often identify social skill deficiencies in managing interpersonal relationships. Appropriate assertiveness can be perceived as aggressiveness. A particular advantage of group, as opposed to individual, treatment is that it provides a non-threatening context for training in various aspects of communication skills.

The importance of regular review

Goal setting is an integral part of pain management and while the patients are in contact with the pain management team goals should be constantly set and reviewed. The patients should set themselves both short and long term goals at the end of the programme. This helps the patient to focus on future attainment and assists the maintenance of change once the formal pain management interventions have been completed (Ch. 14). It should be emphasised to the patient that pain management is a process and that they must continue by themselves, rather than rely only on future attendances at a pain management centre.

TYPES OF PHYSICAL ACTIVITY
Aerobic conditioning

Most patients attending pain management programmes have been physically inactive for a long period of time. Reduced physical activity leads to a reduction in cardiovascular fitness and a feeling of fatigue on the resumption of physical activity. Many patients are discouraged from performing physical activities not only because of the effect it may have on their level of pain but also because of the effects of fatigue on a deconditioned system. Chronic pain is frequently associated with heightened awareness of somatic symptoms, and sufferers may become acutely aware of their bodily sensations. Some patients, particularly those with fibromyalgia, report very high levels of fatigue on the resumption of activity. Although there is some evidence for abnormalities in muscle energy availability in fibromyalgia, increasing levels of physical activity have been demonstrated to reduce the subjective feeling of fatigue if the patient is encouraged to adhere to a regimen where activity is increased gradually. Activities aimed at increasing the range of motion of joints and muscle strength may not address the effect of reduced cardiovascular function. It is therefore essential that an increase in general aerobic physical fitness is incorporated in a pain management programme. Reductions in pain report and increases in physical function on objective testing have been reported for rehabilitation programmes utilising aerobic exercise alone (Burkhardt et al 1994, Martin et al 1996, Wigers, Stiles & Vogel 1996).

Types of aerobic conditioning

Paced walking, stationary exercise cycle, stair walking, use of a stair climber and non-impact aerobic classes have all been suggested as ways of increasing physical fitness in chronic pain patients (Bennett 1996, Bennett et al 1996, Burkhardt et al 1994, Haldorsen et al 1998, McCain et al 1988, Martin et al 1996). The exercises should be performed at least three times each week for best effect. Where possible patients should exercise to 60–70% of aerobic capacity or should pace themselves up to achieve this level of intensity if maximum advantage is to be gained.

The planning of exercise

Endurance exercises need not involve expensive equipment. Stair walking or paced walking around a circuit (either indoors or out of doors) is an excellent form of aerobic conditioning in the early stages of rehabilitation and something that the patient can continue at home. The patient is encouraged to set initial targets and advance these gradually. Although it is preferable if patients set goals based on the attainment of heart rate targets using pulse meters, many will be unable or unwilling to do so because of the restriction imposed by pain or fear of exacerbating their condition. It therefore might be more advisable to set goals based on time, speed or resistance of the conditioning exercises chosen.

Strategies for enhancing compliance

Compliance with exercise is more likely if the individual finds it interesting and rewarding. Exercising in a gym may not be suitable for all. Some people may not have access to such facilities outside of the programme; others may not be motivated by this form of exercise. Developing activities that are patient and family orientated and can be integrated into the normal daily routine will help to improve adherence. Exercise should become part of life not an intrusion into it.

Stretching

Deconditioning from inactivity or restricting joint range to a limited range of motion leads to the reduction in the length of soft tissue structures. This will limit the ranges of available motion in joints and distort the normal body biomechanics. Such distortions can in themselves contribute to nociception or even the risk of further injury.

The influence of injury

Many of the patients on pain management programmes have an initial injury as the precipitating event in their pain history. Scar tissue that develops following injury responds to stresses and mobility by orientating along the lines of stress. Scar tissue formed under the influences of graduated stress and motion is stronger and more pliable than that formed in the absence of movement. This applies also to other non-contractile connective tissue. This makes movement and particularly stretching an essential component of the rehabilitation of deconditioned subjects.

The importance of careful initial assessment

It is not possible to go into detail of the types of problems that may be encountered in specific conditions. Most chronic pain patients have widespread symptoms and often have been particularly avoidant of exercise; hence the problems will affect not only a localised area and generalised stretching exercises will be indicated. The importance of a thorough physical examination must be stressed here. Limited ranges of motion should already have been identified and the problems and areas for improvement discussed with the patient. Although the patients are treated in a group setting the emphasis on treatment targets must be individualised to maximise improvement. Not all patients will be able to achieve the desired starting position for stretching exercises and modification of the positions will be required for some. The therapist should progress the starting position to facilitate improved stretching as increased range is achieved.

Theoretical basis for 'prescription' of exercise

There has been much controversy over the type of stretching exercise that is most suitable to gain an increase in the extensibility of soft tissue. In addition to this there is a further discussion on the need for a 'warm-up' period prior to stretching. Most of the research on the benefits of different types of stretching and the relative benefits of warm-up has been conducted on normal subjects or athletes of varying levels of performance ability. There is still little conclusive evidence to demonstrate that warm-up exercises improve the extensibility of the muscle tendon unit unless the level of exercise is quite vigorous and sustained, something which is not achievable in the group under consideration here. Passive warming with hot packs similarly has little evidence for its efficacy. Some patients may benefit from hot packs prior to exercise but it must be emphasised that this is a means to an end and must not be seen a passive form of therapy by the patient.

Types of stretching

There are at least two main schools of stretching technique. The first favours sustained stretching, where the tissue is taken to its limit and the stretch is maintained for a recommended period of at least 5–6 seconds. Most authorities (Magnusson 1998) suggest longer (greater than 15 seconds) if it can be tolerated. The second is ballistic stretching where dynamic rhythmic, bouncing exercises are performed from the resting length of the muscle to the limit of the range in repetitive movements.

Exaggerated guarding and increased myotatic stretch reflexes have been identified in those with painful muscles (Corderre et al 1993, Mense 1994). Additionally psychological factors have been demonstrated to be closely associated with abnormal guarding patterns of muscle activity (Watson, Booker & Main 1997). (As discussed in Ch. 5, the interaction between psychological factors and guarding may be a key factor in the development of chronic disability.) Such abnormalities of movement could potentially lead to ineffective stretching and at worst injury to the muscle; therefore the ballistic stretching technique is inadvisable.

Sustained stretching, where the force is gradually applied, results in less stiffness in the muscle tendon unit for the same amount of elongation and slow stretches are less likely to trigger a myotatic stretch reflex (Garrett 1996). In addition there is some evidence that the sustained stretch of 6 seconds allows for inhibition of muscle activity in the stretched muscle to occur. This has been attributed to the stimulation of the Golgi tendon organ, which leads to reflexive inhibition of muscle activity (so-called autogenic inhibition) (Hutton & Atwater 1992).

Practice

It is important to be systematic about advice given concerning practice. Stretching exercises should be performed according to quota (number of stretches to be performed) and endurance targets (the length of time for which the stretch is to be held). An example of a stretching regimen is given in the Appendix to this part of the chapter (p. 300).

The initial emphasis is on increasing the length of time the stretch is maintained until the patient can achieve at least a 6-second hold. The number of repetitions as well as length of hold can then be increased gradually. Stretching exercises should be performed at the beginning and at the end of exercise sessions. Introducing regular stretching into daily work and home routines, especially between different activities and after periods of static work, (e.g. reading, typing) is essential. The patient should also identify other times when stretching is beneficial, for instance to break up prolonged static postures as in the goal-setting example given above. Combining the muscle relaxation skills and distraction techniques learned on the programme with stretching will increase the effectiveness of the stretch.

Joint range activities

Motion through complete joint range is required to assist in the nutrition of the cartilage of synovial joints as well as in the maintenance of the length and strength of the soft tissue of the joint such as the joint capsule and ligaments. Repeated motion through a restricted range results in limitation of joint range through the shortening of such structures and an impoverishment of joint nutrition.

Low impact full-range free exercises are an elementary component of a warm-up and warmdown programme in most exercise regimens and this is so in pain management programmes. They should be combined with stretching exercises to capitalise on increased range of motion.

Strengthening and endurance exercises

Theoretical basis

Loss of muscle strength and endurance has been identified in many types of chronic pain patient and it has been suggested that a reduction in the strength and endurance of the muscles, particularly those involved in posture and lifting activities, contributes to the persistence of chronic pain. The evidence for this is still rather tenuous. However, exercises aimed at increasing the strength and endurance of muscle groups is an established component of pain management. Monitoring an increase in strength in particular can be motivating for some patients.

Like most physical-training modalities there are many differing ideas on what is the best way to increase muscle strength. A general rule of thumb is that strength training occurs when the muscles are exercised at an intensity of greater than 40% of maximal force with a relatively low number of repetitions; any lower force than this and a higher number of repetitions would tend to increase endurance. Exercise at greater intensity than this tends to increase muscle bulk and strength. Very high percentages of maximal force (greater than 60%) with low repetitions give the greatest increases in maximal force as an effect of training (Olsen & Svendsen 1992).

Practice

Strengthening exercises can be in the form of free exercises where the starting position is adjusted to increase the load on the muscle groups or can incorporate free weights and weight-resistance equipment. Strengthening exercises should be introduced with caution as discomfort associated with post-exertional muscle soreness and stiffness are inevitable. This is especially true for those suffering from musculoskeletal pain (e.g. back pain, fibromyalgia). Movements should be smooth and fluid. Exercises at highest resistance values or which emphasise the eccentric component of exercise have been demonstrated to be associated with a greater incidence of muscle damage and increased post-exertional soreness and so these are to be avoided.

Like the stretching exercises, strength training will need to be specific to the patient's own problem and generalised to combat the effects of deconditioning. A simple generalised strengthening regimen is given in the Appendix p. 301.

Ergonomics, lifting and handling exercises

Theoretic basis

The principles of good posture and more importantly recognition of risk factors for poor working environments and working practices can be taught in general terms of advice that all should follow (including the healthy) with specific advice for the particular patient group (e.g. low back pain or headache patients). Grossly stressful activities such as bending and twisting of the lumbar spine when the upper body is carrying a load, prolonged task performance or static postures without a break and prolonged exposure to vibration of the lumbar spine have all been demonstrated to increase the risk of developing musculoskeletal pathology

In teaching good lifting and handling and posture the therapist should avoid leaving the impression with patients that a moderately poor posture or inefficient working practices will irreparably damage their musculoskeletal system. There is no convincing evidence to date that it does. Many people work in less than ideal working situations without ever becoming incapacitated or losing significant time from work owing to musculoskeletal pain. In those subjects who already have a significant level of pain such postures and inefficient working positions will lead to an increase in pain in an already sensitised pain system with a consequent risk that they may be unable to perform their work sufficiently well to remain employed. The performance of some tasks is likely to initially increase the patient's level of pain and discomfort. Although the patient should be warned of this, care must be taken. If over-emphasised it is possible to reinforce fear-avoidance behaviour inappropriately

through the provision of artificially strict rules on posture and task performance.

Practice

Patients should become skilled in the appraisal of risk, but the concept of risk needs to be considered carefully. Most movement is not harmful and it is important to reassure patients about this. Patients are given information on good working and lifting postures and the correct execution of movements. They are then asked to consider a variety of practical situations in which they have to identify risk in lifting and handling situations. These are everyday activities such as ironing, carrying shopping, cleaning cupboards, dismantling large items (e.g. a table) and transporting them. The patients are asked to analyse the tasks to identify good and poor postures and make adjustments to the working environment to make the task less stressful. Through participation in a practical task these principles can be linked to pacing activities.

PRACTICE AND PRACTICAL WORK

From Figure 13.3.3 the cycle of education shows that those receiving education must have the opportunity to practise the new information to test its validity and to enhance retention of the

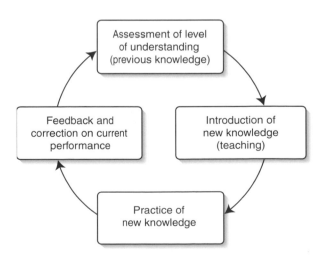

Figure 13.3.3 The cycle of education.

knowledge. This is particularly important in the performance of activities such as specific exercises and pacing. Written examples (or 'paper case studies') can be used to help the patient identify problems with pacing and barriers to goal achievement in a non-threatening way. However, intellectual understanding does not always lead to a practical solution. It is very important that patients practise the skills taught in a way to make meaningful changes in their own personal life.

Practical tasks can be developed during the pain management programme. The groups are given assignments to complete and it is often helpful to videotape sections of these tasks for discussion with the group later. These tasks must be practical and require individuals to pace their activities. Examples of such tasks include emptying a cupboard of equipment and weights and transferring it to another cupboard, or planting up large patio planters with bulbs and plants. The number of tasks depends on the inventiveness of the staff and the group! These practical tasks allow patients to identify tasks within their capability, which they can plan. Examples are shown in Case studies, 13.3.1–3.

CONCLUSION

Reversal of the deconditioning process is an essential part of all approaches to pain management. With long-established 'disuse syndromes' a careful analysis of the pain-associated incapacities is essential. Increase in tolerance for exercise and re-establishment of activities require a planned and systematic approach. Although each rehabilitation protocol must be individualised, the general principles outlined below should be the key features of all physical activity modules within pain management programmes.

KEY POINTS

- Systematic assessment.
- Re-education where necessary.
- Problem analysis.
- Phased re-introduction of increased level and range of function.
- Positive reinforcement of progress.
- Inclusion where possible of significant others.

Case study 13.3.1 ('Mrs D.')

Mrs D. has suffered from fibromyalgia for 7 years and her husband has gradually taken over domestic activities such as cooking and cleaning. Mrs D. has set preparation of the meals as one of her goals. Her husband is concerned that she will be overdoing things and will suffer a setback if she takes this upon herself and is unwilling to relinquish the task.

They come to an agreement that Mrs D. will prepare the evening meal every other evening and will start with simple meals that are relatively quick and easy to prepare, based on some convenience foods. Initially the meal preparation will not require the use of heavy pans. Her pacing strategy includes laying the table for the evening meal in the mid-afternoon, preparing any vegetables required throughout the day and keeping the length of time she is actively engaged in cooking (frying, stirring food) to under 20 minutes. Part of the agreement is that her husband washes up on her cooking days and vice versa. One of the potential barriers identified was the oversolicitous behaviour of the husband. Both agreed that he should be out of the kitchen during the preparation of the meal.

Case study 13.3.2 ('Mr A.')

Mr A. is 63 and retired, he has chronic low back pain. He presents as mildly disabled, highly motivated but tense and frustrated at his lack of progress despite previous treatments. Like many back pain sufferers his pain is very variable and he reports days when the pain is relatively mild. He tries to capitalise on these good days by performing many of the tasks he is unable to do on the days when his pain limits his activity. This leads to an increase in pain to which he responds by increasing his pain relief medication and restricting his activity until the pain subsides. Once the pain subsides he resumes his activities, once again doing as much as he can on good

Case study 13.3.2 Cont'd

days and resting and restricting his activity when the pain increases.

Prior to commencing pain management he is asked to keep a pain and activity diary (see Appendix to this chapter and to Ch. 7, pp. 133 and 134). These demonstrate days of intense physical activity (gardening, washing the car) followed by days of reduced activity (lying in bed, watching television) with an increase in medication consumption. Over time Mr A. has gradually reduced his activities. (A graphic representation of his physical performance is similar to that given in Figure 13.3.2.)

He was asked to write down a list of tasks he wanted to achieve. As a keen gardener many of these were related to the return to this hobby. He then assigned levels of difficulty to each of a series of gardening-related tasks according to the degree to which they might be expected to increase his pain. All were perceived as pain provoking to a different degree. The tasks ranged from planting seed/thinning plants in trays at a bench (low risk); weeding and hoeing (moderate risk) to digging (high risk).

He then assigned times, including rest periods, to each of the tasks that he thought he could comfortably perform. Low risk activities were allowed 15 minutes of activity followed by a series of stretching exercises then 5 minutes of relaxing in a chair. Moderate risk activities were assigned 10 minutes with stretching and 10 minutes of resting. Since he has a tendency to become engrossed in his hobby (and not notice the passage of time) he planned to use a kitchen timer to help regulate rest and activity periods. He also limited the length of time he would engage in gardening (initially for an hour) before he took a prolonged break or went for a gentle walk. The high risk activities were not initially included in the plan but were to be introduced as he gained control of pacing his activity and improved his physical endurance.

Case study 13.3.3 ('Mr B.')

Mr B. has chronic low back pain. He reports a considerable degree of disability and has recently taken to using a wheelchair when travelling out of the house. He has become unemployed because he felt his job as a delivery van driver and lifting boxes of cleaning fluids was injuring his back (since he always had increased pain at the end of a day at work). Gradually he found it difficult to perform his hobbies of playing darts and pool so he stopped and so restricted his social activities. As usual physical activities have become increasingly difficult (because they increase his pain), he has reduced his overall activity level and now spends more time reclining in bed or on the settee to reduce the exercise-associated pain. His wife helps him to dress each morning. He is now very fearful that any activity will increase his pain and is extremely reluctant to perform physical activities and uses a wheelchair if he needs to walk more than 50 metres.

Although Mr B. is now very physically disabled, he is not yet suitable for a comprehensive pain management programme since he requires help in dressing and spends long periods reclining. Following negotiation with the physiotherapist he has identified a programme to be performed at home with targets to be reached.

Long term goals

1. To become independent with dressing—to dress self every day within 2 months
2. To increase sitting tolerance to 1 hour within 2 months
3. To increase walking tolerance
4. To eliminate reclining within 2 months
5. To carry out a regular exercise programme to increase fitness in preparation to attend a PMP

These can be seen in his plan (Appendix p. 299):

His targets were reviewed weekly with the physiotherapist and new goals set. In addition to the exercise plan he aims to reduce the amount of time he spends reclining each day. Currently he spends most of the day reclining on a settee or on the bed. He has agreed to stop reclining on his bed, to restrict each period of reclining on the settee to 30 minutes maximum from immediate effect and to gradually increase his sitting tolerance. He will intersperse the planned restriction of 'downtime' with 'pottering' around the house, and eventually increase his walking distance in his garden. His aim is to eliminate reclining within 2 months and increase sitting tolerance to 1 hour within the same time frame.

In a plan developed in discussion with his wife, he aims eventually to dress himself every day, beginning with having help dressing his lower body only, progressing to having help only with his shoes and socks within one month, and be fully independent within 2 months. If he achieves these goals within the agreed time frame he will then be reviewed for possible inclusion on a full pain management programme.

Present difficulties

Poor fitness/flexibility
Reliant upon wife for help
Poor fitness and tolerance for sitting
Poor fitness and tolerance for walking
Poor sitting/walking tolerance/reduced fitness

REFERENCES

Bandura A 1977 Self-efficacy: towards a unifying theory of behavioral change. Psychological Review 84:191–215

Bengtsson A, Backman E, Lindblom B, Skogh T 1994 Long term follow-up of fibromyalgia patients: clinical symptoms, muscular function, laboratory tests—an eight year comparison study. Journal of Musculoskeletal Pain 2:67–80

Bennett R M 1996 Multidisciplinary group treatment programmes to treat fibromyalgia patients. Rheumatic Diseases Clinics of North America 22(2):351–367

Bennett R M, Clarke S R, Goldberg L et al 1989 Aerobic fitness in patients with fibrositis. A controlled study of respiratory gas exchange and ^{133}xenon clearance from exercising muscle. Arthritis and Rheumatism 32(10):1113–1116

Bennett R M, Burkhardt C S, Clarke S R, O'Reilly C, Weins S N, Campbell S M 1996 Group treatment of fibromyalgia: a 6 month outpatient programme. Journal of Rheumatology 23:521–528

Bucklew S P, Parker J C, Keefe F J et al 1994 Self efficacy and pain behavior among subjects with fibromyalgia. Pain 59:377–384

Burkhardt C S, Mannerkorpi K, Hedenberg L, Bjelle A 1994 A randomised, controlled trial of education and physical training for women with fibromyalgia. Journal of Rheumatology 21:714–720

Corderre J T, Katz J, Vaccarino A I, Melzack R 1993 Contribution of central neuroplasticity to pathological pain: review of clinical and experimental evidence. Pain 52:259–285

Donovan M R, Andrew G 1987 Plasma beta endorphin immunoreaction during graded cycle ergometry. Sports Medicine 17:358–362

Droste C, Greenlee M, Schreck M, Roskamm H 1991 Experiments in pain thresholds and plasma beta endorphin levels during exercise. Medical Science and Sports Exercise 23:334–345

Fordyce W E 1976 Behavioural methods for chronic pain and illness. C V Mosby, St Louis

Garrett W E Jr 1996 Muscle strain injuries. American Journal of Sports Medicine 24(suppl):S2–S8

Gil K M, Ross S L, Keefe F J 1988 Behavioural treatment of chronic pain: four pain management protocols. In: France R D, Krishnan K R R (eds) Chronic pain. American Psychiatric Press, Washington, DC, pp 317–413

Gurevich M, Kohn P, Davies C 1994 Exercise induced analgesia and the role of reactivity in pain sensitivity. Journal of Sports Medicine 12:549–552

Haldorsen E M H, Kronholm K, Skounen J S, Ursin H 1998 Multimodal cognitive behavioural treatment of patients sicklisted for musculoskeletal pain: a randomised controlled study. Scandinavian Journal of Rheumatology 27:16–25

Henriksson K G, Mense S 1994 Pain and nociception in fibromyalgia. Pain Reviews 1(4): 245–260

Hutton R S, Atwater S W 1992 Acute and chronic adaptations of muscle proprioceptors in response to increased use. Sports Medicine 14(6):406–421

Jacobsen S, Wildshiodtz G, Danneskiold-Samsoe 1991 Isokinetic and isometric muscle strength combined with transcutaneous electrical muscle stimulation in primary fibromyalgia. Journal of Rheumatology 18(9):1390–1393

Keefe F J, Beaupre P M, Gil K M 1996 Group therapy for patients with chronic pain. In: Gatchel R J, Turk D C (eds) Psychological approaches to pain management. Guilford, New York, pp 259–282

Locke E A 1967 Towards a theory of task motivation incentives. Organisational Behavior and Human Performance 3:157–189

McCain G A, Bell D A, Mai F M, Halliday P D 1988 A controlled study of the effects of a supervised cardiovascular fitness training program on the manifestations of primary fibromyalgia. Arthritis and Rheumatism 31:1535–1542

Magnusson S P 1998 Passive properties of human skeletal muscle during stretch maneuvers. A review. Scandanavian Journal of Medicine and Science in Sports 8(2):65–77

Martin L, Nutting A, Macintosh B R, Edsworthy S M, Butterwick D, Cook J 1996 An exercise program in the treatment of fibromyalgia. Journal of Rheumatology 23(6):1050–1053

Mense S 1994 Referral of muscle pain: new aspects. American Pain Society Journal 3(1):1–9

North T C, McCullagh P, Tran Z V 1990 Effect of exercise on depression. Exercise and Sports Science Review 18:379–383

Olsen J, Svendsen B 1992 Medical exercise therapy: an adjunct to orthopaedic manual therapy. Orthopaedic Practitioner 4:7–11

Watson P J, Booker C K, Main C J 1997 Evidence for the role of psychological factors in abnormal paraspinal activity in patients with chronic low back pain. Journal of Musculoskeletal Pain 5(4):41–55

Wigers S H, Stiles T C, Vogel P A 1996 Effects of aerobic exercise versus stress management treatment in fibromyalgia: a 4.5 year prospective study. Scandinavian Journal of Rheumatology 25:77–86

APPENDIX: GOAL-SETTING CHARTS AND EXERCISE PROGRAMME

Goal setting

Goal 1

Long term goal

To dress independently within 2 months.

Short term goal

To begin having help with dressing of lower half only. To progress to having help with shoes and socks only within 1 month.

Plan

Key

✓ = help with lower half only
× = help with shoes and socks only
○ = help with shoes and socks, one foot only
☐ = fully independent with dressing

Week one

Mon.	Tue.	Wed.	Thurs.	Fri.	Sat.	Sun.
✓	(full help)	✓	✓	(full help)	✓	✓

Week two

Mon.	Tue.	Wed.	Thurs.	Fri.	Sat.	Sun.
✓	(full help)	✓	✓	(full help)	✓	×

Week three

Mon.	Tue.	Wed.	Thurs.	Fri.	Sat.	Sun.
✓	×	✓	×	×	✓	×

Week four

Mon.	Tue.	Wed.	Thurs.	Fri.	Sat.	Sun.
✓	×	✓	×	×	×	×

Week five

Mon.	Tue.	Wed.	Thurs.	Fri.	Sat.	Sun.
○	×	○	○	×	○	○

Week six

Mon.	Tue.	Wed.	Thurs.	Fri.	Sat.	Sun.
○	×	○	○	○	○	○

Week seven

Mon.	Tue.	Wed.	Thurs.	Fri.	Sat.	Sun.
☐	○	☐	☐	○	☐	☐

Week eight

Mon.	Tue.	Wed.	Thurs.	Fri.	Sat.	Sun.
☐	○	☐	☐	☐	☐	☐

Goal 2

Long term goal

To increase sitting tolerance to 1 hour within 2 months.

- Mr B. must work out his present *baseline* for sitting—that is, how long he can sit for at the moment without overdoing it. Some patients work this out by taking their average ability of the specific activity over several days.
- He must then decide upon the *pacing interval*—that is, exactly how he intends to increase his sitting tolerance in order that sitting can be built up gradually in a paced manner. Making a written plan and recording progress in a chart is helpful (see below). He should set daily targets for 1 week at a time recording this in the 'G' column and make a note of his achievement in the 'A' column.
- At the end of each week he should evaluate his progress. If there is difficulty reaching the set daily targets, the pacing interval may need to be reduced. If daily targets are easily achieved the rate of pacing may be increased.

Goal: to increase sitting tolerance

G = the daily target (min)
A = a record of what is actually achieved (min)

Week one

Goal	Baseline (min)	Pacing interval	Mon.		Tues.		Wed.		Thurs.		Fri.		Sat.		Sun.	
			G	A	G	A	G	A	G	A	G	A	G	A	G	A
Increase sitting tolerance	7	1 min each day	7		8		9		10		11		12		13	

Week two

Mon.		Tues.		Wed.		Thurs.		Fri.		Sat.		Sun.	
G	A	G	A	G	A	G	A	G	A	G	A	G	A
14		15		16		17		18		19		20	

Week three

Mon.		Tues.		Wed.		Thurs.		Fri.		Sat.		Sun.	
G	A	G	A	G	A	G	A	G	A	G	A	G	A
21		22		23		24		25		26		27	

Week four

Mon.		Tues.		Wed.		Thurs.		Fri.		Sat.		Sun.	
G	A	G	A	G	A	G	A	G	A	G	A	G	A
28		29		30		31		32		33		34	

Week five

Mon.		Tues.		Wed.		Thurs.		Fri.		Sat.		Sun.	
G	A	G	A	G	A	G	A	G	A	G	A	G	A
35		36		37		38		39		40		41	

Week six

Mon.		Tues.		Wed.		Thurs.		Fri.		Sat.		Sun.	
G	A	G	A	G	A	G	A	G	A	G	A	G	A
42		43		44		45		46		47		48	

Week seven

Mon.		Tues.		Wed.		Thurs.		Fri.		Sat.		Sun.	
G	A	G	A	G	A	G	A	G	A	G	A	G	A
49		50		51		52		53		54		55	

Week eight

Mon.		Tues.		Wed.		Thurs.		Fri.		Sat.		Sun.	
G	A	G	A	G	A	G	A	G	A	G	A	G	A
56		57		58		59		60		61		62	

Goal 3

LONG TERM GOAL

To increase walking tolerance.

As for goal 2 Mr B. must establish his *baseline* for walking tolerance decide upon the *pacing interval* and gradually increase his walking tolerance in a paced manner. (Week one only is illustrated.)

G = the daily target (min)

A = a record of what is actually achieved (min)

Week one

Goal	Baseline (min)	Pacing interval	Mon.		Tues.		Wed.		Thurs.		Fri.		Sat.		Sun.	
			G	A	G	A	G	A	G	A	G	A	G	A	G	A
Increase walking tolerance	4	1 min every other day	4		4		5		5		6		6		7	

GOAL 4

Long term goal

To eliminate reclining within 2 months.

Short term goal

To restrict each period of reclining on the settee to 30 mins interspersed with walking and sitting.
Mr B. may set himself a plan to gradually reduce the amount of time he spends reclining. He may record his plan in a chart; an example of such a chart is illustrated below. Each time he reclines during the day he should not do so for longer than his planned time limit for that day. (Weeks one and two only are illustrated; G and A as before.)

Week one

Goal	Baseline (min)	Pacing interval	Mon.		Tues.		Wed.		Thurs.		Fri.		Sat.		Sun.	
			G	A	G	A	G	A	G	A	G	A	G	A	G	A
To eliminate reclining	30	Reduce by 1 min each day	30		29		28		27		26		25		24	

Week two

Mon.		Tues.		Wed.		Thurs.		Fri.		Sat.		Sun.	
G	A	G	A	G	A	G	A	G	A	G	A	G	A
23		22		21		20		19		18		17	

EXERCISE PROGRAMME

To improve flexibility and fitness slowly, increase confidence with feared movements and ultimately help in the achievement of specific activity-related goals a structured exercise programme is followed.

Daily stretching exercise programme

Patients are taught a stretching programme and given written instructions in order that they may continue the exercises at home. Patients must take responsibility for carrying out and progressing their own exercises at home. Their progress is reviewed by the physiotherapist usually at weekly intervals.

Instructions

Think of 3 'Ss' when carrying out the stretching exercises: 's' low, 's' ustained and 's' teady.

- Move slowly into the stretching position.
- Sustain (hold) the stretch beginning with a slow count of 5 seconds.
- Steadily release the stretch and return to the start position.
- Repeat each stretch twice only.
- Progress by gradually increasing the length of hold for each stretch up to a maximum of 20 seconds.
- Set your targets at the beginning of each week for the length of hold and record your achievements each day. An example of a record chart is shown below.
- Carry out a gentle warm-up before the stretches as already shown.

Daily stretching exercise schedule

In this example Mr. B. has decided to increase the length of hold by 1 second every other day. A selection of exercises is chosen in consultation with the physiotherapist. Full instructions for each exercise can be found in the stretching exercise patient booklet that is provided. (Week one only is illustrated.)

G = daily target for the stretching programme; this refers to the length of time in seconds each stretch is held

A = record of achievements

Week one

Exercise	Mon.		Tues.		Wed.		Thurs.		Fri.		Sat.		Sun.	
	G	A	G	A	G	A	G	A	G	A	G	A	G	A
Side bend	5		5		6		6		7		7		8	
Arching	5		5		6		6		7		7		8	
Rotation	5		5		6		6		7		7		8	
Knee to chest	5		5		6		6		7		7		8	
Hamstrings	5		5		6		6		7		7		8	
The cat	5		5		6		6		7		7		8	
Knee rolling	5		5		6		6		7		7		8	
Thigh stretch	5		5		6		6		7		7		8	

Strengthening exercise programme

Strengthening exercise may be incorporated into Mr B.'s rehabilitation programme. This may be best introduced at around the third week. At this stage Mr B. will be familiar with the stretching programme and his confidence with exercise may have started to increase. A strengthening exercise programme is selected in joint consultation between Mr B. and the physiotherapist.

- Set your initial exercise baseline (i.e. the number of repetitions you feel you can achieve without overdoing it). It is important to set your initial quota at an easily achievable level to help you gain confidence and reduce fear of injury. Five repetitions is usually a reasonable starting point for most people. Initially set your daily target each day before beginning your strengthening programme. Then after the first week set your daily targets for the week ahead. It is important to follow your exercise programme according to your set plan and not according to pain levels.
- For some exercises it is beneficial to hold for a count of 5 seconds. This is indicated as (H) in the exercise chart. For these exercises it is not necessary to increase the length of hold.
- Progress by increasing the number of repetitions you do up to a maximum of 15 repetitions. You may choose to progress the various exercises at different rates depending upon the fitness of specific areas of your body.

Strengthening exercise schedule

G: daily target for the strengthening exercises; this refers to the planned number of repetitions
A: record of achievements
H: hold this exercise for 5 seconds only

Exercise	Mon.		Tues.		Wed.		Thurs.		Fri.		Sat.		Sun.	
Name	G	A	G	A	G	A	G	A	G	A	G	A	G	A
Pelvic tilt (lying) (H)	5													
Head arms by side, lift (H)	5													
Diagonals	5													
Leg straightening	5													
Wall slide	5													
Leg lifting (lying)	5													
Opposites all fours	5													

PART 4 PSYCHOLOGY COMPONENT

*Helen Parker   Wolfgang Dumat
C. K. Booker*

INTRODUCTION

Without doubt the psychology input to the programme is vital. The psychology input will not only focus on education and teaching of positive skills such as relaxation and problem solving but should also be focused on addressing the psychological and emotional barriers to progress that may be present. A simple exercise programme in itself, without psychological input, is unlikely to produce significant change in patients with chronic pain. Many of the barriers to improvement in physical function are psychological. Specifically tackling these will enable the exercise component of the programme to be more effective. It is vital, therefore, to address the major psychological barriers that will have been identified at assessment (Ch. 10).

DEFUSING ANGER, HOSTILITY AND RESENTMENT

It is not uncommon for patients to express anger during the assessment process. The assessment team will have begun the task of addressing the issues that have given rise to such emotions. However, it is unlikely that all of the issues will have been addressed by the time the patient enters the programme. Keefe, Beaupre & Gil (1996) identify dealing with anger and high levels of emotional distress as one of the most common and important problems encountered when running a group programme. Often much of patients' anger is directed either at their previous treatment and their previous medical advisors or at the benefit or legal system. Such emotions are invariably destructive and do not help patients to adjust to their situation or focus on the rehabilitation process.

It is important, therefore, to hold a session specifically aimed at defusing these emotions at the start of a pain management programme. Dealing with these destructive emotions early on in a programme should potentially help to reduce the chance of their re-emergence later on. The doctor will have attempted to provide an explanation to the patients. However, psychologists will need (in their session) to allow patients to discuss any feelings of anger, hostility or resentment about previous consultations and previous treatments and their general experience within the health-care system. These emotions may also be directed towards the legal system, benefits agencies, employers and relatives.

Perhaps the best way to begin is to present patients with a table of common causes of anger, hostility and resentment, Table 13.4.1. Thus the patients will begin to identify their own emotions and begin to realise the reasons behind them. This may well produce a significant emotional response from the group. Group skills in handling these emotions are essential and the inability to provide straightforward answers should be acknowledged rather than covered up. Patients often cope better with 'don't knows'. It is essential that the team members communicate well. Truthful and *consistent* answers must be

given by each team member. In addition, specific questions may be raised in this session that will need to be addressed by doctors at their next session, or if necessary before the start of the next session.

Despite early clarification these issues may resurface later in the programme. Constantly focusing on the anger surrounding previous treatments or assessments is destructive for both the individual and the group. Regular meetings of the team will enable a consistent stance to be taken. Strong doubts and recurring destructive resorting to medical queries may in some cases represent resentment of the overall management approach and may only be solved by individual sessions.

INTRODUCING A BIOPSYCHOSOCIAL MODEL OF PAIN MANAGEMENT TO THE PATIENT

At the beginning of the pain management programme most if not all patients will still subscribe to the medical model of assessment and treatment of their pain problem. Despite careful counselling by the assessment team they may believe that their pain is a symptom of underlying injury or disease that needs to be diagnosed and then treated by doctors. It is important to move the patient away from this model. The patients must be presented with an alternative model of pain, which acknowledges their suffering and explains continuing pain without ongoing disease or damage. The *natural*

Table 13.4.1   Attributions about objects of anger and appraisals about reasons for anger among chronic pain sufferers

Agent (object of anger)	Action (reason for anger)
Causal agent of injury/illness	Chronic pain
Medical health-care providers	Diagnostic ambiguity, treatment failure
Mental health professionals	Implications of psychogenicity or pshchopathology
Attorneys and legal system	Adversarial dispute, scrutiny and arbitration
Insurance companies; social security system	Inadequate monetary coverage or compensation
Employer	Cessation of employment; job transfer; job retraining
Significant others	Lack of interpersonal support
God	'Predetermined' injury and consequences; ill fate
Self	Disablement, disfigurement
The whole world	Alienation

From Fernadez & Turk 1995 reproduced with permission.

consequences of chronic pain (Ch. 13 part 1) should be outlined and the patients helped to understand the biopsychosocial model of chronic pain. It is also important that from the start of a programme that patients feel that the team understands their problems. It is worth revisiting and discussing the patient traps presented in the opening session as a way to begin to gain patients' confidence; in addition it can help to form common bonds between group members and also provides a useful introduction to a biopsychosocial model of pain.

Describing the development of chronic pain and the biopsychosocial model

The development of chronic pain and disability should be described, with the focus on it being a developing process in which different factors play a significant role at different points in time (Ch. 5). The patients should come to understand that, whether pain onset is insidious or traumatic, a sequence of events is set up that can lead to failed treatment, job loss, immobility, negative emotions and the inability to cope. Patients should realise that some of these factors, such as failed surgery, may not be within their control but that others, such as family relationships, may very well be.

As patients recognise their own history in the description of the development of chronic pain and disability the clinician can then challenge their causal attribution of single, identifiable and treatable somatic factors for their pain. Patients must come to understand that there is no simple treatment which will 'cure' their pain. Understanding of the multiple factors involved in the development of pain and disability should then lead the patient on to the understanding that treatment also has to involve multiple factors.

RELAXATION TECHNIQUES

Relaxation has been demonstrated to be a valuable technique in pain management. It gives patients a skill, that in many cases can quickly lead to significant benefits and also gives them an immediate sense of control. The importance of the latter cannot be stressed too strongly as frequently those attending such groups will, at the outset, feel that they have no techniques at all with which to effectively manage their pain problem. However, it is important to recognise that it is only one of a number of techniques and forms only part of the treatment approach to chronic pain.

There are a number of different relaxation techniques available (Bernstein & Borkovec 1973, Jacobson 1974) and some patients may have previous experience with some of these. It is therefore important to start with a careful assessment of patients' previous experience and any problems that they may have encountered. Any worries, misconceptions or unrealistic expectations need to be addressed. (Details of the specific relaxation techniques follow.)

Ideally relaxation is best taught from start to finish by the same clinician to allow careful monitoring of progress and for the personal preferences of patients to be integrated as far as is possible.

The impact of relaxation should not be underestimated. It has been shown that unresolved psychological traumas may surface during relaxation. Such problems need to be dealt with efficiently and speedily by the psychologist.

Diaphragmatic breathing

One relaxation technique that can be easily demonstrated, learned and applied in almost all daily life situations is diaphragmatic breathing. This method may be the technique of choice for some patients and it is advisable to start relaxation sessions with this technique. Commonly most patients will have some initial difficulties but with repeated practice they can develop the skill quite quickly.

Often the realisation that they have been using chest or shoulder breathing can be an eye-opener for patients and the majority of patients are often unaware of the relationship between poor breathing and psychophysiological arousal.

Progressive muscle relaxation (PMR)

The overall goal of progressive muscular relaxation, or PMR, is to enable patients to become aware of muscle tension and to have the ability to produce muscle relaxation in different muscle groups in daily life. In PMR tensing and relaxing of the muscles are used to achieve an increase in muscle relaxation. All muscle groups in the body that are amenable to voluntary relaxation are systematically relaxed. The general rule is that the first step consists of tensing a muscle for approximately 5 to 7 seconds followed by the second step of trying to relax the same muscle for at least 25 seconds.

Concentration on tensing and relaxing is important because it will both enhance the effect and at the same time help to decrease unwanted intrusive thoughts and images. It is not necessary to tense muscles completely. Two-thirds of the possible muscle tension is sufficient. The purpose of getting patients to first tense their muscles is to raise awareness of the difference between a tense and a relaxed muscle.

General guideline for teaching relaxation exercises

1. Although relaxation training is best done lying down it is also possible to carry out the exercises in a sitting position if lying down proves too difficult. Patients may use a towel or a pillow under their head, lower back and knees if desired.
2. Ideally start off with a few minutes of abdominal breathing.
3. Loose comfortable clothing should be worn.
4. When practising at home patients should schedule relaxation into their daily routine. They will need to find time and physical space where they are able to be undisturbed for approximately 30 minutes.
5. If difficulties are experienced with learning to relax it is important to encourage the patient to continue as most difficulties are of a short term nature. Patients should also be made aware that relaxation may not work every day and that forcing it through may have detrimental effects on motivation and self-efficacy. It is important to develop a relaxed approach rather then simply applying a technique.

Initially the patient should start off with full PMR. Once this has been sufficiently mastered the patient should progress to combining muscle groups. One of the advantages of this is that relaxation can be applied in a shorter period of time with the same effect. Following this, patients can then progress to the use of relaxation without tensing.

As much time as individuals need should be allowed for them to reach this position, although with regular practice 4–6 weeks should be sufficient. At this stage the patient omits tensing muscle groups and instead simply concentrates on the different muscle groups without tensing and simply concentrating on the feeling of relaxation.

Applying relaxation in daily life

It is important that patients get into the habit of using relaxation as part of their everyday routine. Patients can be advised to practice in the following ways:

1. Normal relaxation. This is just practising relaxation for 15 to 30 minutes, at least once a day. As far as possible this should be kept up despite difficulties although if other stressors make this very difficult then a short break is acceptable.

2. Brief relaxation. This means a relaxation of about 5 to 10 minutes during the day when activities are deliberately stopped. This can be done in almost any position, sitting or standing and it should be done several times a day in real life.

3. Mini relaxation. This is relaxing for anything from a few seconds to a few minutes and should be done as often as possible. It will help to make relaxation a habitual skill in almost any situation. Patients should be encouraged to identify particular 'trouble spots' for muscular tension and to focus particularly on these areas.

Imagery techniques

Once patients have mastered diaphragmatic breathing and PMR and have shown good insight into the application of these techniques within pain management, it is possible to enhance the effect of relaxation by introducing techniques such as guided imagery and visualisation. Such techniques take the process of relaxation a step further by introducing elements of hypnotherapeutic interventions, which can be used effectively in pain management. These can improve the quality of the relaxation experience, increasing perceived self-control and self-efficacy. Such methods can be introduced by explaining that they are techniques aimed at enhancing mental relaxation. It is advisable that such techniques are initially practised on their own and then combined with the physical relaxation methods.

Problems that may be encountered with teaching relaxation

1. Initially patients may feel self-conscious or embarrassed when practising exercises as a group. This should be acknowledged before the start of teaching and a certain amount of embarrassed 'giggling' expected.

2. When practising PMR some patients may experience pain when tensing a muscle. When this occurs it may be because too much tension is being applied or the muscle is already on a high level of tension and any slight increase will cause pain or muscle spasm. As relaxation skills improve these problems should subside. If, however, pain persists then focusing on the tensing without actually tensing the muscle may be used.

3. One frequent complaint of patients is that after practising for two or three sessions they declare that 'the exercises don't work'. The importance of regular practice should be stressed; it can be useful here to use the analogy of learning to drive. Just as you don't expect to be able to go out and drive on a motorway in the rush hour after two or three driving lessons so you cannot expect to master relaxation after a short period of time.

4. Patients may complain of lack of time in which to practise relaxation; such problems need to be discussed in detail and often a problem-solving approach to time management is helpful. However, there are instances where personal difficulties and family issues may need to be addressed. Lack of assertiveness may also be responsible. Generally speaking, patients will need to address the issue of practising skills as part of the overall changes they are making to their lifestyle if they want to manage their pain successfully.

5. Some patients may have the unrealistic expectation that by religiously practising relaxation that this will lead to automatic success (i.e. pain relief and control of pain-related problems). Such beliefs need to be tackled at the outset and relaxation should be presented as one part of a series of techniques, which will be used by them to manage their chronic pain problem.

6. There may be confusion between deep relaxation and sleep and the difference between the two states should be explained. Those patients who find that they consistently fall asleep during relaxation (a problem that tends to occur when relaxation is practised at the end of the day) should be encouraged to practise at a time of day when they are less tired.

7. Some patients can have problems with imagery techniques, particularly in the generation of images. One useful strategy is to ask them to spend a few minutes looking at a painting or picture and then shutting their eyes and trying to describe it to themselves.

STRESS, PSYCHOPHYSIOLOGICAL AROUSAL AND CHRONIC PAIN

The ability to cope with chronic pain in daily life could be rephrased as the ability to cope with stress. Pain and the problems it can lead to (e.g. work loss leading to financial difficulties) are major stressors. Many patients will also have other non-pain-related stressors in their lives. In order to develop effective stress management techniques the patient first needs a basic understanding of the psychophysiological stress reaction and its influence on cognitive, emotional and behavioural functioning.

Stress experiment

To demonstrate psychophysiological arousal and its consequences patients can be put through a stressful event that provokes physical, mental and behavioural reactions strong enough for them to be able to describe their experience.

This can be done in the group by introducing a relaxation exercise with a built-in anticipated stressor such as a performance task. This task, introduced in such a fashion during the initial stages of pain management, is enough in some cases to provoke quite a strong stress reaction. The psychologist must therefore be prepared to deal with the possibility of having to debrief some patients and rebuild constructive group participation. This procedure will generally successfully lead into an in-depth discussion of stress responses, which are usually very familiar to the patient but so far have often been unexplained.

Explaining the stress response—the 'fight or flight' reaction

One very useful method to explain the stress response is by describing it in terms of the 'flight or fight' response. This includes giving the patient a basic understanding of sympathetic and parasympathetic nervous systems and the roles that they play in this response. Individual differences in reactions will need to be explained carefully along with the effect that stress can have on coping mechanisms. Knowledge and understanding will in itself alleviate some of the patients' worries and enable them to put symptoms within a more appropriate context. It will also increase their awareness of their own personal responses to perceived stressors. Using this approach patients are given the opportunity to understand their symptomatology fully with regards not only to the physical but also the mental and behavioural consequences.

The ABC of stress

Knowledge and understanding of stress are the basis of being able to implement changes and progress to more appropriate coping styles. A major goal of pain management lies in the ability to change unhelpful or negative thinking (cognitive restructuring). In order to achieve this patients are best helped by making use of the ABC of stress (antecedents, beliefs, consequences, (these may be emotional or behavioural). This simplified model of understanding the role of unhelpful cognitions and the effect they can have on emotions and behaviour gives patients a first insight into the effects of stress and allows them to start self-monitoring. Distorted or negative thinking patterns are then open to appraisal and change.

Illustrating the ABC of stress

Ellis's simplified therapeutic technique (Ellis 1962) has several advantages. It matches patients' daily experience and is easy to understand. It provides a tangible skill to change a patient's appraisal of a stressful event and consequently the emotional and behavioural responses.

An example of the technique is as follows:

- **A** — patient doing some gardening experiences an increase in pain
- **B** — patient believes that the back has been harmed thinks 'I can't cope with this pain, I'm useless, I'll never be able to get back to doing the things I used to do'.
- **C** — patient rests, takes painkillers, feels depressed.

The dangers are that the complexity of the problem is often underestimated and implementation into daily life often takes persistent application and the ability not to be demoralised by making mistakes.

Once patients have developed the ability to identify the ABCs they can then move on to the final stage, which is disputing or challenging their beliefs.

COGNITIONS (THOUGHTS) AND CHRONIC PAIN

Typical cognitive errors within chronic pain

Clinicians working with depressive or anxious patients have identified a number of typical thinking errors such as 'all-or-nothing thinking' or 'expecting the worst to happen'. With regard to chronic pain patients there are a number of distorted and/or negative cognitions that need to be addressed.

A major goal of pain management is to teach patients to change unhelpful or negative thinking (cognitive restructuring). Patients need to learn to recognise that their thoughts about their pain and themselves can affect not only their levels of stress and mood state but also their behaviour.

Catastrophising and negative thoughts

The tendency of chronic pain patients to 'catastrophise' (i.e. expect the worse to happen—see Ch. 2, p. 20) and the negative effect that this has on psychological functioning (particularly in its contribution to depressed mood) has been demonstrated by numerous studies (see Jensen et al (1991) for a review). If this is pointed out, patients readily accept and acknowledge this difficulty. There may be erroneous expectations of decline, increased disability and insurmountable pain at some future time. Past medical treatment failures may well have enhanced such thoughts.

'All-or-nothing thinking' may be equally frequent as it represents patients' expectations within a medical model approach. Common thoughts include: 'Unless the pain can be cured nothing will be of any help' and 'Unless I can return to how I used to be or how I should be then nothing will be of benefit'.

Patients may hold a number of erroneous beliefs about their pain that affect their behaviour (Ch. 2 Specific beliefs about pain, p. 000). For example the belief that 'hurt = harm' is very commonly held by patients with chronic pain and can lead to reduction and avoidance of activities.

Identifying cognitive thinking errors and incorporating them within stress and pain management

The ability to identify thinking errors and the effect that these have on both their emotional and behavioural responses should enable patients to be able to change dysfunctional cognitive coping styles in general. Based on other elements of the programme such as education about chronic pain, patients may be in a position to adopt a management approach on the basis of the biopsychosocial model rather than remaining on the treatment approach based on a medical model. This is particularly important for patients who perceive pain management as a further 'treatment' that is simply enhanced by a few helpful skills such as exercise and relaxation.

Patients may well vary in their initial abilities to identify their own cognitive-thinking errors. When teaching patients how to identify such errors it can be of value to start with case examples. Once the ability to recognise the major types of errors made then the patients can proceed to identify their own errors in thinking and the effects that these have on both their emotional functioning and behaviour. Techniques that can be of value here are diary keeping, where patients record their activities, thoughts and mood, and asking patients to recall the types of thoughts that they have when having a flare-up or dealing with stressors.

PROBLEM SOLVING

Using a case study

Problem solving has been identified in many studies as a valuable approach and is a major treatment component in many pain management programmes. The aim of problem solving is to enable the patient to use effective coping strategies to deal with the problems identified.

Patients are best made familiar with the technique by confronting them with a 'case study'

Box 13.4.1   Problem solving

- Step one   Decide which problem to tackle
- Step two   Describe and break down the problem into small parts
- Step three   Pick one part to work on
- Step four   Think of as many ways as possible of dealing with part identified
- Step five   Evaluate how realistic each way is; look at both the positive and negative consequences for each way
- Step six   Pick the method that you decide is the best
- Step seven   Plan how you are going to put this into action
- Step eight   Carry it out
- Step nine   Evaluate how successful you were

---

that demonstrates the most common problems that chronic pain patients develop. The advantage of using a hypothetical case study is that this is not perceived as threatening by the patients. It is often easier to 'solve' someone else's problems than one's own.

When working on such a case study, patients should work together in small groups. This adds another important dimension to the course. It builds mutual trust and enables patients to realise that discussing even personal issues within a group setting may prove to be beneficial.

Principles of problem solving

Having identified problems using a case study, patients should then be introduced to the stages of problem solving (Box 13.4.1).

Application of problem solving

The first stages of problem solving (steps one to seven) should initially be practised using case examples as this will be less threatening to the patients. Patients may initially need considerable help with this, particularly in breaking problems down and in generating solutions. Hawton & Kirk (1989) suggest that one way to aid a patient to generate solutions is to use 'brainstorming': as many potential solutions as possible, no matter how unlikely they seem, are generated; the authors also suggest that if the therapist

proposes solutions that are obviously inappropriate this can help to facilitate patients' involvement. Once patients feel comfortable with the method they can then generate their own problem lists and start working on their own solutions.

ASSERTIVENESS AND COMMUNICATION

Introduction: passive, aggressive and assertive styles

Pain management skills are skills that patients need to apply in daily life both within their family and their working environment. In order to be successful, assertiveness and good communication are essential. Most patients will describe difficulties in these areas, as they have become passive and withdrawn or angry and disaffected. Feelings of guilt with regard to those close to them may also impair good communication.

It is important that patients learn to recognise the difference between expressing what we feel and think to others in an aggressive way, a passive way and an assertive way. Assertiveness should be stressed as one way in which patients can feel that they are more in control of situations and less helpless.

Sessions relating to these topics should be placed towards the end of a course. The group will need to develop a degree of trust between the members if these sessions are to be of value. The topic is best introduced as a further skill that will help to put pain management into practice rather than a personal deficit. Describing different styles such as the aggressive or passive communication style may give patients a good opportunity to discuss and assess their own difficulties in these areas.

Role play of assertiveness techniques

Simple exercises such as 'repeated refusal' or 'repeated request' will provide a simple understandable start for role plays. Initially patients may feel inhibited about participating in such role plays. To overcome these initial difficulties only volunteers should be used and the clinician may need to function as a role model and to participate in the majority of role plays.

One way of practising role-play techniques is as follows:

1. Explain each role and the situation in very concrete terms.
2. Split the group up and give the members observational tasks such as the non-verbal communication of participants.
3. Participants are allowed to feed back their experience first with particular emphasis on how they felt during the role play. Audience and clinician should then feed back after this.
4. Make sure that all difficulties that may have occurred are resolved.

Role play should be aimed at giving the patient the opportunity to try out new or different behaviours in a supportive situation. Every role play should conclude with a general discussion emphasising the points learned.

As the group increases in confidence the participants should be invited to contribute any particular situations that they would wish to role play. Assertiveness practice can be usefully combined with problem-solving sessions as many solutions to problems will require assertiveness to put them into practice.

THE PARTNER SESSION

Partners' and family members' behaviour is likely to influence chronic pain patients' coping behaviour. Solicitous behaviour will reinforce maladaptive coping strategies as much as neglect or withdrawal by disaffected spouses. Partners and family members are not to blame as they are reacting in a way not dissimilar to patients; their often unhelpful responses are in most cases well meant and may be based on a poor understanding of the process of chronic pain. For example spouses who believe that 'hurt = harm' are likely to tell partners to avoid those activities that provoke pain and to advise them to adopt coping strategies such as increasing medication and resting.

Partners should ideally be present at the initial assessment (Ch. 7). During the feedback given at the end of the assessment it needs to be made explicit that if a place is offered on a programme then partners are expected to become involved and to attend for certain sessions. Only if patients and partners become aware of the seriousness of this part of the programme will they make an effort to participate.

For pain management to be applied successfully in daily life both partners and family members need to have an understanding of the approach. In addition flare-ups and setbacks may be dealt with more efficiently and without resorting to use of health-care resources if this support is available from the partner. A partner session is therefore a vital element of any pain management programme.

Structure of partners' session

Ideally 2–3 hours should be set aside for this session. Partners are best seen by the team by themselves for up to 1 hour. This should preferably take place in the same setting as the main programme.

The time should be devoted to individual questions from the partners who will by this time have formed some impressions of how the programme has affected their spouse. This part of the session should also give the team the opportunity to observe partners' understanding and commitment to pain management and to identify any potential problems with particular couples.

As a next step partners and patients should meet informally during a break and then meet with the whole team. A final discussion, facilitated by the team, should aim to start the process of making the expectations and the understanding of both patients and partners explicit and correcting any misconceptions.

How to get partners involved

One of the great challenges of the partners session is how to get partners involved. In order to avoid passive reception (i.e. expecting an informative lecture from the clinicians) techniques that have been shown to be successful in other group work or group settings should be used.

One such technique may be to let partners answer a simple questionnaire regarding their expectations after the patient has participated in a pain management programme (see Appendix to this chapter, p. 313). This questionnaire must be filled in anonymously and should be returned to the clinical psychologist who will prepare and lead the session. In most cases questions will reveal unrealistic expectations and poor knowledge about the rationale of pain management. The answers may then be summarised and presented on a flip chart to both patients and partners. Patients will then be given an opportunity to comment on the expectations and hopefully correct the obvious errors. In most instances this sparks off a discussion amongst patients and partners although careful facilitation will be necessary.

CONCLUSION

The psychological component is a vital component of the programme. It is not possible to run a cognitive–behavioural rehabilitation programme without skilfully presented psychological sessions. Many of the barriers to progress that might initially appear to be physical or practical in nature have significant psychological aspects. By working in close collaboration with the physician and in particular the physiotherapist such barriers may be more readily identified and addressed. Finally there are specific psychological skills that patients will need to acquire if they are to be successful in maintaining their progress and continuing to improve when they have completed the programme.

KEY POINTS

- Psychological input aims to educate, to teach positive skills for coping with pain and to address barriers to progress.
- Issues of anger, hostility and resentment need to be addressed.
- Relaxation techniques, identifying cognitive-thinking errors, problem solving and assertion training are all valuable techniques that need to be incorporated within the group programme.
- It is of great importance that partners are involved in the group.

REFERENCES

Bernstein D A, Borkovec T D 1973 Progressive relaxation training: A manual for the helping professions. Research Press, Champaign Il

Ellis A 1962 Reason and emotion in psychotherapy. Lyle Stuart, New York

Fernandez E, Turk D C 1995 The scope and significance of anger in the experience of chronic pain. Pain 61:165–175

Hawton K, Kirk J 1989 Problem solving. In: Hawton K, Salkovskis P M, Kirk J, Clark D (eds) Cognitive behavioural therapy for psychiatric problems. Oxford Medical, Oxford, pp 406–426

Jacobson E 1974 Progressive relaxation. Midway reprint. University of Chicago Press, Chicago Il

Jensen M, Turner J A, Romano J M, Karoly P 1991 Coping with chronic pain: a critical review of the literature. Pain 47:249–283

Keefe F J, Beaupre P M, Gil K M 1996 Group therapy for patients with chronic pain. In: Gatchell R J, Turk D C, (eds) Psychological approaches to pain management. Guilford, New York, pp 259–282

APPENDIX:

Partner session—Manchester & Salford Pain Centre

Re: partner session

Dear partner, family member or friend,

As explained during the assessment, we would like you, as the partner/friend/relative of a programme participant, to come in on the **Friday afternoon of the second week of the programme**.

This session will be dealing with the content of the programme and the patient's progress. It is also an opportunity for you to ask the members of staff questions about the programme and about realistic expectations for change after the programme.

In order to prepare this session we would like you to answer a few questions for us and to return your answers without your name and address before next **Wednesday**.

It might also be valuable not to discuss your answers with your partner and not to let him/her see your answers. That will be something that you can do after the partner session. Do not refer to 'him/her' but to 'my partner' in your answers.

Please put your answers in a sealed envelope and let the patient give it to **Karen** or **Sandy**.

Please answer the following questions:

(using a separate sheet of paper)

How would you like your partner to change after the programme:

1. with regards to pain?
2. with regards to activities?
3. with regards to family life?
4. with regards to mood?
5. with regards to future use of the health-care system (seeing doctors/further treatment/using medication)?

The answers will be used **anonymously** (so please do not mention your name or your partner's name on your envelope) during the partners' session to discuss the possible difficulties of pain management.

Thank you very much for your cooperation.

The M & SPC team

PART 5 GENERAL ISSUES AND CONCLUSIONS

Chris C. Spanswick   Helen Parker

CONSISTENCY OF APPROACH

Although the content of the group programme has been dealt with in different chapters this has been done for pragmatic reasons. It is important to understand that the running of the programme is very much a team effort. There are many issues and topics that cross the boundaries between the various professions of the team. Consistency of approach is vital and will enable patients to link psychological issues and physical activity.

There must be regular scheduled time for team members to meet to discuss the progress of individuals and the group as a whole. Problems can then be identified and important issues raised can be addressed as soon as possible, if necessary allowing patients' concerns to be addressed individually.

Regular 'handing over' of sessions will contribute to presenting a consistent approach. Adopting a 'Kardex' or written record of the group's and individual's progress is of great help in keeping all members of the team informed and helps in the formulation of the discharge letter at the end of the programme. Each team member should record the content of their session with the group and write comments in the individual's record if appropriate.

HOUSE RULES

It important to have a written set of 'house rules' (see Appendix to part 1 of this chapter, p. 267).

These should be given to patients prior to their agreeing to opt into treatment. The rules should be reinforced at the first session of the programme. The purpose of the rules is to make both the staff's and patient's responsibilities explicit. Such rules protect the staff and allow for a more objective means of assessment of the patient's behaviour in cases where either compliance or disruptive behaviour threatens the group.

MONITORING PROGRESS

Throughout the group programme the patients' progress is monitored, both by the team and by the patients themselves. The need to monitor progress is made explicit from the very beginning of the programme. Patients attend the centre just prior to the first session for completion of various questionnaires and assessments of physical function. The need to collect outcome data is stressed to patients and they must agree to participate in this as a condition of attending the programme.

The patients are asked to bring a loose-leaf file with them. This will enable them to keep a written record of their progress including charting their exercises and progress towards their declared goals. They are encouraged to make notes during the teaching sessions and keep the various handouts from team members in their file. Thus they are able to develop their own handbook to which they can refer later.

Individual review

Each patient is interviewed at the end of the first week by the team. This may seem a little daunting for the patient, but is done in as relaxed a manner as possible. Patients are invited to give their own assessment of their progress and to identify any specific problems or barriers (Box 13.5.1). The team members feed back their view of the patient's first week offering support,

---

Box 13.5.1 Potential problems on the programme
• Patient does not understand model • Patient not convinced of the pain management model • Patient still considering other treatments • Difficulty in coping with pain • Acute flare-up of pain • Difficulty in concentration • Patient's anger unresolved • Socioeconomic factors • Overprotective partner • Partner undermining confidence or gains • Patient failing to observe 'house rules'

---

advice and praise where it is appropriate. Occasionally it is clear that the patient is making no progress or progress is very slow. The team will try to identify the specific barriers with the patient and come to a conclusion as to whether the patient should continue with the group or if there are appropriate alternatives (individual management).

Patients may be given advice as to how to tackle their problem and their progress will be reviewed at the end of the second week. Rarely patients are destructive to the cohesion of the group or non-compliant and may be invited to leave.

If a patient has to leave the group for any reason, it is important to discuss this with the group after the event to ensure that the group understands the reasons and does not lose its morale. Frequently the group members anticipate patients dropping out, as they are aware that that patient was not engaged.

Task assignment

During the second week of the programme the group is set the task of putting pain management techniques into practice. A session is set aside during the third week. The patients have to decide upon a task, which they will do 'as a group'. It must incorporate activity that demonstrates the need for planning, pacing, physical activity and patients monitoring their own performance. Although some guidance may be given, essentially the group must decide what it wishes to do. Such task assignments have varied from 'American line dancing' to a major gardening project. The purpose of this is to place responsibility firmly with the patients and allow them to put their knowledge into practice in a very practical way.

Group review

At the end of the second week and at the end of the final week the patients' progress is reviewed in a group setting. In particular the issues surrounding the 'task assignment' are discussed and feedback on performance is given. Commonly problems do occur with the task assignment. It is important for the patients to use this as a learning experience upon which they can build.

THE END OF THE PROGRAMME

It is important to impress upon the patients right from the very beginning that the purpose of the programme is for the patients to develop the necessary skills to manage their pain for the rest of their lives. They should not regard their treatment as being completed at the end of the programme. The programme is simply an opportunity to learn and develop lifelong skills. Perhaps the most important period is that in the first 6 months after the end of the programme when they should be implementing all that they have learned. They will, of course, need to continue with such skills indefinitely.

The patients must have committed themselves to the follow-up sessions at the very beginning of the programme as a prerequisite for inclusion on the programme. It is vital that the later sessions concentrate on getting patients to identify the specific goals they wish to achieve by the time they come for the follow-up session. They should be directed not only to picking realistic goals but also to identifying the difficulties and barriers to reaching their goals. They should

---

> **Box 13.5.2** Patient plans
>
> - Targets for exercises and physical activity
> - Planning for relaxation and exercise
> - Management of tablets and medicines
> - Involvement of partner/significant other and family
> - Managing acute flare-ups
> - Planning middle and long term goals

have specific plans as to how they are going to address and overcome the barriers that they have identified (see Appendix, to this part of the chapter, p. 319).

Finally the patients must receive feedback on their performance on the programme. This should be honest and include an analysis of the good points and any specific weaknesses or worries the team may have about the patient. Although it is important to boost the patient's confidence, this should be done with a degree of realism. The patient otherwise will leave the programme on something of a 'high' and will not be adequately prepared for the reality of life without the immediate support of the team or the other participants.

By the end of the programme all patients should have explicit goals and targets for the next 4 weeks (Box 13.5.2). They should have plans for managing an acute flare-up of their pain should that occur.

DOCUMENTATION AND DISCHARGE LETTERS

Adequate documentation of patients' status prior to commencing the programme, their progress and status at the end of the programme is vital. Time should be allocated for the team to meet after the programme to discuss the content of the discharge letter. Patients' GPs should be given a summary of their progress and any potential problems that may be anticipated. They should also be given details of the aims and objectives of the pain management programme together with the patient's specific goals (Ch. 14).

KEY POINTS

- An integrated approach to the delivery of a pain management programme is essential.
- Individual team members' responsibilities must be explicit.
- Frequent informal meetings of the team members will ensure early identification of problems both with individual patients and with the group as a whole.
- Close team working will produce a consistency in approach and avoid mixed messages.
- Clear goal setting with the patients by the end of the programme will prepare the patients for the future and should be the focus of the follow-up sessions.
- Detailed discharge letters are vital to helping the patient's GP support the patient in the community and avoid unnecessary use of the health-care system.

APPENDIX: RECORD OF ACHIEVEMENTS, PLANS AND BARRIERS

Name: _____

My achievements so far:	
My plans for the next 3 months:	
Barriers to achieving my goals:	

14

Maintenance of change and skill enhancement

Paul Watson   Chris C. Spanswick

INTRODUCTION

In patients who have responded positively to pain management, it is important to address the issue of maintenance of treatment gains. Marlatt & Gordon (1995) identified four steps in relapse prevention. The essence of their recommendations is shown in Box 14.1. They include such techniques in an 'emergency-card', which patients have developed at the end of the treatment programme.

Bradley (1996) addresses the issues of high risk situations and relapse prevention, and notes that nearly all CBT interventions in patients with rheumatoid arthritis (RA) include some element of relapse prevention training (Bradley et al 1987). He cites Keefe & van Horn (1993) who suggest: 'relapse tends to occur when patients' symptoms increase in intensity, their perceived abilities to control symptoms are compromised, and their psychological distress is magnified'. If patients stop their effort at coping in response to setbacks they are likely to experience a major decline in pain control, functional ability or

---

Box 14.1   Steps in relapse prevention

- Stopping and paying attention to cues that a setback is occurring
- Keeping calm and using relaxation to prevent an over emotional response
- Reviewing the circumstances leading up to the setback
- Implementing appropriate coping strategies

---

psychological status. It is suggested that there are critical components designed to help patients cope with a relapse. They identify four phases of treatment:

- practice in identifying high risk situations that are likely to tax patients' coping resources
- practice in identifying early signs of relapse such as increases in pain or depression
- rehearsal of cognitive and behavioural skills for responding to these early relapse signs
- training in self-reinforcement for effective displays of coping with possible relapse.

Indeed there is a substantial emphasis on relapse prevention in the Salford programme. At the conclusion of the pain management programme the patients will have been required to identify their own specific goals for the immediate and long term future (see Ch. 13). These will have addressed specific areas including medication use, management of acute flare-ups, use of the health-care system, targets for exercise and relaxation, return to social and family activities, the potential for the return to gainful activities (return to work) and other areas specific to that patient (e.g. improving communication with partner).

It is important to prepare the patients on the pain management programme for their return to home. Most patients comment upon the loss of immediate support upon return home, even if the programme has been a largely out-patient based programme with attendance only once or twice per week. The patients gain a great deal from the mutual support and camaraderie on the course from their fellows as well as the obvious support and encouragement they gain from the staff. By the end of the programme the patients have usually become good personal friends and provide each other with significant moral support, particularly when difficulties are encountered. Patients often describe that they leave a programme on a 'high'. This may be to the extent that they have not adequately addressed how they are going to manage on their own at home.

Others do become more anxious about their ability to manage on their own at home, but fail to plan for this. The mutual support of the group may even distract them from focusing their attention on the necessary plans for the future. It is vital, therefore, to help the patients on the programme to plan how they will manage their return to their home (and possibly work) environment.

In addition to the issues of relapse prevention contained within our actual teaching programme, there are a number of other key features which should be addressed during the postprogramme period. They are shown in Box 14.2.

ADVICE TO THE PATIENT AND FAMILY

The programme will have helped patients to focus on their own specific problems. Patients will have been set the task of identifying the problems they anticipate and how they propose to manage or solve them. They will have set specific targets that they expect to achieve and the time-scale in which they propose to do this (Fig. 14.1). Patients should therefore have explicit written plans that they have agreed. It is important that the patients are the main instigators of this and that the staff do not coerce or dictate the agenda.

At least one session of the programme will have been devoted to the partner (significant

---

Box 14.2 Key features needing to be addressed after the programme

- Advice to the patient and family
- Advice to the referring agent and GP
- To follow up or not?
  - the purpose of follow-ups
  - frequency and timing of follow-ups
  - content and organisation of follow-up sessions
- Management of 'cries for help'
- Postprogramme support groups
- Accessing return to work
  - barriers to return to work
  - preparation for return to work

PACED EXERCISE CIRCUIT

NAME OF EXERCISE	MONDAY		TUESDAY		WEDNESDAY		THURSDAY		FRIDAY		SATURDAY		SUNDAY	
	G	A	G	A	G	A	G	A	G	A	G	A	G	A

KEY
G = The goal—how many exercises you plan to do   CENTRE FOR PAIN MANAGEMENT
A = Achievement—how many exercises you actually do   SALFORD ROYAL HOSPITALS NHS TRUST

Figure 14.1   Example of patient's targets form.

other) (Ch. 13). The prime objective is to educate the partner, improve communications between the partner and the patient and enable the couple (patient and family) to plan how they will manage at home without the immediate support of the group. It is vital that the partner understands the need for the patient to retain control and not to take over managing the patient's pain and other related problems. Written instructions for the partner may be helpful but it is more important that the patient and partner work on the ground rules themselves. A failure to educate partners of how they should behave may lead to patients losing control and returning to unhelp-ful strategies including seeking further cures for their pain.

How things can go wrong

Case study 14.1 illustrates the potential for problems to ensue if patients have not planned their progress at home carefully and in some detail. It also illustrates the importance of educating the patient's partner. Neither the patient nor the partner had plans for how to manage acute flare-ups. They both therefore resorted to previous behaviour (calling the GP for more help) in the panic and stress of the acute situation.

Case study 14.1 A problem after the programme

Mrs G. is a 48-year-old housewife with a 7-year history of low back pain. She had seen a large number of specialists in a search for an explanation of her ongoing pain and a cure. Scans had not revealed any structural cause and she felt reassured by the team's explanation of her ongoing pain. She attended all of the sessions of the pain management programme and made substantial progress both physically and emotionally. She felt that she had gained a great deal from the programme but was fearful of how she would manage at home. Her husband was often away from home for extended periods of time and she had few friends locally.

Mrs G.'s husband had noticed a major improvement, but was fearful of her 'overdoing it'. He was unable to attend the partner session. He tended to be overprotective when at home insisting on doing everything (although he felt quite resentful).

Mrs G. had made only vague plans by the end of the programme. For example, she expressed a wish to walk more without specifying any detail or how she was going to achieve this and monitor it. She had not discussed any of her plans with her husband.

When at home Mrs G. suffered an acute flare-up. Her husband had to return home and he arranged with her GP for her to be admitted to the local hospital.

Box 14.3 Advice to patients

- Have written plans for managing acute flare-ups
- Practise these regularly
- Make sure that you have discussed this with your partner (family)
- Explain exactly how your partner/family can help
- Have plans (time and space) for your exercises and relaxation
- Have specific short term targets (e.g. increase walking tolerance to 15 minutes by 1 month's time)
- Plan for moral support (e.g. involve friends, family or keep telephone contact with group)
- Visit your GP and explain what you are doing
- Ask for GP's support and help (not more medicines or referrals)
- Translate gains into something pleasurable/useful (e.g. going out for coffee)
- Plan to do something to keep the mood and morale up (e.g. go to pictures, visit friends)

Box 14.3 summarises advice that may be given to patients.

ADVICE TO THE REFERRING AGENT AND GENERAL PRACTITIONER

In addition to the discharge letter at the end of the programme both the referring agent and in particular the patient's GP should be sent specific guidelines to help with the further management of the patient after the programme (Box 14.4). The guidelines should include the philosophy, aims and objectives of the programme. Such guidelines simply outline the purpose of the programme and the general principles of management in the community after the programme. Any specific detail that relates to a particular patient should be included in the discharge letter (e.g. detail of the gradual withdrawal of medication).

Sending such detail to referring agents is important, to indicate to them not only how the patient has done but also how the patient should manage the future and avoid unnecessary further evaluations and treatments. Communication with the patient's GP is, however, vital. It is the GP to whom the patient is likely to turn in event of an acute flare-up. Therefore GPs must be given the rationale and details of the long term plan if they are to be actively involved in the patient's management. It is vital that the patient does not get 'mixed messages'. GPs must have details of what the team members have told patients and what is expected of them.

GPs must also be given an understanding of what the long term plans are and precisely what their role in these are. The outline of the general principles of pain management will be useful as well as specific instructions relating only to their patient. For example GPs must be involved in managing any changes in medication. They must be informed as to what changes are to be made, how they are to be made and the rationale behind this. Only then is their cooperation likely to be achieved.

Despite communicating with GPs problems can still occur. If GPs are not convinced that pain

---

Box 14.4   Advice to GPs on how they can support their chronic pain patients in management of their pain

Management of flare-ups
1. Short period of rest is acceptable for a maximum of 48 hours
2. Check pacing
3. Look for other stressors
4. Accept that explanations may not always be possible
5. Prevent the patient relapsing into models of pathology as causes of pain
6. Encourage gradual increase in activity
7. Medication may be increased on a time contingent basis for short periods to enable restoration to normal levels of activity as soon as possible

General advice
1. Reinforce that what has been learned at the pain centre should be exploited for an *unlimited* length of time
2. Avoid return to medical model:

— emphasise no structural or pathological cause for the pain
— emphasise no specific medical intervention will cure pain
— emphasise hurt does not indicate harm
3. Encourage continued activity and pacing of activity; use exercise programme taught at pain centre and avoid prolonged rest
4. Actively encourage continuing use of stress reduction and relaxation training techniques
5. Encourage continued medication reduction:
— avoid opioids (alone or in combination) for long term use
— avoid hypnotics and benzodiazepines
6. Avoid artificial aids to mobility (e.g. walking sticks, corsets, etc.)
7. We would not anticipate putting the patient through a further full programme but occasional top-ups may be available according to clinical indications at the time

---

management is appropriate or, for example, that reduction of medication is sensible in the face of chronic pain then they are likely to unintentionally undermine the patient's progress. This is far more likely to occur if they have not been given specific guidelines and reasons for pursuing this line of management.

It should be remembered that the care of the patient rests with the GP. They may be under considerable pressure (from the patient or the family) to do something in the event of an acute flare-up. It is very difficult to resist in the heat of the moment unless the team has given explicit (written) support. All patients should therefore be given a copy of the guidelines that are to be sent to their GPs. This ensures that there are no misunderstandings and gives explicit permission to the GP to remain firm in neither prescribing inappropriately nor referring the patient for further specialist appointments or treatments that are not clinically indicated.

The guidelines will also give the GP the confidence to refer the patient to a specialist if 'new' pain problems arise that are clearly different from the 'chronic' and long-standing problems. The clinical decision rules, therefore, become explicit. The pain management team, the patient and the GP will share an agreed understanding of the specific reasons for further

investigation or the appropriate refusal of this if indicated.

TO FOLLOW UP OR NOT?

Most pain management programmes include some form of follow-up sessions as an integrated part of their programme. It is essential to have some assessment of longer term progress of patients if the purchasers are to be persuaded that pain management programmes are a worthwhile investment. In addition the team cannot audit either outcome or the content of the programme without some evaluation of the patients' progress other than that demonstrable at the end of the programme.

The purpose of follow-up

Monitoring patients' progress

The patients will have set themselves specific goals and targets at the end of the programme with the help of the team members. The prime purpose of at least the first follow-up session should be to monitor the patients' progress in achieving their goals, identifying any problems and helping the patients to plan how to overcome these and set their targets for the future.

Despite warning patients that they will come across problems when they are at home, setbacks often come as a shock and can be very demoralising. Many patients leave the programme on a 'high', often buoyed up by the support of the group, thinking that they have got on top of their problems. They expect to make continuous improvement and do not anticipate any setbacks. Setbacks should be regarded as normal, however. The patients must be encouraged to learn from their experience, identify specifically what went wrong and why. They should then plan how they will manage such problems in the future and anticipate what other problems may occur.

Trouble shooting

'Trouble shooting' is often done in a group setting. This enables other members of the group to offer a different perspective on problems identified. It will demonstrate that setbacks are common and group members may well come up with the solution to the problem. This is an essential part of the programme and can be done only after the patients have had a chance to practise their skills on their own at home. It is the only way of assessing how much patients have learnt and is an integral part of the learning process on the programme.

Auditing outcome

Follow-up sessions present an opportunity to measure outcome. This may be done formally by asking patients to fill out questionnaires that they will have completed prior to starting the programme. Patients may be asked to keep medication diaries for the week prior to follow-up sessions and comparisons may be made with preprogramme measures and with the patients' declared goals. Finally physical measures may be performed (e.g. timed walk) to indicate performance of specific tasks. Such data is vital to audit not only the performance of individual patients but also the efficacy of the programme as a whole. Changes in outcome may then be investigated to determine whether there have been changes in case mix, programme content, programme delivery or clinical decision making.

Auditing the programme

Whereas auditing outcome is vital to maintaining standards the content and style of delivery should also be audited. Patients should be encouraged to give constructive criticisms of both some time after the programme. This may be done anonymously by questionnaire. The team may also identify specific problems arising after programmes at the follow-up sessions that can alert them to specific weaknesses in either content or delivery. Thus follow-up sessions should include time for team debriefing in order to audit the session and the programme. Changes can then be made and the effect monitored in successive programmes.

Frequency and timing of follow-ups

There is no absolute rule. Clearly it is not possible nor desirable to follow up groups indefinitely. It would seem to be counter to the ethos of the programme of teaching patients to become less dependent upon others to manage their pain and other associated problems.

Some form of patient contact is vital at about a month after the programme. This is when problems are likely to emerge and leaving these for too long can be counterproductive. It enables the patients enough time to test out their skills, identify problems and weaknesses and get help within a reasonable time. There are no scientific data to support this view, but our experience has shown that leaving the first follow-up for too long can lead to patients failing and becoming demoralised or catastrophising. It is then much harder to help them regain control.

At the time of writing follow-up sessions are arranged at 1 month, 3 months and at 6 months at Salford. This is partly for pragmatic reasons. All the follow-up sessions are regarded as an integral part of the programme. Patients are asked to commit themselves to coming to all the follow-up sessions at the beginning of the programme.

Attendance at the 1 month follow-up is usually good. This is not too far away from the programme itself and the patients regard it as simply another session. The number of drop-outs from the programme increases at the 3- and 6-month follow-ups.

Content and organisation of follow-ups

All follow-up session times and dates are given to patients when they accept the invitation to treatment. The patient is asked specifically to agree to come to all the sessions of the programme, the preprogramme assessment and all of the follow-up sessions.

The follow-up sessions should be staffed by the same team members as the programme itself. There are occasions when this is not possible (e.g. sickness or holidays). There must be at least one member of the original team at these sessions. It is not appropriate to have an entirely different set of staff. The group will have developed good rapport with the staff and this cannot be established quickly at a single session.

One-month follow-up

The 1-month session should follow a similar pattern to sessions on the programme itself (Fig. 14.2). All of the team members should be involved. The purpose will be to monitor progress and to ask for feedback from the

9.00–10.30	Introduction and problem-solving review (psychologist + physiotherapist)
10.30–11.00	Break
11.00–11.30	Problem-solving review (cont/d) (psychologist + physiotherapist)
11.30–12.30	Relaxation (psychologist)
12.30–1.30	Lunch
1.30–3.00	Medical issues (doctor)
3.00–3.30	Break
3.30–5.00	Exercise and goal setting Speed walk (physiotherapist)

Figure 14.2 Timetable for 1-month review group.

patients regarding any specific problems they have had.

The doctor may have to reassure some of the patients if they have concerns about the cause of any increase in pain or any new symptoms that may have emerged. It is important not to be dismissive but take such problems seriously. On occasions it may be necessary to re-evaluate patients (including re-examination) in order to reassure them and be very positive in reinforcing the notion that in their case hurt does not mean harm. The doctor should review the patients' progress with medication reduction and encourage them to continue towards their goal of drug reduction.

Occasionally patients may have experienced problems with the health-care system. The doctor should reinforce the patients' avoidance of further assessments, treatments and emergency use of the health-care system unless there is clear indication to do so. For example, it is appropriate to consult their GP if a new pain or symptom emerges, but further consultations because they have had a exacerbation of their usual pain not only will not be helpful, but may lead them into further and repeated assessments and unhelpful treatments.

Both the physiotherapist and the psychologist should run very similar sessions. They should assess progress so far (as a group) highlighting the positive and allowing the other members of the group to offer solutions to problems that patients may bring up. Essentially the session is one of reinforcing patients' problem-solving skills, and helping them to set their goals for the next 3 months. In addition the psychologist should revise relaxation skills with the group and the physiotherapist will revisit specific and general exercises. Finally the opportunity should be taken to perform some physical measures of performance, for example the speed walk, to provide some outcome data.

Subsequent follow-ups

The follow-up sessions at 3 and 6 months should allow a gradual change of emphasis (Fig. 14.3). There should be a gradual reduction in the

9.00–10.30	Introduction and problem-solving review (physiotherapist + psychologist)
10.30–11.00	Break
11.00–11.30	Problem solving review/physio review (cont/d) (physiotherapist + psychologist)
11.30–12.30	Relaxation (psychologist)

Figure 14.3 Three-month booster session timetable.

medical input as the programme itself progresses and likewise with the follow-up sessions. Therefore by the 3-month follow-up the sessions should include only the physiotherapist and psychologist. The aim of the sessions at this stage is to facilitate the patient's self-management. The above table shows the outline of a 3-month booster. As can be seen the time allocated is reduced to half a day and emphasis should be placed on maintenance of change and long term goals.

The 6-month follow-up should include specific time for patients to complete questionnaires and other tests to allow audit of outcome. By emphasising the importance of outcome data patients are usually compliant in attendance and cooperation.

MANAGEMENT OF 'CRIES FOR HELP'

Cries for help immediately after the programme are not common. They usually indicate that the patient has panicked or catastrophised following a flare-up. Although it is important to encourage patients to take responsibility for their own pain and related problems it is better that they be allowed access to the team rather than risk being lost in the health-care system. Most patients are aware that following the programme they should take control of their pain and associated problems. A small number lack confidence in doing so. Problems that do arise can usually be managed by advice given over the telephone. Rarely the patient may need to attend the centre for a physical check to ensure that a 'new' problem has not arisen.

Most centres will not have resources to allow continuous unlimited follow-up. Allowing such access would eventually flood the centre with follow-up patients and no time could be given to new patients. Patients often do not understand this. The patients must, therefore, learn to manage their problems in the future without continuous reference to the staff at the centre. Limited access should be allowed as the dangers of unhelpful treatment or management (as has usually happened in the past) is very likely. Both the patient and the GP should therefore at least seek advice from the centre if there are clear problems that the patient is not managing well.

The commonest reason for problems arising is the failure of patients to maintain the skills and techniques they have learned on the programme. This is more likely to be the cause with patients who develop problems some time after the end of the programme (e.g. 1 to 2 years later). Occasionally such patients may return to the centre via other departments to whom they have been referred. An example is given in Case study 14.2.

It can be seen from this actual case that the patient ultimately was rescued by good fortune. Patients and their GPs should be encouraged to seek advice from the centre before being referred back into the health-care system. The GPs should be encouraged to check that the patient has been able to continue with all of the advice from the centre before referring elsewhere.

POSTPROGRAMME SUPPORT GROUPS

There is little evidence in the literature to support the efficacy of postprogramme support groups in helping patients to maintain progress (Linton, Hellsing & Larson 1997). Commonly patients who have benefited from the social contact wish to continue after the programme. Patients who have been able to incorporate the skills learned on the programme in their normal life usually do not wish to be involved in such groups. Many self-help groups tend to be attended by those patients who have made the least progress in changing lifestyle. They are at risk of focusing on

---

Case study 14.2   A rereferral to a pain centre

Mrs W. had been referred to the pain centre by the department of rheumatology for a lumbar sympathetic block. She had a long history of back pain and continuing sciatica which had not been helped by decompressive surgery some 8 years previously. A diagnosis of neurogenic pain had been made and it was felt that a sympathectomy should be attempted. Rather than simply act as technicians and perform the block without further evaluation the pain centre decided to review the patient.

At interview it became apparent that the leg pain was not of major importance to the patient but that her back pain was the major problem. She had become very disabled and despondent. On further questioning and introduction to the potential for self-management (pain management techniques) Mrs W. revealed she had been on a pain management programme elsewhere and had benefited greatly from it, but now did not have the control she had had.

Following the 'apparent' failure of these techniques her GP had referred her to a number of other specialists who had instituted further investigations and repeated treatments to no effect. In desperation she had been referred to a department of rheumatology at a teaching hospital that was linked informally to a pain management programme.

Only when referred to the pain centre did it emerge that she had attended and made good initial progress on a pain management programme. She explained that she lived in an isolated village and had not managed to remain in contact with other members of her group nor had she been able to motivate herself to keep up with her exercises and relaxation. When it was put to her that she might benefit from returning to the original programme for a booster and to institute workable plans for managing at home she was anxious to take up the offer.

She was duly seen by the original pain management team, included on a booster programme and made good progress.

---

pain and mutual support in their invalidity and failing to address the need to focus upon return to useful activity.

Not all support groups are unhelpful. Some are well focused on helping their members keep out the health-care system and are truly focused on maintenance of change. It has to be said that such successful groups are not common. They require a dynamic person with substantial time and energy to lead them. Burnout among the leaders is common as some group members make unrealistic demands upon the leaders.

Any formal arrangements with such groups should be taken on only with considerable care. The groups should be independent. Support in the way of occasional talks to encourage members to keep active and reinforce self-reliance is wise. Any further participation is likely to be counterproductive. A number of self-help groups have arisen at Salford. Most have not lasted very long and only a few seemed to be firmly focused on helpful activities.

Finally, there is a danger that support groups may be used as a 'dumping ground' for patients who have either failed on the programme or are not suitable. This is unreasonable, as the members of the group will potentially be faced with patients who are least likely to benefit from

any encouragement to change their lifestyle. Such groups may ultimately become a 'mutual moaning society', of little value to the members or the centre.

Not all support groups are so disastrous. Some provide good emotional and physical support for patients with long term pain and disability. Support must be given to the leaders of such groups in order to prevent burnout and help maintain a group that is of significant help to the centre.

ACCESSING RETURN TO WORK

Return to work as an outcome measure has been suggested by many as the true measure of successful pain management. Despite this there are very few studies that demonstrate that pain management programmes assist people in returning to work. This may be because those attending pain management, in some centres at least, are so disabled and deconditioned that return to work is not an achievable goal. Others may contend that return to work should be the focus of pain management only where patients identify it as one of their own desired goals.

It is an often repeated statistic that those not working because of low back pain for 2 years have, statistically, no chance of returning to work

(Waddell 1998). This apparently gloomy statistic must be taken in a broader context. Statistically, anyone out of work for 2 years for whatever reason has a very low likelihood of regaining employment. This group has frequently been referred to the 'hardcore' unemployed by governments. Evidence from a few studies that have looked at the rehabilitation of those with long term work loss due to chronic pain suggests that a return to work is feasible (Jordan, Mayer & Gatchel 1998; Kendall & Thompson 1998; Main & Watson 1995) provided the patient is given the right help and environment.

There is evidence that countries are no longer prepared to support large numbers of people on state benefits of whatever kind. In the UK the government introduced the 'all work test', a medical assessment designed to identify who is fit for work using a series of criteria that are more stringent than previous tests. In addition to this, all people who are not employed are required to attend individual interviews to assist them in returning to work. Continued receipt of the 'Job Seekers' Allowance' benefit is contingent on attendance at these interviews. This includes those who have recently been denied incapacity benefits following the all work test. There are no accurate figure for the number of people who are not working because of a chronic pain problem. Those with chronic pain may be in receipt of unemployment-related benefits rather than sickness or incapacity benefits and therefore will not appear in the official figures for benefits associated with incapacity to work.

Barriers to return to work

There are five distinct but connected problems in assisting people make the transition from benefits to work; these are:

- overcoming psychological dysfunction that accompanies chronic pain
- improving functional limitation due to physical deconditioning
- access to training for developing the skills to facilitate return to work
- access to employment
- retention in sustainable employment.

Resources

In a study for the North-West Disability Services in 1994 Burns et al found that chronic low back pain was the single biggest cause of referral to local disability employment advisers (DEAs). Despite this there was no programme available (such as was available for people with some other specific disabilities) to assist these people back into work. This is still the case in most parts of the UK. Local health-care based rehabilitation services are not able to offer the specialist rehabilitation and vocational advice required by those wishing to return to work. Until a coordinated programme linking health-care rehabilitation services, vocational guidance and retraining programmes is developed, pain management programmes will have to work with the services that are available locally.

Contact with employers

Continued contact with the employer is the most influential predictor of re-employment. Those who remain in employment and are still 'on the books' or who remain in contact with their previous employer are much more likely to regain employment even after a long absence from work. There will be many people attending pain management who have not worked for long periods and have lost contact with the employment market.

Physical function

The role of physical function testing in predicting success in return to work and in specifying which occupations are most appropriate for individuals has had mixed results. Consequently its additional value over and above routine clinical and physical assessment in assisting vocational decision making is currently unclear and it is unlikely to assist most centres. Counselling about the type of work that is inappropriate to the individual's condition may be required. Patients who have had extensive surgery or have significant physical limitations, or both, may not be able to return to physically demanding occupations and a change of career may be indicated. However clinicians must be sensitive to the employment prospects of the patients concerned when making suggestions about changes in career. A person who has worked as a labourer in the building trade for most of his life, and who has few transferable skills, is unlikely to be able to access other employment easily.

Practical barriers

The common, practical barriers to return to work identified by patients (Goldsmith & Mills 1998) are:

- outdated skills or requirement for new and different skills
- lack of experience in job interviews
- uncertainty about changes to benefits on commencing employment
- lack of recent employment history
- employer prejudice and assumption of poor work record
- availability of suitable employment.

In the UK DEAs can be accessed through most government agency job centres. Their role is to give help and guidance to people with disabilities to access employment and retraining opportunities. Those who have been out of work for a long period of time may often feel that they do not have skills that will enable them to return to work. In the modern employment market skills can become outdated very quickly. Skills required by employers are greater than those associated with a specific occupational skill. During their time out of work patients may have developed other skills, however, such as running support groups or fund raising. They may also have been caring for children or relatives. These skills should be identified and incorporated into the individuals' CV of skills.

Employers

Employers are often reluctant to take on people who have no recent employment record. They feel people who have been out of the employment market are an unknown quantity. Participation in training, education or work experience, especially if the hours of attendance are comparable to working hours, can be used as evidence of the patient's ability to perform an occupation.

For this reason engaging in an educational programme or retraining is a useful initial step towards employment. The employer must be convinced that the patient is capable of returning to normal working practices, which includes good time keeping, punctuality and an ability to commit to a regular working schedule. The Salford pain management programme is deliberately run from 9.00 a.m. to 5.00 p.m. each day to simulate a full working day and all patients are required to sign a consent form confirming that they will adhere to the requirements of good punctuality and full attendance.

Preparation for return to work

Positive steps towards employment, which could be made during the pain management process, are:

- identification of personal gains and barriers to work
- identification of possible work opportunities
- interview skills and techniques
- positive disclosure of health problems
- learning from interview experiences.

Some people may have become so isolated from the work environment that they no longer see themselves as potential employees. Helping the patient to identify the positive aspects of returning to work may help to motivate them to start setting goals towards this eventual aim. Few people on incapacity benefits and disability are likely to be financially better off on these benefits than they would be if they were able to gain employment. The patient may not see the risks of trying to regain employment (fear of reinjury, fear of rejection) as worth the increase in income, especially if the increase is modest. Helping them view work in a broader context of increased social contacts, reduction of social isolation and a sense of achievement and increased self-esteem may be sufficiently motivating to some individuals.

The job market

Increased volatility in the employment market may mean that patients' previous occupations no longer exists in the vicinity and they must look towards alternatives. This requires that people identify the transferable skills that they have (those skills that may be relevant to other occupations) and review the local employment opportunities regularly to see which skills are most commonly required in their areas. This will also help them to identify training needs.

It could well have been a long time since these patients attended a job interview and they will need coaching in how to present themselves positively in an interview situation. In some cases specific interpersonal skills training is required through practice and role play. Return to work is unlikely to be smooth; setbacks and rejections are inevitable. This needs to be discussed beforehand and people need to develop strategies to cope with rejection. Discussing the interview or application following a rejection can help put it into perspective and can be an important learning experience.

Convincing the potential employer

At an occupational interview, or in the process of applying for employment, people with chronic pain will inevitably be asked about their health. Attempting to mislead the employer may have serious consequences in the future and a policy of honesty is recommended. People must be clear about their previous health record when asked but should not give an overly negative impres-sion of their condition. They should focus on their current activity levels and achievements rather than their previous level of incapacity, telling the prospective employer what they can do and how they get around things they find difficult if asked. Role play is a useful tool; the patients play the interviewer and the intervie-wee. During this they can identify positive and negative statements about health and try to give a more positive view of their current function and abilities.

The return to work is complex and depends on many factors outside the patients' and the clinician's control.

CONCLUSION

Pain management should be regarded as a process rather than a single event. The patients, their partners and the treating team should be focused on the maintenance of change after the group programme has finished. Patients should be made aware of their commitment to all of the follow-up sessions prior to commencing the group programme. From the very beginning of the programme the patients must commit to planning short, middle and long term goals. They must, with the help of the team, identify the barriers to continued progress and plan in detail how they will address them. Others, including their partners, (potential) employers and GPs, will need to be recruited to assist.

KEY POINTS

- Relapse prevention and management should be addressed both on the pain management programme and at subsequent follow-up sessions.
- Specific advice with regard to both prevention and management of relapse should be given to patients, their families and their GPs.
- Advice should include specific details of the planned management of any 'flare-ups'.

- Follow-up sessions should be regarded as an integral part of the pain management programme.
- Follow-up sessions should be focused on maintenance of skills and 'trouble shooting', and include audit measures.
- Adopt specific plans to manage 'cries for help'.
- Offer support for those who wish to return to work.

REFERENCES

Bradley L A 1996 Cognitive–behavioural therapy for chronic pain. In: Gatchel R J, Turk D C (eds) Psychological approaches to pain management: a practitioners handbook. Guilford Press, New York, ch 6, pp. 131–147

Bradley L A, Young L D, Anderson K O et al 1987 Effects of psychological therapy on pain behavior of rheumatoid arthritis patients: treatment outcome and six-month follow-up. Arthritis and Rheumatism 30:1105–1114

Burns A, Main C J, Ratcliffe M, Watson P J 1994 From back pain to employment. Employment Services Publications, Department of Employment, London

Goldsmith C, Mills B 1998 Evaluation of a prevocational programme for ex-incapacity benefits clients. Employment Services Publications, Manchester UK

Jordan K D, Mayer T G, Gatchel R J 1998 Should extended disability be an exclusion criterion for tertiary rehabilitation? Socioeconomic outcomes of early versus late functional restoration in compensation spinal disorders. Spine 23(19):2111–2116

Keefe F J, van Horn Y 1993 Cognitive–behavioral treatment of rheumatoid arthritis pain: maintaining treatment gains. Arthritis Care and Research 6:213–222

Kendall N A S, Thompson B F 1998 A pilot program for dealing with the co-morbidity of chronic pain and long-term unemployment. Journal of Occupational Rehabilitation 5–26

Linton S J, Hellsing A L, Larson I 1997 Bridging the gap: support groups do not enhance long-term outcome in chronic back pain. Clinical Journal of Pain 13(3):221–222

Main C J, Watson P J 1995 Screening for patients at risk of developing chronic incapacity. Journal of Occupational Rehabilitation 5:207–217

Marlatt G A, Gordon J R 1995 (eds) Relapse prevention. Guilford New York

Waddell G 1998 The back pain revolution. Churchill Livingstone, New York p 111

Issues in delivery and evaluation

SECTION CONTENTS

In this section of the book three critical aspects of pain management are addressed if a pain programme is to be established and maintained. In Chapter 15, clinical service delivery is addressed from the strategic point of view. It is necessary to identify and develop the necessary patient pathways needed to meet the clinical needs of the patients, and also the requirements of the other key 'stakeholders' such as family members, employers or purchasers of heath care. In Chapter 16, competencies in delivery of pain management is addressed in terms of the skills needed for key staff to deliver a pain programme. (The issue of competencies is currently a matter of much debate among the professions involved in pain management and so our recommendations should be regarded as suggestive rather than definitive.) Finally in Chapter 17 the important issue of outcome evaluation is addressed from both a clinical and a methodological perspective.

15

Clinical service delivery (the organisation of the pain management programme)

Chris C. Spanswick   Helen Parker

INTRODUCTION

The purpose of this chapter is first, to outline how to go about describing the service in detail to facilitate discussions with managers aimed at either establishing or expanding a pain management programme and, secondly, how to build and maintain an interdisciplinary team.

Delivering the clinical service requires substantial input from all of the team members. It will require as much energy to maintain the service as it does to build and develop a service in the first place. The importance of team building and team maintenance cannot be overemphasised. No one person will have skills in all of the areas necessary to keep the clinical service functioning. It is essential that team members be chosen to fulfil specific roles within the team and subscribe to the central philosophy and goals of the team.

It is important that the clinical team members should be allowed to concentrate on clinical activity without distraction. That is not to say that they should not be involved in any administrative work or managerial duties. However, the day-to-day running of the clinical activity must be well organised so that the clinical team members can perform efficiently, effectively and to their best ability. A well-organised clinical system must therefore be in place.

Most pain management programmes are started by enthusiasts in their own spare time using any resources they can find at the time. Clinics and programmes often end up being run on an ad hoc basis with little or no administrative support. If a reasonable level of service is to be provided then adequate time, personnel and financial resources must be made available for the efficient and effective running of the service. The very nature of the patient population or case mix demands the focused and undistracted attention of the clinical staff. Such patients have often been through multiple ineffective and inefficient health-care provision. They frequently become angry and sensitised to further mistakes (either administrative or clinical). It is vital therefore that the administrative part of the system runs smoothly and is able to respond rapidly to any errors that occur.

This chapter describes the important stages in setting up a service and offers some guidance as to how the service may be organised and financed.

KEY PLAYERS

Key players include:

- referring agents e.g. GPs, specialists
- managers of the hospital unit
- purchasers of health care e.g. insurers, health authorities (UK).

There are three main groups of people that have to be convinced of the worth of the pain management programme if it is to have any chance of long term survival. These include the potential clinical colleagues who will refer to the programme, including both GPs and specialists; the managers in the hospital/unit in which the programme will be located and, finally, the purchasers or insurers who will be paying for the treatment. Further groups may emerge as the pain programme becomes more established and demonstrates its clinical effectiveness. These include patient support groups. They are usually concerned with specific problems—for example, back pain, complex regional pain syndromes, etc.

Referring agents

Most clinicians can readily identify a group of patients in their practice in whom they perceive

that the organic features do not explain the whole of the patient's complaints. They often appreciate that psychological factors play an important part. However, they also frequently recognise that they do not have the skills, time or the resources to assess such patients in detail, nor are they able to offer helpful treatment. Most clinicians, either GPs or specialists, find this group of patients difficult to deal with. The patients tend to return repeatedly to their clinics dissatisfied with their treatment, still with substantial pain and disability, often distressed, demanding and occasionally angry. In such circumstances clinicians are usually only too willing to hand their care over to another service, especially if that service is offering treatment for such patients.

Giving clear guidance on how to identify suitable patients for pain management will ensure that the programme does not become a dumping ground for *all* 'difficult' patients. Agreeing on referral criteria and methods of identifying suitable patients will not only protect the pain management programme from inappropriate referrals but will provide a 'link' between the programme and other services providing a more efficient system and one in which the referral agent feels at least part ownership. It is important to have explicit agreed referral criteria so that the occasional inappropriate referral may be returned without the risk of destroying clinical cooperation.

The potential referring agents should be made aware of the aims and outcome of the pain management programme. This will enable the patients to be counselled appropriately (over-selling the programme is common) as well as ensuring that the referring agent also has realistic expectations. In some units (hospitals) the setting up of a pain management programme may result in removal of resources from one department to another, or be possible only if this happens. This can be threatening to some other departments unless they can see some benefit to themselves. It is therefore important to portray the programme as an extension of good clinical practice, which will not only provide help for the difficult patient but also the beleaguered referring agent. Demonstrating the potential benefits to the referring agents will help gain their support. These benefits will, of course, include not only providing more appropriate help for the patients but may also free up more time for referring agents enabling them to spend more time on patients they *can* help. It is essential to have substantial clinical support before attempting to persuade the local hospital management.

Hospital/unit management

Local hospital managers are unlikely to have come across pain management programmes before and are unlikely to know the aims, objectives and outcome of a programme. Time must be spent in persuading local management and ultimately the purchasers of health care to invest in the clinical service. There will already be an established pattern of health-care purchase and the managers of both the hospital and the purchasers will have to be convinced to direct financial resources to a new service. It may well mean moving financial and other resources from other areas in order to invest in pain management. The arguments must, therefore, be well prepared and convincing. It will be necessary to spend time in preparing and presenting information to the managers as well as the clinicians within the hospital. It is of particular importance to liaise with other clinical teams, especially those who are likely to refer patients or to whom the pain management service itself may refer. Managers are more likely to take notice of other clinicians pressurising for the establishment of a service. Without both clinical and managerial support it will not be possible to convince purchasers to invest in the service. Once the local managers have been convinced, they will be a useful ally in convincing the purchasers.

The purchasers

Although the systems of funding of health-care delivery may vary from country to country many involve an organisation that is responsible for finance. In the UK 'purchasing authorities' are responsible for purchasing health care on behalf of the local population, although at the time of writing this is soon to change. In other countries (e.g. USA, New Zealand, Germany) the cost of health care is provided by insurance companies who 'purchase' health care for the patient. Claims are usually made at the time of use, although insurance companies may well not cover all treatment. Some treatments may not be covered at all and some may only be partially funded.

The purchasers (insurers) should not be approached until the local clinicians and managers have been convinced and are signed up to the development of the centre. The local managers will give guidance on how to approach the purchasers (insurers) and what will stimulate their interest. It is not adequate just to say that the service is needed. It has to fit in with the purchaser's (insurer's) priorities and the case will have to be argued financially as well as clinically. The purchasers (insurers) will require hard clinical outcome data and a business plan. The business plan will have to detail the costs of the service including the costs of the individual components. Justification for each part of the service will have to be made both clinically and financially.

The development of the new service will have to be shown to link well with current services (e.g. links with orthopaedics or spinal services) and address other areas (e.g. the community) for which the purchasers are responsible. The purchaser (insurers) will require the proposed service to demonstrate control over referral as well as efficacy. They will be anxious that any money allocated is used explicitly for the appropriate patient group and that it is not wasted on groups of patients who will not benefit from the proposed treatment. Key points in the development are listed in Box 15.1.

ASSEMBLING THE ARGUMENTS

The service must have clear and explicit plans regarding what care it will deliver, how it will be delivered and how the efficiency and effectiveness will be monitored. Audit and the measurement of

---

Box 15.1 Key points in the service development

- Assembling the arguments:
  — description of case mix, assessment process and treatment options
  — expected outcomes and their measurement
  — supporting literature
  — clinical pathways
  — administrative needs
  — links with other services
- Convincing colleagues
- Meeting with management
- The purchasers agenda
- The team approach:
  — team building
  — team maintenance
- Potential for development

---

outcome are (Ch. 17) in vogue at the time of writing. However, outcome measures are of little value unless there is an adequate description of the starting point. There is otherwise a danger that the pain management service may be inappropriately compared with other services that treat much simpler cases (back schools or back education classes aimed at patients with acute back pain).

Case mix

A careful description of the case mix is vital. Most administrators and managers in the health-care system have little understanding of the types of patient seen in pain clinics or in pain management programmes. They are likely to equate the service to other medical specialist clinics (e.g. orthopaedic spinal clinics, headache clinics). It is important to emphasise the complex nature of the patients' problems, both in terms of medical aspects and with regard to physical functioning and psychological status. A description of one or two 'typical cases' outlining the length of the clinical problem and the repeated referral from specialist to specialist will help give an indication of the costs to the system and the potential costs to the patient (both financial and emotional). The prime purpose of such information is to give administrators/managers an understanding that such patients simply cannot be assessed quickly, given a simple treatment and then discharged.

A case mix example is as follows:

- patients with chronic low back pain (history greater than 6 months):
  — average length of history 10 years
  — ranges from 12 months to 30 years
- complex medical problems:
  — 30% of patients have had previous spinal surgery
  — 55% have seen two or more previous specialists
- significant psychological distress:
  — measures of distress show that 70% of patients are very distressed
  — less than 5% of patients in an average orthopaedic clinic fall into this group
- high medication use:
  — 20% of patients are using medication in excess of the recommended dose
  — no demonstrable effect despite high levels of medication use
- poor level of functioning:
  — high scores on disability measures (compared with other clinics)
- employment status:
  — high level of unemployment
  — employment status related to pain complaints.

The above information outlines the nature of patients attending the centre at Salford. These represent only a small proportion attending an average orthopaedic out-patient clinic. However, they consume much more in the way of resources (Watson et al 1998). The case mix in smaller pain clinics in the UK is little different. The larger centres tend to attract a higher proportion of distressed patients, but nevertheless smaller clinics still have a significant proportion of distressed patients.

The managers will wish to know what resources, if any, are currently available for the management of this group of patients and how effectively those resources are being used. They need to be given an understanding of what happens to such patients if they are not treated in the way that is envisaged. This should include both the clinical implications and the financial implications for the health-care system.

Having made the clinical case for the service the next step is to negotiate adequate resources. These should include clinical, administrative and physical resources (i.e. space, equipment, etc.). Care should be taken with this. An inadequate level of administrative support is common and can lead to additional stress on staff who are delivering the clinical care. A careful list should be made of staff, space and equipment that are required. This will need to be in some detail and arguments may well be required for each component. Needs should not be understated. It should also be remembered that teamwork is vulnerable to one person being away. In practice this means that work load should be planned on the basis of 40 weeks per year. (Normally calculations are made on the basis of 46 weeks per year.)

The list of space requirements in Box 15.2 is neither exhaustive nor necessarily appropriate for smaller programmes. It is intended as an aide mémoire. Access to most of the items should be available and if a separate unit is envisaged then it should at least include them.

Finally, it is rare that finances permit unlimited resources. An assessment of other available resources should be made. Linking with other relevant services (e.g. spinal services or rheumatology) may allow sharing of some. In addition it may enhance links and working with other departments.

Points for managers to attend to are listed in Box 15.3.

The evaluation system

The nature of the case mix should lead logically to the type, style and delivery of the assessment process. It should be assumed that both other clinicians and in particular managers have little or no background information. The assessment process should be explained in detail and cogent arguments for each component of the process must be given. This should include justification of the need for the depth and breadth of the interdisciplinary evaluation, and its relationship to the clinical decision-making process. Making use of the case examples, emphasis should be made on the complex nature of the patient's medical

---

> **Box 15.2** Space requirements
>
> - Adequate number of rooms for assessment process including large room for feedback to patients and their partners
> - Dedicated rooms for individual treatments
> - Dedicated large room for the programme
> - Day room for patients, including tea/coffee-making facilities
> - Changing and shower rooms for patients
> - Toilet facilities for patients
> - Waiting area
> - Adequate number of rooms for secretarial and administrative staff
> - Offices for team members
> - Meetings/seminar room for team
> - Staff room
> - Changing and shower rooms for staff
> - Toilet facilities for staff
> - Quiet/study room with library facilities

> **Box 15.3** Points for managers
>
> - Identify patient population to be assessed/treated (case mix)
> - Describe case mix (complexity of medical and psychological problems)
> - Explain need for careful, broad-based assessment
> - List resources required
> - List resources currently available
> - Outline clinical and financial consequences of *not* setting up a pain management programme

---

problems and the effects of this upon the patient's level of physical functioning and psychological status. A careful description of the interaction between the different factors will help reinforce the importance of the broad-based assessment and the need for interdisciplinary treatment.

The nature of the assessment clinics and the programme is so unlike any other hospital-based service that managers may have some difficulty in understanding the complexity of these patients' problems. Inviting the relevant manager to observe clinics and parts of the programme directly can often be helpful. Only then will they gain an understanding of the nature of the problems the patients present with and the need for careful assessment. It will

---

Box 15.4 Points of emphasis for managers

- Complex nature of the patient's pain and associated problems
- Need for availability of other information (scans, etc.)
- Time essential for good communications with patient
- Management of patient's pain and associated problems *begin* at the first point of contact
- Need for interdisciplinary assessment (especially psychological and physical function assessment)
- Need for individual treatment/management prior to inclusion in a pain management programme
- Significant proportion of patients are not willing/appropriate for pain management programme

---

Box 15.5 Examples of treatments offered

- Out-patient pain management programme (20 sessions spread over 6 weeks)
- Individual physiotherapy preprogramme
- Individual psychology intervention preprogramme
- Medical follow-up to manage medication problems and address other medical issues
- Follow-up programme (1 day) at 3 months and 6 months
- Joint clinics to address specific patient problems

---

become apparent that a significant amount of information from other sources is required (e.g. notes from other hospitals, previous X-rays and scans, etc.) in order to complete the assessment. In addition it should also become clear that the treatment and management of the patient begin during the assessment process itself.

In principle the administrative, management and economic arrangements should follow best clinical practice rather than vice versa. It is only by carefully outlining the details of the assessment and treatment process that the argument may be won. Points that require emphasis are listed in Box 15.4.

Treatments to be offered

Interdisciplinary pain management does not consist of a pain management programme alone. Few patients are suitable for immediate inclusion in a programme. Most patients will need some individual treatment or management prior to the programme even if only to complete the evaluation and prepare or persuade some patients. At the Salford centre less than 25% of new referrals take up a place on a programme. Most of the remainder are offered some form of individual pain management. This is usually taken on by one of the team members as the lead clinician, but frequently additional support is needed from one or more other members of the team. Individual treatment/management is time consuming and specific protected clinical time must be allocated to this. There is great temptation for team

members to perform such treatment in 'flexible' time. Such work should be scheduled and audited to evaluate the service and protect the individual professional. Some example treatments are listed in Box 15.5.

Having described the potential patient population one should plan carefully what treatments are to be offered (Ch. 13). It is essential to be explicit about inclusion and exclusion criteria and what rules are to be used in clinical decision making (Ch. 12), and not to be over-optimistic about outcome. It is also necessary to ensure that there are clear links with other relevant services and that these links have been agreed with those departments. These might, for example, include orthopaedic surgery, physiotherapy and clinical psychology. An explanation should be given of how the treatments offered differ from those provided in such departments, as should a rationale, and details of how the new service will link with these other departments.

It should not be assumed that others have an understanding about pain management programmes. Most other medically trained people and other health-care professionals have little idea about the philosophy and nature of pain management. Managers are even less likely to have any knowledge. They may have even been sensitised against pain management by other health-care professionals' misunderstandings. A careful detailed plan of the treatment process should be made (Ch. 12), with an explanation of the reasons for each part. It is worthwhile including some references to relevant papers in support (see Further reading, p. 356).

Publicity

The profile of the pain management programme within the hospital is important. Clinical case presentations at postgraduate meetings are a useful forum to increase the profile of the programme. This gives an opportunity to publicise the service as well as the inclusion/exclusion criteria for the programme, thus giving other clinicians guidelines on who to refer, who *not* to refer and how to refer. The managers within the hospital will naturally take advice from others within the hospital. Time invested in convincing colleagues of the worthwhile nature of the pain management programme is well spent.

Expected outcomes

Hard outcome data will be required. At the time of writing, evidenced-based medicine is in vogue. It will be necessary to outline specific anticipated outcomes of treatment. There is a major potential for misunderstanding as other clinicians (including the patient's GP), managers and purchasers may have different expectations of the programme (e.g. pain relief). If there are hard data available then these should be presented. In the absence of this then reference to published studies should be made.

It is worth while explaining the factors that will influence outcome. Some of these are outside the control of the team—for example patient motivation, or concurrent major psychological problems. It may be necessary to emphasise the fact that one of the purposes of the assessment process is to identify such factors. This enables clinical resources to be used more effectively. Perhaps the best model to use in explaining the pain management approach is that of alcohol treatment programmes. In such programmes the outcome is as dependent on the motivation and willingness of the patient as it is on the input from the treating team. Most purchasers seem to understand this model well. This model places significant emphasis on assessment in order to identify those patients who are more likely to

make progress. The purchasers will be seeking reassurance that resources will be used to best effect.

Care should be taken in choosing a range of outcome measures (Ch. 17) to ensure that undue emphasis is not made of any one particular outcome. Generally speaking, neither managers in hospital nor purchasers know what measures should be used. So the pain management service has the opportunity of ensuring appropriate and realistic outcome measures are employed. Measures should not be used if the programme does not address the issue or does not have the resources to influence outcome. For example, return to work should not be used as a measure if there are no links with employers and the local department of employment. It is far better to use measures that reflect the breadth of the assessment and treatment.

Supporting literature

Arguments for resources should be backed up with as much evidence as possible. There are a number of useful references outlining the efficacy of pain management programmes.

These should be used in support of the proposed service and carry significant weight with both hospital managers and purchasers (see Further reading, p. 356).

Clinical pathways

The treatment offered cannot exist in isolation. Managers will want to know how and on what basis patients are to be selected for this treatment and what will happen to those who are deemed unsuitable. They will want to see a method of auditing the process as well as the outcome of treatment. The clinical pathways (see Ch. 13) will help give an indication of what resources will be required and how this service will link with others. This is important in the financial negotiations with managers that inevitably follow. It will not be possible to argue for resources unless there is a clear detailed plan of what is being offered and how the service is to be delivered.

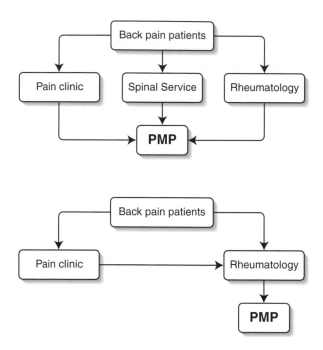

Figure 15.1 Potential relationships with other services.

This will have to include the impact of the service on other departments (e.g. orthopaedic surgery, radiology) (Fig. 15.1).

Differing programmes will have different relationships with other departments. Some programmes, for example, may be linked closely with a pain clinic, whereas others may be linked to an orthopaedic spinal service. Some may be independent of any other clinical services, but work closely with a number of other departments. The exact nature of the relationship and flow of patients should be explained.

Having established the rationale for treatment and the proposed clinical pathways an administrative system that supports the clinical team must be organised. This will have to ensure the smooth running of the assessment clinics, track individual patients through the system to ensure they receive the planned treatment and timetable the running of the programmes. The administrative system should follow the needs of the patient and the team rather than dictate the clinical pathways or treatment. This cannot therefore be planned until after the clinical pathways have

been agreed. There will be constant adjustments to the system as clinical needs are identified and as the pain programme develops.

Figure 15.2 is not exhaustive, but indicates the complexity of the service offered and need for specific administrative support in order to ensure efficient clinical activity. Against each activity an estimate of the amount of time required will have to be made. This will enable a bid to be made for an appropriate amount of administrative support as well as the correct mix of administrative skills.

Clerical and secretarial staff are an important part of the team. If the administrative system does not work well, the clinical team can become paralysed into inactivity. It is often the most ignored part of the process. The clinical team must be able to focus totally upon the patients and its work. It should not become distracted by administrative problems. Care must be taken in describing the administrative needs of the team and the patients in detail so that cogent arguments may be put forward in support of administrative resources.

Clinical pathways   Staff involved

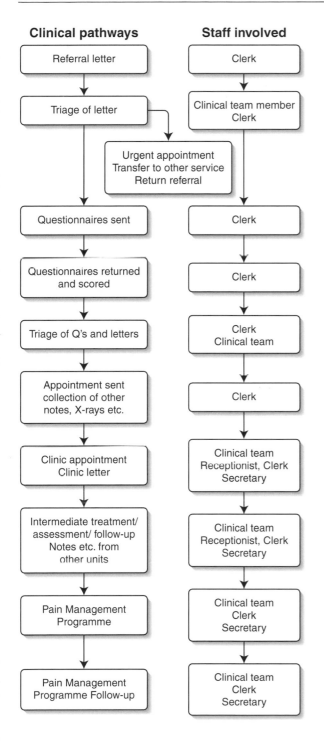

Figure 15.2 Clinical pathways and staff involved.

For example, most patients attending a pain management programme will have been seen by a significant number of other specialists, some of whom will work at other hospitals. It is important to see the notes related to those consultations. This will require a significant amount of administrative time in chasing notes and test results to ensure they are available for the assessment. The level of administrative support is far greater than might be expected for many other clinics.

The administrative system needs to be led by a single person who should be responsible for coordinating all clinical and administrative activity. This person is one of the 'key players' in the running of the service, and should understand the philosophy of the team and be an integrated member of it. In successful departments there is no separation of administrative or managerial members and clinical members of the team. All members of the team must have ownership of the service. There is no room for hidden or other 'agendas'. That is not to say that there should not be robust discussion and constructive argument, but the ultimate goal must a shared one of producing and maintaining the best possible service with an emphasis on quality rather than quantity.

Box 15.6 gives some idea of the complexity of the administration of a pain management

---

Box 15.6   Administrative requirements

- Good communications with patients (phone)
- Assist in triage (collating of notes, referring letter and questionnaires)
- Organising assessment clinics (timetabling team members, ensuring notes/investigations from other hospitals are available)
- Typing of all clinical letters from all team members (clinics, follow-ups, end of programme, etc.)
- Tracking patients' planned treatment, or further assessments and treatments from other departments
- Running waiting list for the pain management programme and intermediate treatments
- Timetabling programme and follow-up sessions
- Liaising with other departments, hospitals and GPs
- Patient literature and teaching materials for the programme
- Collecting and recording audit data
- Preparation of audit and outcome data
- Link with hospital management and purchasers

programme. Both clinicians and managers usually underestimate such requirements. Persons leading this part of the team must be able to use their own initiative and present any problems and potential developments at the team meetings concisely. If the service is to run a significant number of programmes there will be sufficient work for more than one person allocated to administrative and secretarial duties.

Links with other services

Links with other services will vary from centre to centre and will depend to a large extent on what other services are available locally. Most clinical departments can identify patients with chronic pain problems within their own case mix. A substantial proportion of such patients would benefit from pain management techniques.

Links with other services should be cultivated. First, it enables some degree of protection by ensuring a continuous supply of referrals. Secondly, close clinical links will ensure that, largely, only appropriate referrals are made and the centre is not used as a dumping ground. Thirdly, the other departments can become a useful resource for clinical opinions or referring on when necessary.

Links with other services therefore are not a luxury but an essential. Constant contact with other clinical services will facilitate the development of the pain programme. Maintaining links will enable the development of clinical pathways that ensure that patients receive the treatment/management that they need. For example, a clinical pathway for patients with back pain referred to the hospital can be developed ensuring consistent assessment and treatment irrespective of the department to which they were originally referred. There is a danger, otherwise, that the treatment patients receive is dependent upon whom they see or to which service they were initially referred (see Fig. 15.1).

MEETING WITH MANAGEMENT

Once all of the information about the service has been collated then an approach should be made

to the hospital or unit management to state the case for setting up the service. All of the supporting literature should be available together with a plan of how the service will start and how it will develop. It will be necessary to provide for or develop with the managers the costs of establishing the service. The costs of *not* setting up the service should also be outlined.

It will be necessary to convince the hospital (unit) management of the need and the viability of the service before an approach can be made to the purchasers of health care. Provided that the hospital managers have been convinced of the clinical need (Box 15.7) and the viability of the proposed service they will be of invaluable help in preparing the necessary arguments and documentation to present to the purchasers. They may also recommend changes of emphasis to fit in with the prevailing local political climate. With their special knowledge of other local services and local health-care politics they may suggest additional clinical links or sources of money to help set up the service. They may also provide ideas regarding the potential development.

The meeting with the hospital management should not be regarded as a battle, but in essence no different from meetings with clinical colleagues. The aim is to establish a good working relationship, which is mutually beneficial. The clinical and management team must share the same objectives. Only then should an approach be made to the purchasers. This will need to be a joint approach. Just as the lack of support from other clinical teams will lead to failure so lack of local hospital/unit management support for the proposal will inevitably lead to failure.

Box 15.7 What will local managers be looking for?

- Appeal to GPs and purchasers
- Clearly stated health outcome and critical success
- Contribution to avoiding hospital stay
- Cost-effectiveness criteria
- Income generation potential
- Marketing and presentation
- User satisfaction
- Role in a strategy for the care of the chronically ill

Box 15.8 Data for the purchasers

- Clinical need for service
- Case mix
- Referral controls
- Outcome data
- Supporting literature
- Resources and costings
- Cost controls
- Cost of not setting up the service
- Emphasis on links with other services
- Future development
- Relationship of service to the purchasers objectives

Box 15.9 What are the purchasers looking for

- Value for money
- Clearly defined service
- Proven outcome
- Integration with other services (e.g. back pain)
- Links with community
- Case control
- No overall increase in expenditure

THE PURCHASERS' AGENDA

All of the background work must have been completed by the time an approach is made to the purchasers. A joint document (clinical and managerial) outlining all of the relevant data (Box 15.8) should be prepared.

The purchasers will have their own objectives for health care in the locality, which may or may not include pain management. Their objectives are unlikely to specifically include 'pain management' but may include, for example, 'services for back pain'. The presentation will therefore have to be adjusted in such a way as to be seen to address at least some of these objectives. Collaboration with other clinical services is therefore absolutely vital and should be emphasised. The hospital managers should have advised on the type and style of approach as they will be aware of the purchaser's agenda. It will be necessary to check on policy documents that the purchasers have published recently to assist in the preparation of the presentation. This will give an indication of their priorities and will enable the presentation to be aimed (as far as possible) in the right direction.

The purchasers' duty is to provide the best possible health care in a large number of different areas for the least cost. They will have an entirely different perspective on matters (Box 15.9) and may be judging pain management against other totally unrelated needs of the community (e.g. mental health). It is important to point out the costs of *not* funding the proposed service and the potential for reducing ineffectual

and unhelpful other treatments. They may be attracted by early intervention.

They will be anxious to see not only a clinical justification of the service (with explicit support from other departments) but also some mechanism of controlling costs. Emphasis should therefore be made of the assessment system, which will identify the patient group who will benefit from pain management, and the links with referral services to ensure appropriate referrals are made. This will indicate control over referrals and costs of the service.

There has been a move by purchasers recently to cut costs as much as possible. This has on occasions been to the extent of purchasing only parts of pain management. Outcome data are therefore vital. It is important to point out to purchasers that failing to address all of the problems that prevent chronic pain patients from rehabilitating is simply wasteful. There is therefore a minimum level of intervention that is required to produce meaningful changes in patients with chronic pain. Although this may be regarded as a risky argument (the purchasers may decide that no treatment is the cheapest option) it is important to explain that cutting corners is counterproductive. Full justification for each part of the assessment and treatment packages must therefore be provided. A list of important points when dealing with purchasers is given in Box 15.10, and pointers for approaching purchasers in Box 15.11.

THE TEAM APPROACH

Pain management requires a *team approach* to both the assessment and treatment of patients. There are three main types of team: multidisciplinary, transdisciplinary and interdisciplinary.

Box 15.10 Important points when dealing with purchasers

- Emphasise case mix (data)
- Explain model of care
- Be honest about limitations
- Reason each component of service
- Show outcome data

Box 15.11 Approaching the purchasers

- Joint approach with trust management
- Crisp clear presentation
- Good documentation
- Background literature
- Emphasise benefits and costs of not investing
- Agree monitoring and audit

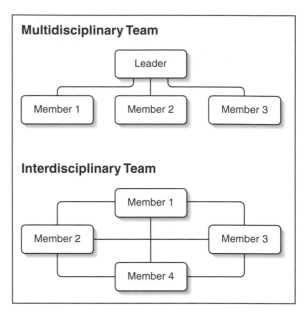

Figure 15.3 Communication within the multi- and interdisciplinary team.

The multidisciplinary team

Melvin (1980) gave the following definition of the multidisciplinary team: 'This refers to activities which involve the efforts of individuals from a number of disciplines. These efforts are disciplinary-orientated and, although they may impinge upon clients or activities dealt with by other disciplines, they approach them primarily through each discipline relating to its own activities' (Melvin 1980, p. 379). As this definition implies, in a multidisciplinary team, that members of each discipline will be working towards their own individual goals for the patient and in general there is little or no overlap between the team members.

Melvin (1980) has pointed out, that when such an approach is used the results achieved for a patient are 'the sum of each different discipline providing its own unique activity'.

Members of multidisciplinary teams tend to work in physically separate departments from each other, communicating more with their own colleagues rather than with other team members. They can function as part of a multidisciplinary team without explicit knowledge of the skills of other disciplines.

In general, multidisciplinary teams are led by a member of the medical profession (usually of consultant level) and team meetings involving the different professionals will, in general, consist of members of the different disciplines making reports to the doctor regarding a patient's progress in their particular therapy. All communication will be channelled through the team leader (Fig. 15.3)

A classic example of the multidisciplinary team meeting is the traditional ward round. Within the team some coordination may be achieved, such as agreement with regard to reduction of medication, but the team's ability to coordinate treatment is otherwise limited. In certain settings the only time members of different disciplines meet will be at team meetings.

The key features of the multidisciplinary team are as follows:

- the team is usually medically led
- communication is directed via the team leader
- individual team members work towards their own individual goals for the patient
- members tend to work in physically separate areas
- an explicit knowledge of the skills of other disciplines is not required.

Problems with the multidisciplinary approach

There are a number of problems with the multidisciplinary approach to the assessment and treatment of pain. The main problems are as follows:

1. Lack of effective communication between disciplines may lead to a lack of awareness of problem areas. For example, the physiotherapist may be unaware that a patient has an alcohol problem.

2. There may be fragmentation of the approach to treatment and assessment, in which the patient is treated as a series of problems rather than holistically. One consequence of this is that the patient then comes to view the different professionals as having clearly defined roles (e.g. the doctor deals with medication, the physiotherapist with exercise and the psychologist with emotional aspects of pain). This in turn will make it difficult for the professionals concerned to give advice or attempt to assess areas that the patient perceives are not within their remit.

3. Duplication of certain parts of the assessment process is common in a multidisciplinary team. For example, all disciplines may obtain details from the patient about duration of pain, length of present episode of pain, medication and previous treatment. Such duplication can lead to two main problems. First, it is time wasting for the professional involved and, secondly, it can lead to patients feeling frustrated or annoyed (or both) that they have to answer the same questions on a number of different occasions within a short space of time.

4. Different management strategies may be employed in dealing with the same problem.

5. Patients and their relatives may receive conflicting information from different disciplines leading to confusion on their part about which approach should be adopted.

6. In certain cases manipulative patients can 'play off' one team member against other members, specifically seeking advice on the same problems from different members and if the advice received is conflicting to confront the professional with this information. The implication obviously is that the professional is incompetent.

7. As a consequence of the restricted communication that occurs within the multidisciplinary team, professionals involved may feel a sense of isolation and lack of support. This is a particular problem if the team is physically separated/or there are no colleagues from your own discipline working in the same area (or both).

The transdisciplinary team

In the transdisciplinary team all borders are broken down between individual professionals and there is a lack of role differentiation.

Diller (1990) gives the following description of the transdisciplinary team: 'In this approach, one member of the team acts as a primary therapist, with the other members feeding information and advice with regard to management through a single primary person' (p. 277). As Diller (1990) notes such an approach is most useful when patients' condition means that they would find it very difficult to tolerate a shift in therapists, for example patients with severe head injury.

The interdisciplinary team

In the interdisciplinary team (Melvin 1980, p. 379):

… individuals not only require the skills of their own disciplines, but also have the added responsibility of the group effort on behalf of the activity or client involved. This effort requires the skills necessary for effective group interaction and the knowledge of how to transfer integrated group activities into a result, which is greater than the simple sum of the activities of each individual discipline. The group activity of an interdisciplinary team is synergistic, producing more than each individually and separately could accomplish.

A further description provided by Diller (1990) indicates that the interdisciplinary approach 'involves timely and anticipatory communications, engaging in interactive problem solving, and ability to translate technologic findings to people who are untrained in the techniques which are used' (p. 277).

Two differing patterns of cooperation within the interdisciplinary team have been described (Finset et al 1995). In the *coordinated interdisciplinary team* mutual goals are set and the individuals from each discipline attempt to work on these goals in their individual sessions. In the *integrated interdisciplinary team* mutual goals are worked on in joint treatment sessions with members of different disciplines participating in the sessions. The treatment could not be carried out by individual members of the team alone. Instead of being medically led the team leader is usually a clinician, experienced in working with pain patients, ideally the leader should also be experienced at working with teams and in resolving the problems that can occur within teams.

The key features of the interdisciplinary team are as follows:

- the team shares common assessment and treatment goals
- the main task of all members of the team is to deliver treatments that are dependent on the patient's needs, not on the constraints of the individual disciplines involved
- unlike multidisciplinary teams, interdisciplinary teams are not necessarily led by a member of the medical profession. They are most likely to be led by an experienced clinician who has knowledge not only of working with patients with chronic pain but also of working in a team
- there are core areas of specialty unique to each discipline but these are secondary to the goals of the team as a whole
- team members will have explicit knowledge of the skills of other disciplines involved in the team.

- communication occurs between all team members (Fig. 15.3)
- all team members have equal status within the team
- decisions are arrived at after considering input from all team members.

A comparison between multidisciplinary and interdisciplinary teams is presented in Table 15.1.

TEAM BUILDING

The philosophy of the team—the policy document

The philosophy of the team should be made explicit to all members and this should be contained within a written policy document (sometimes referred to as a 'mission statement'). This document will also include details relating to the working practices of the team (including sanctions if team members fail to adhere to the team philosophy), the objectives of the team and the roles and responsibilities of each team member (Hastings, Bixby & Chaudry-Lawton 1988). Such a document should be produced by the joint efforts of the team and should not be regarded as being written on tablets of stone as it will most probably be necessary to adjust and adapt the policy over time, especially if membership of the team changes, or there are changes in external conditions (e.g. sources of funding), or both.

Table 15.1 The multi vs. the interdisciplinary team

	Multi	Inter
Leadership	Medical profession	Experienced clinician, leadership may be joint/multi or rotating
Formal communication	Team meeting/ward round; 'report back to leader	Team meeting (clinical and business); exchange of ideas
Informal communication	Infrequent	Frequent
Status of members	Hierarchical	Equal status for all members
Skills knowledge	Limited to own discipline	Extended to other disciplines
Goals	Formulated by individual disciplines	Jointly set by team
Decision making	By leader	By team
Role of patient and family	Passive recipients	Active participants
Outcome of treatment	Equal to sum of individual treatments	Synergistic

Staff training

This is a vital area in the development and growth of a team. Effective training will aid in the development of the team and also will help to foster respect for the skills of other disciplines. Topics of value to cover are:

- processes within groups
- teaching on the core skills required for the team
- education regarding the work of other disciplines.

This teaching can be achieved through a variety of methods that include: visiting other institutions where there are established teams working with the same or a similar patient group, observing other disciplines at work (either by direct observation or by use of video), lectures, seminars and workshops.

Communication channels

Communication is vital to the effective running of the team and a considerable amount of time should be spent on this area. Communication between team members can be at either an informal or a formal level.

The most common formal channel for communication within an interdisciplinary team is the team meeting. Such meetings may be further subdivided into two major categories: the business meeting and the clinical meeting. Different meetings may be led by different members of the team. Such meetings will differ from the multidisciplinary team meeting in that they are not simply an opportunity to 'report back' to one person who is 'in charge' who them makes the decisions, they should involve the exchange of ideas and information leading to decision making by the team.

Team meetings are expensive; therefore it is of importance that they are conducted efficiently and for maximum effectiveness.

- All meetings should be held for an explicit purpose and not simply because 'we always have a meeting every Wednesday'.
- If appropriate, there should be a written agenda, circulated well in advance of the meeting in order that members have time to prepare for the meeting.
- All meetings should start and end on time, with time limits being set for each area to be discussed.
- Effective, firm leadership may well be needed to ensure that members stay on the particular area being discussed and that the discussion does not drift off into other areas.
- The leader should also ensure that all members participate in meetings and not allow them to be dominated by a few to the detriment of the many.
- As one of the roles of a meeting is to make decisions and take action it is important that these are made explicit in the meeting (with explicit time limits being set if necessary) and reinforced in writing as soon as possible. This will help to overcome the problem of team members being either unaware or forgetting that they were supposed to carry out certain task/activities within a certain period of time.

Informal channels of communication take many forms and are likely to be in part dependent on the physical location of team members. For example, team members may agree to meet regularly for lunch or at the coffee break.

It is of importance to note that the larger the team the harder it will be to maintain effective communication. For example, in a team of three there are only three possible communication channels; in a team of 15 this rises to over a hundred.

Additional areas

Confidentiality

Furnell, Flett & Clark (1987) comment that within a team setting it is necessary to share clinical information about patients with other team members; this means that complete confidentiality cannot be observed. It is therefore of great importance that this is explicitly explained to the patient and that consent is given for information to be shared. If the patient refuses to give consent then obviously this must be respected but the patient should then be informed that this may place limits on both the assessment and any treatment options that can be offered.

Legal implications of working in a team

Furnell, Flett & Clark (1987) point out that claims of 'primacy' (i.e. when one team member claims to have overall responsibility for the team) are untenable and incompatible with the tort of negligence. The consequence of this is that it would appear that team leaders cannot be held legally responsible for the negligence of another team member 'except in part by negligent delegation or referral'.

Encouraging commitment to the team

Team members should have a sense of commitment to the team; within social psychology this is referred to as 'group cohesiveness' and is most likely to take place under the following conditions:

- when there is frequent communication between group members
- if membership of the group is a rewarding experience
- if there is an absence of disturbing personalities in the team
- the smaller the group the greater the cohesiveness; within large teams 'splinter groups' and subgroups may develop reducing the level of cohesiveness
- the physical proximity of the team.

TEAM MAINTENANCE

Problems in working in an interdisciplinary setting and some solutions

Most professionals will be used to working as part of a multidisciplinary team and the majority of organisations will be familiar with the concept of and workings of the multidisciplinary team. When different disciplines set up and work as an interdisciplinary team this can give rise to problems in the following areas: managerial, organisational and interpersonal.

Managerial

These problems will be encountered when there is discord between the philosophy of the team and its working practices and that of management. The types of problems that may be encountered include the following.

1. Management may not see the need for a psychologist, physiotherapist and consultant anaesthetist to be working together on the assessment of one patient, viewing this as costly and an inefficient use of resources (i.e. they may have the attitude that the three professionals could be dealing with three patients rather than one).
2. They may desire clearer role identification between the disciplines.
3. They may fail to perceive the importance of spending time on meetings and team building, seeing this as a waste of time, money and resources that could be spent seeing more patients.

Some possible solutions to these problems include:

- involving management during the early stages of planning and development of the team
- discussion with management of the policy document, including why specific working practices are required
- documenting outcomes to show to the management the value of the programme.

Organisational

Time management and time wasting. Time can be wasted:

- in meetings
- in duplication of records/assessments
- if patients fail to turn up for appointments.

Some suggested solutions are as follows. First, unstructured, poorly organised teams are inefficient teams; there must be an effective working structure that is adhered to. At the simplest level if team meetings are due to begin at 10 a.m. then the team should ensure that this happens.

Secondly, it is advisable that all records, notes, etc. are kept together within one file as opposed to individual disciplines having their own files.

This reduces paperwork and duplication (the latter will also be avoided by explicit documentation of roles and responsibilities) and also means that professionals will not waste time looking for a specific piece of information.

Thirdly, efficient clerical support and organisation of working practices can reduce time wasted by patient non-attendance. For example, when appointments are sent out for an initial assessment then patients should be asked to confirm that they will be attending for the appointment. They should be notified in the appointment letter that if they do not respond within a given time period that it will be assumed that they do not wish to attend and that the appointment will be allocated to someone else.

Finally, there should be a specific policy for giving further appointments to patients who fail to attend for their appointment. Consideration should be given to the following:

- After a non-attendance by patients will positive attempts be made to contact them (e.g. by telephoning them to ask why they did not attend)?
- Are patients who repeatedly fail to attend for appointments showing ambivalence or poor motivation?

Fragmentation of the team and formation of 'splinter groups' within the team. Some solutions to this problem include:

- ensuring good communication occurs between all team members
- controlling the size of the team
- encouraging cohesiveness by using team-building techniques.

Interpersonal

Interpersonal problems may arise within the team for the following reasons:

1. there may be problems if the commitments of team members bring them into conflict with other members of their discipline who are not part of the team (e.g. line managers)
2. areas of professional overlap may lead to conflict between different disciplines

3. new team members may find it difficult to adapt to working in an interdisciplinary team approach
4. old team members may be resistant to the introduction of new ideas from newer members of the team
5. there may be a lack of respect among team members and professional rivalry, including a lack of respect for others training or qualifications; some members of the team may perceive themselves are being more important than others, or that they contribute more towards the assessment/treatment process
6. working with patients with chronic pain and their relatives can be very stressful This stress can lead to professionals experiencing burnout; there may be high staff turnover with high levels of sickness.

Some suggested solutions are as follows:

1. There must be effective communication between team members. This can be encouraged by a skilled team/programme leader. Any communication or interpersonal problems between team members need to be dealt with as early as possible.
2. When introducing new members to the team a 'probationary period' may be extremely useful. Considerable time must be spent when introducing new members to an established team to ensure that they fully understand the way in which the team works, their specific roles and responsibilities and the team philosophy.
3. There must be acceptance of others and the skills that they have. This can be encouraged by staff observing each other during therapies across disciplines to gain further understanding of the skills that different disciplines have.
4. There should be time set aside specifically for team development and team building. This is particularly important in the early stages of forming an interdisciplinary team, but should not be abandoned once the team has been set up and is functioning. All members of the team need to acknowledge the need to develop and to recognise that team development

should be explicit and that it takes both time and effort.

5. There must be support systems available to help team members cope with the emotional pressures that can occur when working with such a demanding group of patients.

Potential for development

No clinical service of any kind should remain static. It is incumbent upon all members to improve their own service. This requires constant questioning and reappraisal by all members of the team (audit), making best use of links with other clinical services, auditing outcome and the process of pain management itself to seek further improvements. Attending scientific meetings, peer review, and keeping up to date with the journals and clinical research will stimulate debate within the team and help identify areas for improvement, or areas into which the service should expand or improve.

The first areas in which further development should be sought are with those departments who already refer to the service. It is important to make sure that current working relationships are working well before seeking new ones. Make sure the clinical and administrative links work smoothly. Do not simply start up new links without carefully looking at the implications to the current service and the potential impact on areas that may be vulnerable. For example most centres have limited resources for 'individual' pain management. There is little point in starting up a new service (for CRPS patients for example) that will put even more pressure on staff to provide 'individual' management. Such a development must be planned, staffed and budgeted.

However, if, for example, the local department of orthopaedic surgery, which frequently refers patients to the service, wished to improve the clinical service and have expressed a willingness to collaborate on a joint assessment system, it would be worthwhile pursuing this further. It is likely to be of significant benefit to both parties and ultimately to the patients. In addition it may

not take much if any more input of resources to implement the changes.

Such collaboration as above has the potential to disseminate skills. This is to be encouraged. First, it will improve the clinical decision making and the subsequent referral pattern. Secondly, it will allow exchange of skills in both directions thus allowing the orthopaedic team to gain more insight into the aims of pain management and types of patient that might benefit. The team will also gain a better understanding of the orthopaedic surgical team's perspective. Such collaboration does not just happen, but needs time to be set aside for joint clinical meetings to ensure there are no misunderstandings, also that the two teams share the same objectives and that plans for evaluation are set. The meetings should culminate in an agreed document, which will be revised in light of continuing audit.

Primary care

Links with primary care are perhaps the most important of all links. Most patients referred to pain clinics or pain management programmes have a very long history. There is good reason to believe that earlier intervention may prevent the development of chronic pain problems. Developing links with primary care should be an important long term goal. Links with primary care should enable the team to give guidance to GPs about how to manage difficult pain problems in the community and how to support patients after they have completed a pain management programme. It should also provide advice for GPs to help with preparing patients for pain management.

It will not be possible to develop close links with every GP. It is worth liaising initially with those who already refer to the centre and offering an opportunity to meet up with that particular primary care team to establish common assessment and management plans. This can be extended to other primary care teams as and when they express interest or refer patients to the service. There will be considerable benefits to both the pain management service and in particular to the primary care team (Box 15.11).

Box 15.11 Benefits to referring agents

By outlining the aims and objectives of 'pain management', agreeing referral criteria and assessment details, together with advise on managing the 'difficult patient', the following advantages will follow:
- Assistance in selecting appropriate patients for referral (assessment guidelines)
- Fewer patients with unmet expectations following pain team assessment (nature of treatment/management explicit to both patient and referrer)
- Specific guidelines for management of the patient while awaiting pain team assessment
- Specific guidelines for management of patient following assessment whether listed for pain management or not
- Specific long term management plans for patients following pain management

---

CONCLUSION

The delivery of a clinical service is very complex. This is even more so with an interdisciplinary team. Choosing the right team members is vital, as it is possible for individual members to disrupt the whole team if they do not subscribe to the team philosophy.

Make clear plans for the development of the service and allocate areas of responsibility to each team member to ensure 'ownership' of the service. It is important to allow enough protected time to develop clinical pathways, maintain the morale of the team and perform audit. Constant evaluation of the team's performance and outcome of the programme will allow adjustments to be made early on rather than as a response to a crisis. Anticipate the future by developing links with other services and referring agents.

KEY POINTS

- Assemble the data and information to sell pain management to the 'key players'.
- Understand the 'key players' agendas.
- Plan the shape of the service carefully and in detail.
- Be sure to identify clinical pathways and the necessary space and administrative support to institute them.
- Choose team members with care.
- Invest time in team building and maintenance.
- Continuously reappraise clinical activity and service delivery.
- Search for potential areas of development with other services.

REFERENCES

Diller L 1990 Fostering the interdisciplinary team, fostering research in a society in transition. Archives of Physical Medicine and Rehabilitation 71:275–278

Finset A, Krogstad J M, Hasen H et al 1995 Team development and memory training in traumatic brain injury rehabilitation: two birds with one stone. Brain Injury 9:495–507

Furnell J, Flett S, Clark D F 1987 Multi-disciplinary clinical teams: some issues in establishment and function. Hospital and Health Services Review 83:15–18

Hastings C, Bixby P, Chaudhry-Lawton R 1988 Superteams: a blueprint for organisational success. Fontana, London

Melvin J L 1980 Interdisciplinary and multidisciplinary activities and the ACRM. Archives of Physical Medicine and Rehabilitation 61:379–380

Watson P J, Main C J, Waddell G, Gales T F, Purcell-Jones G 1998 Medically certified work loss, recurrence and cost of wages compensation for back pain: a follow up study of the working population of Jersey. British Journal of Rheumatology 37(1):83–86

FURTHER READING

Bonica J J 1990 Multidisciplinary/interdisciplinary pain programs. In: Bonica J J The management of pain, 2nd edn. Lea & Febiger, Philadelphia, ch 9, pp 197–208

Evans R 1997 In-patient v. out-patient pain management programmes that adopt a cognitive behavioural approach. DEC report no. 70. NHS Executive, South and West R & D Directorate *www.epi.bris.ac.uk/rd/publicat/dec70.htm*

Flor H, Fydrich T, Turk D C 1992 Efficacy of multidisciplinary pain treatment centres: a meta-analytic review. Pain 49:221–230

Gatchel R J, Turk D C (eds) 1996 Psychological approaches to pain management; a practitioner's handbook. Guilford, New York

Gatchel R J, Turk D C (eds) 1999 Psychosocial factors in pain; critical perspectives. Guilford, New York

McQuay H J, Moore R A 1998 An evidence-based resource for pain relief. Oxford University Press, Oxford

McQuay H J, Moore R A, Eccleston C, Morley S, Williams A C de C 1997 Psychological approaches. Chapter 19 in: Systematic review of outpatient services for chronic pain control. Health Technology Assessment 1(6)

Main C J, Parker H 1989 The evaluation and outcome of pain management programmes for chronic low back pain.

In: Roland M, Jenner J R (eds) Back pain—new approaches to rehabilitation and education. Manchester University Press, Manchester, pp 1–137

Morley S, Eccleston C, Williams A C de C 1999 A systematic review and meta-analysis of randomised controlled trials of cognitive behaviour therapy and behaviour therapy for chronic pain in adults, excluding headache. Pain 80:1–13

Malone M D, Strube M J 1988 Meta-analysis of non-medical treatments for chronic pain. Pain 34:231–244

Peters J L, Large R G 1990 A randomised controlled trial evaluating in-patient and out-patient pain management programmes. Pain 41:283–293

Peters J L, Large R G, Elkind G 1992 Follow-up results from from a randomised controlled trial evaluating in and out-patient pain management programmes. Pain 50:41–50

Williams A C de C, Nicholas M K, Richardson P H et al. 1993a Evaluation of a cognitive behavioural programme for rehabilitating patients with chronic pain. British Journal of General Practice 43:513–518

Williams A C de C, Richardson P H, Nicholas M K et al 1993b Inpatient vs. outpatient pain management: results of a randomised controlled trial. Pain 66:9–13

16

Competencies for clinically orientated pain management programmes

*Paul Watson   Chris C. Spanswick
Chris J. Main*

INTRODUCTION

Throughout this book we have tried to make the case for an interdisciplinary team rather than a multidisciplinary team (Ch. 15, p.337). In a multidisciplinary team the team leader is usually a doctor, individual team members work towards their own individual goals for the patient and often work in physically separate areas. Furthermore, knowledge of the skills of other disciplines is not required.

This may give rise to problems such as lack of effective communication between disciplines, which may lead to a lack of awareness of problem areas. For example, the physiotherapist may be unaware that a patient has an alcohol problem. This may lead to fragmentation of the approach to treatment and assessment in which the patient is treated as a series of problems rather than holistically. Duplication of certain parts of the assessment process is common in a multidisciplinary team. For example, all disciplines may obtain details from the patient about duration of pain, length of present episode of pain, medication and previous treatment. In certain cases manipulative patients can 'play off' one team member against other members, specifically seeking advice on the same problems from different members and if the advice received is conflicting to confront the professional with this information.

In the interdisciplinary team, as detailed in the previous chapter (p. 337):

individuals not only require the skills of their own disciplines, but also have the added responsibility of the group effort on behalf of the activity or client involved. This effort requires the skills necessary for effective group interaction and the knowledge of how to transfer integrated group activities into a result which is greater than the simple sum of the activities of each individual discipline. The group activity of an interdisciplinary team is synergistic, producing more than each individually and separately could accomplish (Melvin 1980, p 379).

CORE DISCIPLINES INVOLVED IN THE TEAM

So far we have looked at the mechanics of the development of chronic incapacity and the delivery of a pain management approach to increasing physical and psychological functioning. The selection of patients for different clinical paths based on their individual experiences, expectations and individual attributes has been discussed in some detail. The one missing part of the equation is the staff. What should be the required training, attributes and competencies for those responsible for delivering pain management?

The Pain Society has published a document 'Desirable criteria for pain management programmes' (Pain Society 1997), which addresses the issue of which professions are key personnel required for the provision of a pain management service, as opposed to pain treatments (Loeser 1991). The aim of this document was to outline the minimum skill mix appropriate to run pain management programmes. Unfortunately, although it identifies the doctor, physiotherapist and psychologist as the key staff, it gives no indication of the individual competencies required. Competencies required may be divided into general (i.e. those required by all members of the team) and professional skills specific to individual team members.

Although the Pain Society identified the above professions as the minimum to provide a pain management programme ideally the programme would have input from other professionals (Pain Society and Association of Anaesthetists of Great Britain and Ireland 1997). It is not possible to review the skills required by every profession that might be involved. This chapter will review the core skills and give indications for the level of

---

Box 16.1   Classes of skills used by team members

- Those relating to required clinical practice and procedure, for example the need for confidentiality
- Certain practices/procedures that are restricted to persons with specific professional qualifications/training; for example, only medical practitioners may prescribe drugs
- Areas of expertise that are expected of or are basic to one particular professional group rather than another—although there is no formal restriction on such skills; for example, the development of a paced exercise programme by the physiotherapist
- Skills that are (or should be) common to all team members; for example, history taking and communication skills (these will be referred to as 'core skills')

---

certain minimum competencies of these key personnel.

Furnell, Flett & Clark (1987) identified a number of different classes of skills utilised by team members (Box 16.1). These are essentially skills that are required to work in any clinical team. Without adherence to this basic minimum set of skills the team cannot function efficiently or with any confidence. In addition to the above, 'skills that are specific to working in the area of pain management' should be added.

Patients with chronic pain are commonly very distressed and often feel they have not been dealt with non-judgementally. Such patients have often been 'damaged' by the health-care system and become sceptical about further assessments and treatments. There are, therefore, an additional set of 'core skills' that are needed for those involved in pain management programmes. These are outlined in Box 16.2.

CORE KNOWLEDGE

The International Association for the Study of Pain (IASP) has published a number of core curricula (Fields 1995), (see also IASP web pages listed on p. 362). These include an outline of the core knowledge for all professionals involved in the assessment and treatment of patients with pain as well as a number of core curricula relating to specific professions (medicine, dentistry,

---

> **Box 16.2**   Core skills required by all professionals involved in pain management teams
>
> * Demonstrate an empathic approach to patients and relatives
> * Demonstrate excellent communication skills with patients, relatives and other staff
> * Demonstrate good, active listening skills in clinical interviews
> * Be able to translate complex information into a form readily understood by patients of different educational levels and experience
> * Skilled in the recognition of non-medical barriers to progress
> * Be non-judgemental in the interpretation of non-medical barriers to progress
> * View chronic pain from a biopsychosocial perspective

---

nursing, psychology, pharmacy, and occupational and physical therapy). At the time of writing a number of professions and disciplines have identified the need for specific training in the assessment and treatment of patients with pain (Pilowsky 1988, PPA 1998, RCA 1996, 1999). The change has been so rapid that readers are directed to their own professional body to check on the current training requirements.

INDIVIDUAL PROFESSIONAL COMPETENCIES

Medical profession

It is not the place of this book to dictate the minimum training requirements. This is the duty of the various professional bodies, for example the royal colleges (e.g. Royal College of Anesthetists (RCA) 1996, 1999). We do, however, make certain recommendations in the light of our own experience and that of others.

In the United Kingdom most consultants involved in medical rehabilitation specialise in neurorehabilitation. In the United States there are specialists in musculoskeletal rehabilitation called physiatrists. These are virtually unknown in the UK.

The medical practitioners most likely to be involved in pain management programmes are from the areas of anaesthesiology or rheumatology, or both. We recommend that they should be employed at consultant level. This does not exclude other disciplines but simply states the current status. It does not matter from which specialty doctors are from provided they have completed the appropriate higher professional training and have clinical experience in the patient group being treated. The doctor should be familiar with the current standard methods of medical assessment of patients and have an understanding of the criteria for further investigation or referral of the patient. For example, a spinal surgeon (of either neurosurgical or orthopaedic background) could be expected to have the necessary skills to be involved in a programme for patients with chronic low back pain, whereas a neurologist might be more appropriate for a programme with headache patients.

Pain programmes are commonly headed by anaesthetists who have undergone specific training in the assessment and treatment of patients with chronic pain (RCA 1996). It is important to have good general medical skills in addition to any specialised skills as a significant number of patients with chronic pain also have other concurrent medical problems. It is very useful to have medical specialists from more than one discipline involved in the programme. It is essential to be able to call on other specialist opinions (e.g. orthopaedic surgery, neurosurgery, neurology) as necessary. Close working relationships with colleagues in other disciplines are therefore vital. It is highly recommended that the medical specialist has undertaken training in an interdisciplinary approach to pain management as well as having received specialist professional training. Pain management is at the time of writing a subspecialty of anaesthesia and the RCA (1999) have published criteria for centres wishing to offer training.

Physiotherapy

In the United Kingdom standards for physiotherapists working in pain management have been developed by the Physiotherapy Pain Association (PPA) (1998).

The physiotherapist should be of at least senior I level, have been qualified for 4 years or more and have specific experience of working with chronic pain patients with a broad range of diagnoses. Where physiotherapists have undertaken extra specialist postgraduate training in pain management and perform a significant amount of the clinical interview, examination and clinical decision making without supervision of a doctor, it is recommended that they should be employed at clinical specialist level.

Specialist training in a biopsychosocial approach to patient assessment and management is an essential prerequisite or should be undertaken immediately on commencing work in the pain clinic. There are a few specialist training and education centres in the UK who offer this and the PPA also offers training in this area or can give information about how such training can be accessed. The PPA also produces a yearbook of collected papers on the subject of pain and the management of those with painful conditions, which is an excellent resource for physiotherapists.

Experience in working with disabled patients in a group setting is essential. Specialist training in the skills of examination of patients with musculoskeletal pain problems (usually the greatest proportion of patients seen in a pain clinic) is also considered highly desirable.

Physiotherapists must be familiar with standardised measures of impairment, disability and functional capacity evaluation. They should be able to perform and interpret these tests competently. It is advantageous if the physiotherapist has some experience of occupational rehabilitation, although this is not essential.

The physiotherapist should be able to develop a functionally orientated physical rehabilitation plan, which includes education about fitness and deconditioning, pacing of exercise and goal setting for patient groups and individuals.

Psychology

We recommend strongly that the psychologist on the team should have undertaken a recognised clinical training programme. If working without the support of a senior clinician, the psychologist should have at least 2 years post qualification experience, which should include working with chronic pain patients using a cognitive–behavioural model. Proven ability to work within a multidisciplinary or interdisciplinary team is essential.

Psychologists must be familiar with the administration and interpretation of psychological tests for the assessment of general distress, cognitive coping strategies, fear avoidance and pain behaviour. In addition to this they must be able to carry out an individual interview to identify important psychological and social barriers to successful rehabilitation.

They must be able to offer clinical management of patients in both a group and an individual basis. The role of the psychologist will vary from programme to programme but they must be able to design and deliver an educational programme on the psychological sequelae of chronic pain at a level appropriate to the understanding of the patient group. The ability to organise and deliver a range of stress reduction techniques, both physiologically and cognitively based approaches, is essential—as is the ability to foster in the individual patients, a problem-solving approach to chronic pain and disability.

Currently there are initiatives under way to develop a clearer framework for addressing the specific competencies required by psychologists.

CONTINUING PROFESSIONAL DEVELOPMENT

This is a vital area in the development and growth of a team. Effective training will aid in the development of the team and also will help to foster respect for the skills of other disciplines. Training should cater for the needs both of the team and of the individual members. It is essential that team members keep up to date, not only with interdisciplinary pain management issues, but also with unidisciplinary, specialist skills within their own profession.

Interdisciplinary training

Interdisciplinary education can be achieved through a variety of methods. These include:

visiting other institutions where there are established teams working with the same or a similar patient group, observing other disciplines at work (by either direct observation or use of video), lectures, seminars and workshops.

It is important for the team to allocate time for constant evaluation and training in the core skills. For example, all team members will need skills in motivating patients to make changes. The psychologists in the team can help in training their non-psychology colleagues by giving them a general understanding of the psychosocial aspects of illness and in the specific skills of motivational interviewing. This will be of enormous value to the team as a whole and enhance clinical effectiveness.

Unidisciplinary training

Although this book strongly advocates an interdisciplinary approach to the management of chronic pain, all team members must remain up to date in the skills of their own profession through specialist training. There may be concern in some individuals that in accepting an interdisciplinary approach to pain management they may become 'deskilled' in their own profession. The strength in an interdisciplinary approach comes from the variety of skills that come from those involved. It is counterproductive if a doctor does not keep abreast of new techniques in physical or pharmaological interventions, or if the physiotherapist does not take to opportunity to learn and critically appraise new approaches in manual therapy.

It is recommended that professionals involved in the team regularly work (this need not necessarily be frequently) with their peers to ensure that their individual professional skills are kept up to date. This is also a useful way to enhance working relationships with colleagues who either refer patients or may be used for second opinions.

It is important to remember that in using a biospychosocial approach to the management of chronic pain the practitioner must not ignore the biomedical needs of patients.

CLINICAL GOVERNANCE AND PEER REVIEW

The principle of clinical governance are outlined in the paper Clinical governance; quality in the new NHS (NHS Executive 1999).

Although continuous training and professional development should automatically ensure that skill levels are maintained there must be some form of regular peer review of the clinical performance of both the team as a whole and individual professionals. At the time of writing this has become an important topic. The precise methods of formal peer review and clinical governance have not been published and the process is still under debate.

Audit of team working

The team should audit clinical cases regularly. It is useful to take either a fictitious case or a real case and ask all team members to outline how the patient should be treated. This may be performed openly to the group or anonymously and the findings presented to the team. If this task is set for all team members then it will be possible to identify the variations in opinion amongst team members. It will allow for discussion and enable the team to develop an agreed policy as to how the case should be handled.

It might appear that this would stifle individual clinical opinion. In practice it should promote discussion and necessary peer review. Individuals will need to justify their opinions to their peers and colleagues from other disciplines. Finally it should promote some consistency of approach to all patients and reduce the potential for esoteric treatments.

Individual skill review

Individuals must check their skills against their peers. This can feel threatening but is an essential part of clinical governance. Time should be allocated for joint working. For example, this will enable cross-checking of skills in physical examination for both the doctors and physiotherapists. The psychologists might jointly interview patients to assess the level of agreement on assessment and planned treatment.

CONCLUSION

Patients should be able to expect a minimum level of competence of both the team as a whole and individuals within the team. This should be at least at the level of the average practitioner in their own field. It behoves the team and the individuals in the team to display high levels of skill in their own field and in that of pain management. It is also essential that there must be explicit methods of continuous professional development and monitoring peer review.

KEY POINTS

- All clinicians should have pre-established competence in individual clinical assessment and management as part of their professional accreditation.
- Specific experience with pain patients should be a prerequisite for becoming part of an interdisciplinary pain management team.
- New members of staff may require a degree of 'apprenticeship' from a member of their own profession before exerting clinical independence.
- In addition to specific training, a minimal level of skill in communication with patients is required. With new members of staff, appropriate 'skill-based learning' should be provided.
- Additional specific skills are needed for interdisciplinary team working.

REFERENCES

Fields H L (ed) 1995 Core curriculum for professional education in pain, 2nd edn. IASP, Seattle

Furnell J, Flett S, Clark D F 1987 Multi-disciplinary clinical teams: some issues in establishment and function. Hospital and Health Services Review January: 15–18

Loeser J D (for IASP) 1991 Desirable characteristics for pain treatment facilities: report of IASP taskforce. In: Bond M R, Charlton J E, Woolf C J (eds) Proceedings of the VIth world congress on pain. Elsevier, Amsterdam, ch 50, pp 411–417

Melvin J L 1980 Interdisciplinary and multidisciplinary activities and the ACRM. Archives of Physical Medicine and Rehabilitation 61:379–380

NHS Executive 1999 Clinical governance; quality in the new NHS. NHS Executive, London

Pain Society 1997 Desirable criteria for pain management programmes. Pain Society, London

Pain Society and Association of Anaesthetists of Great Britain and Ireland 1997 Provision of pain services. Pain Society and Association of Anaesthetists of Great Britain and Ireland, London

Physiotherapy Pain Association (PPA) 1998 Standards for physiotherapists working in pain management programmes. Chartered Society of Physiotherapy, London

Pilowsky I 1988 (Editorial) An outline curriculum on pain for medical schools. Pain 33:1–2

Royal College of Anaesthetists (RCA) 1996 Training in and curriculum for anaesthetists wishing to specialise in pain management. RCA, London

Royal College of Anaesthetists (RCA) 1999 Criteria for pain management units seeking approval from the Royal College of Anaesthetists for subspecialty training in pain management. RCA, London

The following are available as web pages on the IASP web site (http://www.halcyon.com/iasp/):

Proposed outline curriculum on pain for dental schools
Outline curriculum on pain for schools of nursing
Outline curriculum on pain for schools of occupational therapy and physical therapy
Outline curriculum on pain for schools of pharmacy
Curriculum on pain for students in psychology.

17

Evaluation of outcome

George M. Peat

INTRODUCTION: THE IMPORTANCE OF ASSESSMENT OF TREATMENT OUTCOME?

Modern health-care delivery systems require sophisticated systems of data collection of increasing complexity. Information available on patients is collected for a variety of purposes ranging from simple patient indexing, to patient scheduling, health-care usage expenditure, triaging through patient pathways to monitoring of progress. Purchase of health care is, however, becoming increasingly dependent on results. Evaluation of outcome of treatment has become a essential component in health-care delivery. In this chapter, the evaluation of outcome of pain management is considered from both a methodological and a practical point of view.

EVIDENCE-BASED MEDICINE

Clinicians in every field of patient care are usually aware of the need to evaluate the outcome of their interventions. Attending to treatment outcome forms part of clinical experience. In turn this is used to influence decisions on when and how to intervene with future patients. Unfortunately, the use of clinical judgement in an unstructured, case-by-case way to assess treatment outcome can provide misleading and biased appraisals of our effectiveness.

In recent times, there have been increasing calls for sound clinical experience, knowledge of the individual patient, and patient choice to be complemented by so-called evidence-based medicine (EBM): the use of current empirical evidence ('best evidence') in making decisions about the care of individual patients (Sackett et al 1996). Melzack & Wall (1996) suggested some criteria for such studies in psychological approaches to chronic pain management:

1. treatment must demonstrate superiority over placebo
2. changes, both in magnitude and duration, must be *clinically* significant
3. changes must be transferable to the patients' normal day-to-day environment
4. skills acquired by patients must have long term effectiveness.

Systematic reviews and large randomised controlled trials (RCT) can offer the most powerful and compelling evidence for the true effectiveness of treatment (McQuay & Moore 1998). In the field of interdisciplinary pain management programmes, results are now becoming available from such reviews and trials conducted in a number of settings with different patient groups and a variety of different treatment approaches (McQuay et al 1997). Some aspects in the quality of these may have been criticised but the gradual improvement in quality over recent times gives grounds for optimism and the real prospect of applying their findings for the benefit of patients.

BEST EVIDENCE AND CLINICAL REALITY

Best evidence can be incorporated into clinical decision making—steering patients towards effective treatments and away from ineffective or harmful approaches. Establishment of clinical guidelines and standards of service for the content and design of treatment does not necessarily guarantee effectiveness. Outcome depends also on the referral and selection procedures, which may differ amongst pain management programmes (Turk & Rudy 1990). Factors such as the proportion of patients who are long term unemployed can have a powerful influence on

likelihood of returning to work after rehabilitation and the proportion of patients suffering significant comorbidity may have a specific limiting effect on the range of therapeutic objectives that can be set. Unlike prescribing medication, the treatment in question (pain management programme) is not rigidly standardised, nor has it a fixed dose that can be administered. The skills of staff, how they interact with patients, group dynamics, the available treatment options, patient compliance and adherence to treatment all complicate attempts to generalise from research findings.

Despite an encouraging number of recent high quality outcome studies, clinicians are usually required to evaluate outcome within the constraints of routine practice. It is just not feasible to conduct randomised trials in each clinical setting on each treatment. The prospect of having to do so to generate meaningful answers to questions on effectiveness can be discouraging. The gulf between RCT standards and routine outcome measurement in pain clinics is still great (Price & Prosser 1998). Nevertheless, there is a growing recognition that this is an important aspect of patient management.

The purpose of this chapter is to prepare clinicians for the inevitable questions on treatment outcome that they will either face from others or ask themselves (see Appendix to this chapter). Detailed consideration of outcome measurement can be found in Fitzpatrick et al (1998). This chapter will outline an approach to routine outcome measurement of chronic pain management that improves upon reliance on clinical judgement alone but acknowledges the constraints of clinical practice. Such an approach emphasises:

- multiple perspectives on treatment outcome (including the participation of the patient in setting outcome priorities)
- multidimensional outcome domains
- valid, reliable and responsive measurement instruments
- acknowledging bias and taking steps to minimise it

- acknowledging the ambiguity of uncontrolled observations and trying to minimise this.

The points discussed relate to evaluating outcome in cohorts of patients participating in treatment. Single-case designs have been discussed in detail by Kazdin (1982).

ADVANTAGES OF SYSTEMATIC ASSESSMENT

Despite methodological problems, routine, systematic and comprehensive assessment of treatment outcome has several advantages over clinical judgement alone.

1. *Criteria for successful outcome can begin to be clearly expressed.* This has been a neglected area in pain management outcome studies (Turk, Rudy & Sorkin 1993) and yet it is essential to the process of defining clinically significant improvements and of measuring individual patient outcomes.

2. *Comparisons of treatment outcome (and baseline) can be made between patients.* This is a process that is intuitively performed by clinicians when rating outcome (or initial severity) but is made more explicit by a systematic approach.

3. *Comparisons with treatments in other settings can be made.* This includes comparison with pain management programmes run in pain centres elsewhere in the country or even abroad. This is likely to be a major consideration for purchasers. It requires consensus between different centres on which measures to use (Ch. 15).

4. *They can provide a candid appraisal of the adverse effects of treatment.* Most treatments, even placebos, carry the risk of adverse or detrimental effects. Pain management programmes are no exception. Some of the effects of failed treatments (discussed in chronic pain centres with the benefit of hindsight) also apply to failed pain management (Ch. 5). Patients and clinicians alike may be reluctant or unwilling to identify these in the usual clinical setting.

5. *Clearer formulation of hypotheses.* By examining outcome in a systematic and comprehensive way clinicians can begin to look for patterns in outcome and to speculate on associations.

Hypotheses can later be formally tested using appropriate methodological frameworks.

6. *The information can be used for patient feedback to reinforce change.* Evidence on the changes made following treatment can be used for feedback. This includes identifying individual priorities for further (self-)management. In some circumstances, measures can be administered during the course of treatment to provide individual 'progress reports'. The information can then be used to direct individual intervention or reinforce patient change (Fig. 17.1).

Patients are often more readily persuaded of change when presented with this sort of evidence than on the basis of staffs' assertions alone. In some respects, those who purchase pain management on behalf of patients are no different. There has been a gradual shift from simple number counting of throughput towards increasingly sophisticated evaluation of outcome and cost–benefit analysis. Purchasers are becoming increasingly demanding of credible information on patient changes following treatment. Empirical support for assertions that the treatment 'works' is likely to be a prerequisite for negotiations over treatment funding.

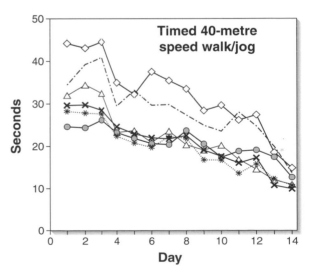

Figure 17.1 Graphing daily progress to reinforce patient changes. Each patient is represented by a line. Time on each of the days of the 3-week pain management programme was recorded. Note that the group differences reduce by the end of the pain management programme.

A summary of these points is given in Box 17.1.

Box 17.1 Mini-summary: systematic assessment

- Assessing the outcome of routine clinical practice is unlikely to satisfy the rigorous methodological standards required for best evidence of treatment effectiveness
- Reliance on clinical impressions and judgement alone can give misleading and biased appraisals of effectiveness
- It is possible for clinicians in pain management to evaluate treatment outcome in a manner that can fulfil a number of desirable objectives of clinical practice and satisfy basic methodological requirements

---

THE OUTCOME 'STAKEHOLDERS'

Who is concerned about the outcome of pain management?

Consider vignette 17.1.

Pain management is a service whose outcome affects, or is of interest to, a number of different parties (Fig. 17.2). In planning how to evaluate the outcome of pain management important questions to ask early on are:

- Whose outcome are you interested in?
- How will success be measured from their perspective?

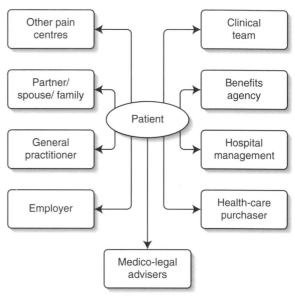

Figure 17.2 Whose outcome? Parties with a direct or potential interest in the outcome of pain management.

Vignette 17.1

A team of clinicians established intensive 3-week pain management programmes 1 year ago. Having run the programmes for a year, clinicians were then asked to estimate their rate of success. After weighing up the available evidence, they felt that 70% of cases had resulted in a successful outcome. Patients were then asked. Surprisingly, only half those referred to the programmes rated the outcome a success. This number included some patients whose outcome clinicians had pronounced a failure. Patients' partners and family occasionally arrived at a different conclusion still, as did the GP.

What reasons were behind this disparity? On closer questioning the factors became clear. The different parties were basing their judgement on different definitions of success. Clinicians were responding to the number of patients who told them at their end of programme review that they were greatly satisfied with their treatment and had also made significant reductions in unnecessary medications and improvements in functional tests. Patients based their decision on attaining pretreatment goals. Some, who had hoped for a significant reduction in their pain as a result of learning coping techniques and exercise, were disappointed to find that in spite of their efforts it was still present. In making functional progress in spite of pain some had jeopardised their benefits without feeling ready for a return to work. They didn't think this was success. Others, who made little change in their medication or functional test performance, were none the less delighted with their newly acquired skill of pacing and as a result had begun to enjoy social activities again. Others had felt reluctant to tell the clinicians their true feelings because although the results had been a letdown they were none the less grateful for the time and effort spent on them. Some partners complained about the amount of time the patient was engaged in exercise and relaxation during the week. They wondered at the end of the day if their partner still had pain whether it was all really worth it. Others agreed with the clinicians that reducing medications was the most important point. A number of GPs felt that there had been no plan for advising them or giving them practical arrangements for how to keep patients on the right tracks with self-management. Others felt that the doctor–patient relationship had been helped by the fact that their patients were no longer pressing them for another referral for investigation or treatment.

By asking these questions one begins to see the diversity of possible outcomes of interest: some of these will be genuine targets, and others substitute endpoints (see later).

Patient and their families are the central figures in any consideration of treatment outcome following pain management—a fact underlined by the emphasis on negotiating programme aims with each patient. The clinician may have a clear idea of what would be a reasonable outcome for a particular patient and this should be specifically addressed both in terms of likely outcome (e.g. improved functional ability) and unlikely outcome (e.g. complete pain relief). Referring agents, GPs, hospital managers and health purchasers also need to know these judgements. It is of most importance, however, to the patient and their family. Patients who opt into pain management with unrealistic hopes and unachievable targets are liable to be disappointed. Such possibilities must be addressed as part of the clinical decision-making process (Ch. 12).

A final word of warning: the situation in which clinicians are encouraged by their local funding bodies to set up pain management programmes with a short (e.g. 1-year) trial period to decide whether it works is becoming all too familiar. The emphasis on empirical proof is normally sufficient to induce a frantic search for measurement instruments that will provide the necessary evidence. Leaving to one side concerns about whether such a time period or pressured situation allows a clear and proper appraisal of their effectiveness, you are left asking what proof is sought? If this question can be clarified this is worth doing. Often it cannot. It is then up to the clinicians to seek the relevant outcome studies and consult peers to decide which areas of outcome to measure and what instruments to use.

Box 17.2 is a summary of the above points.

WHAT OUTCOMES?
Potential outcome domains

It has been acknowledged that pain management programmes can have a diverse range of potential benefits for patients and their families

---

Box 17.2 Mini-summary: outcome stakeholders

- There are often several parties with a direct or potential interest in treatment outcome following pain management
- As a result, outcome measurement can be assessed from a variety of perspectives; each of which may put emphasis on different outcome domains
- By identifying whose criteria for successful outcome you are trying to satisfy you can start focusing on certain areas of outcome
- Patients and their family are central to outcome assessment although it may be necessary to outline to them (and other interested parties) what is realistic

---

(and other interested parties). A helpful classification of these domains of outcome measurement has been described by Morley et al (1999) in their systematic review. Box 17.3 illustrates the major outcome domains and offers examples of tests currently in use in the Manchester and Salford Pain Centre (MSPC).

A glance at the outcome literature confirms the diversity of domains for evaluating outcome and highlights the divergence of opinion that exists between different centres with regard to measurement of outcome.

It is impossible to measure everything and so it is desirable to identify at an early stage which measures will be given priority and relied upon in evaluation.

Narrowing the remit for outcome evaluation

A few simple reminders can prevent an overinclusive approach to outcome evaluation.

1. *Choose outcome domains that specifically meet the programme objectives.* The primary aim of pain management programmes is to reduce disability and distress. From the above list, self-rated interference, pain behaviour and affect will be priority areas for outcome evaluation.

2. *Use patient-preference approaches to prioritise outcome domains.* Not all domains of outcome are of equal concern to patients (and their families). Asking them to rate the importance of different domains gives them an opportunity to express what it is important for them to achieve on a pain

Box 17.3 Outcome domains

Outcome domain	Description of content	Current MSPC assessment
1. Pain experience	Pain intensity, quality, temporal pattern	Short Form McGill Pain Questionnaire (Melzack 1987)
2. Affect	Commonly related to psychological distress and depression	Distress and Risk Assessment Method (Main et al 1992)
3. Cognitive	Beliefs and attitudes about pain and cognitive coping styles	Fear-Avoidance Beliefs Questionnaire[1] (Waddell et al 1993) Tampa Scale of Kinesophobia (Kori, Miller & Todd 1990) Pain-Related Self-Statements (Flor & Turk 1988) Pain Self-Efficacy Beliefs Questionnaire (Nicholas 1989) Pain Locus of Control (Main & Waddell 1991)
4. Pain behaviour	Split into active (normal) behaviour (e.g. walking distance) and abnormal pain behaviour (e.g. observation systems for quantifying verbal and non-verbal pain behaviour)	5-minute walking distance; 20-metre speed walk; Timed step-up test; Waist–knee maximum lift; Observational method for pain behaviour
5. Biological measures	Physiological and physical fitness measures (e.g. SEMG, trunk muscle endurance)	Occasional SEMG; physical fitness tests; pain tolerance and threshold for specific research protocols
6. Self-rated interference	Social role interference and limitation of basis functional activities (e.g. sitting, standing)	Roland & Morris Disability Questionnaire (RMDQ)a (Roland & Morris 1983); Oswestry Disability Questionnaire (ODQ)[1] (Fairbank et al 1980)

Additional domains reported in published outcome studies include:

7 Health-care use	Consultations; treatment episodes; investigations; analgesic intake	GP postal study piloted but poor response rate
8. Patient satisfaction		
9. GP satisfaction		

[1]Specifically for low back pain.

management programme. An alternative approach is to use patient-specific goals and objectives. The information is often valuable and individually relevant but can be difficult to use in comparisons amongst patients. This approach is becoming increasingly popular.

3. *Don't play the substitute game.* The practice of choosing outcomes that are 'substitutes' or 'surrogates' for the real target of treatment has long been lamented (Feinstein 1989) yet is common in medicine. As an example, the effectiveness of treatments that were designed to reduce respiratory distress have been judged by vital capacity tests, and anticoagulants have been evaluated by mortality rates or blood samples rather than the incidence of thromboembolism. In each case the outcome

chosen probably correlates with the real target, but it is an imperfect substitute.

The weakness of surrogate outcome measures can be understood by watching a football game on TV. Coverage of the game is now supported by an impressive array of statistics. At the end of a game you can be told the amount of possession, the number of corners, the number of shots on goal ad nauseum. But how many feel consoled by the fact that their team won more corners than the other side, had 90% of the possession, and had twice as many shots on goal, after being beaten 1–0?

The increasing use of audit and standard setting has also introduced surrogate measures of outcome to ensure that treatment adheres to minimum, desirable, or even exceptional standards in content and delivery. However: 'When the process is successfully carried out, we may congratulate ourselves on reaching the goal, while overlooking the appropriate target that should have been hit, and was not' (Feinstein 1989, p. 301).

If the primary aim of pain management programmes is to reduce disability and distress then, 'outcomes' such as changes in beliefs and attitudes, or physical fitness, or treatment compliance are not primary targets that will determine the outcome of the programme but are substitute endpoints. True, changes in these factors may herald a change in disability and distress. Then again they may not! A randomised trial of educational interventions with a clinic nurse in general practice for back pain found that they increased patient satis-faction, perceived knowledge and exercise participation but were no better than usual treatment in altering symp-toms, functional status or health care use (Cherkin et al 1996). In the same way that sophis-ticated statistics can obscure the outcome of a football game, using substitute endpoints can obscure the effectiveness of treatment. The point is illustrated with data from the back pain management programme in Salford (Vignette 17.1).

The reason for displacing the target is often found in clinicians' preferences for 'hard' data,

---

Data from Vignette 17.1

Twenty-four patients with chronic lower back pain who had completed the pain management programme were identified at 6-month follow-up review. All were still reporting high levels of functional limitation (RMDQ scores greater than 15 out of 24) that were essentially unchanged since the start of the programme. However:

— 5 had improved more than 20 degrees on straight-leg raise
— 8 reported a substantial increase in their use of active coping self-statements
— 9 showed a substantial reduction in fear-avoidance beliefs about physical activity
— 11 had improved by more than 50% on a timed step-up test.

---

the lack of a clear objective, or a preoccupation with treatment process and ancillary goals rather than the end result.

There is a proper place for questions, data collection and analysis regarding *why* patients' levels of disability and distress may fall after being on a pain management programme. However, for those seeking to narrow the scope of their outcome evaluation, substitute outcomes can be an unhelpful distraction.

4. *Consider composite measures.* A number of self-report measures have been developed that contain several scales to represent multifactorial outcomes of interest such as health, the impact of pain or the pain experience itself. Table 17.1 shows the factor structure of three of the most

Table 17.1 Three composite self-report measures used in evaluating the outcome of pain management

SIP[1]	SF36[2]	WHYMPI[3]
Ambulation	Physical functioning	Interference
Body care	Social functioning	Support
Mobility	Bodily pain	Pain severity
Emotional behaviour	Role: physical	Life control
Social interaction	Role: emotional	Affective distress
Alertness	General health	Negative responses
Communication	Mental health	Solicitous responses
Work	Vitality	Distracting responses
Sleep and rest	(transitional index)	Household chores
Eating		Outdoor work
Home management		Activities away from home
Recreational activities		Social activities
Scores combined into physical, psychosocial, and other dimensions	Each scale is scored to give a total 0–100% (the higher the score the better the health)	Each scale is scored to give an average out of six An additional scale—general activity—is the average of last four scales above

[1]Bergner et al 1981
[2]Ware & Sherbourne 1992
[3]Kerns, Turk & Rudy 1985

extensively used and validated instruments. These have been reported in outcome studies of pain management and so have a good track record. Their wide appeal makes them suitable for comparing different treatment centres. The WHYMPI (Ch. 5, p. 92) has also been used to classify chronic pain patients into distinct subgroups (Turk & Rudy 1992). Some researchers have warned, however, that composite measures 'risk obscuring more than they reveal' (Williams 1995a). Some can be quite time consuming to complete (e.g. the SIP contains 136 questions). In contrast shorter indices have constructed scales from very few items (e.g. the role: emotional scale of the SF36) and it is unlikely that such scales act as good indicators for individual change. Calculating scores on some of these indices can be complicated and time consuming. Despite their drawbacks, they remain a substantial improvement over the many poorly validated unidimensional measures. Efforts to construct meaningful indexes of physical tests have had little success—there is simply no consensus on how to weight and amalgamate them.

5. *Remember the outcome 'stakeholder'.* The preferences of both patients and their families have already been highlighted. If an important other party has identified a specific outcome (e.g. return to work) the clinician should be sure to include it in the evaluation or be prepared to explain the reasons for not doing so.

A summary of the above points is given in Box 17.4.

HOW DO YOU GET THE INFORMATION?
Approaches to data collection

General approaches to assessment have already been discussed in Section 2 of the book. Each approach has its strengths and weaknesses. The principal types of outcome measure are listed in Box 17.5.

Patient questionnaires can be used to generate standardised scores for complex constructs such as depression. There may be no alternative to patient self-report for some information (e.g. pain quality). Questionnaires are often easy to administer, since they do not require a lot of time and no special equipment or facilities. This approach is often preferred in busy clinical settings.

Relying on patient self-report brings the potential for inaccurate information. Some patients with chronic pain do not appear to provide consistent or accurate information about their condition (Jensen 1997). Some of these issues relate to recall bias of past events or experiences—for example, current level of pain seems to influence recall of previous levels of pain (Jensen 1994). Others relate to the reporting of current status. Where inaccuracy due to poor understanding of the questions is suspected, interview techniques may be useful. How prevalent inaccurate self-report information is and whether it is conscious or unconscious is not within the scope of this chapter. The problem of overreliance on patient self-report is mentioned

---

Box 17.4 Mini-summary: Outcome domains

- A diverse array of outcome domains exists for pain management programmes. There are no agreed guidelines on which to choose but all of them cannot be covered. Reducing disability and distress are the primary objectives in chronic pain management
- Narrow your remit. Select those areas of outcome that are directly related to your programme objectives. Be wary of using substitute measures. Use patient-preference approaches if necessary to reflect your patients' priorities. Consider using a composite measure
- Don't forget to include information that important parties will demand at a later date

---

Box 17.5 Types of outcome measure

1. Patient self-report:
   — questionnaire
   — interview
   — diary
2. Physical test performance
3. Clinicians' ratings
4. Behavioural observation
5. Activity monitoring (e.g. uptime)
6. Third-party ratings (e.g. GP, spouse)
7. Written records (e.g. hospital notes)

here as encouragement for clinicians not to overlook other methods of obtaining information to evaluate outcome.

Behavioural observation techniques and physical test performance can be used to compare a patients' self-report with how they actually perform. This has been the incentive behind the development of a battery of physical tests designed specifically for evaluating chronic pain patients (Harding et al 1994). It should be remembered, however, that variations in behaviour and performance can be consciously or unconsciously modified by variations in effort and responses to the test conditions (Peat 1998).

Written records may be very useful. Complete medical or GP records can give information on patients' consultations following pain management. Extracting the information and verifying its quality can, however, be problematic.

A summary of the above points is given in Box 17.6.

WHAT MAKES A GOOD OUTCOME MEASURE?

The perfect outcome measure would provide meaningful and accurate information. Scores would be relatively invariant in patients whose condition was stable (good reproducibility). When the patient's condition truly changed, even if only by a small but clinically important amount, the measure would be able to detect this (responsiveness). Scores would also closely reflect the purpose that they were intended to fulfil and not some other factor (validity).

Of course, the perfect measure does not exist. It is important therefore to know how to identify the best measures for a particular situation.

Reproducibility

All measures have some random error. In patients whose condition is unchanged the extent to which scores vary will indicate the reproducibility of the measure. In a sense this can be regarded as background 'noise'. Figure 17.3 illustrates variability in functional status measurement in a subject whose actual level was stable.

In measurements that require the rating of an observer, the scores obtained by different examiners of the same stable patient will be important (interrater reliability).

Responsiveness

Over and above the 'noise' of random measurement error it is important to identify the signal that indicates a true change in the patient.

Box 17.6   Mini-summary: approaches to data collection

- Different approaches can be used to obtain outcome data. The most commonly used is patient self-report questionnaires
- Overreliance on self-report outcome data can give a biased and inaccurate appraisal of treatment effectiveness
- It is important to complement patient report with measures of behavioural change. Sources for this include observational methods, physical tests, third party ratings, and written records like hospital notes. These measures will typically involve more time, effort and resources

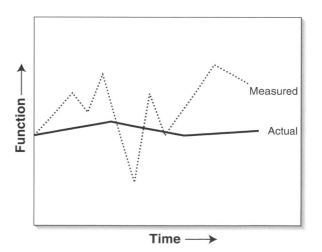

Figure 17.3   Poor measurement reproducibility.

Measures with poor responsiveness may fail to detect clinically important change. Figure 17.4 shows the example of measuring work status as the only measure of functional limitation. It may be reproducible but it fails to detect improvements in the patients' status. There are many statistical ways of summarising how good a measure can detect clinically important change including standardised effect sizes and standardised response means. Almost all are based on this concept of the ratio of signal to noise.

A comparison of functional limitation measures in chronic low back pain patients completing the 3-week back pain management programme is shown in Table 17.2. Although the different statistics yield slightly different results for the responsiveness of each measure the overall picture is clear: the RMDQ total score and all

the functional tests have a similar responsiveness (these figures would be classed as highly responsive). The ODQ score is not so responsive to change.

A more detailed account of measurement responsiveness is provided by Guyatt, Kirschner & Jaeschke (1992) and Stratford, Binkley & Riddle (1996).

In assessing response to treatment, it is important to distinguish between clinically important change that has resulted from the treatment and naturally occurring variability. Case study 17.1 is a typical clinical example.

In this case, the change between pre- and postprogramme performance is unlikely to be due to random error or even to a learning effect but more probably to simple variability in his condition. Strategies for distinguishing between normal variability and true change are discussed later.

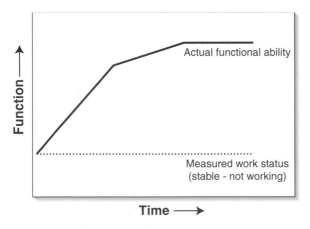

Figure 17.4 Poor responsiveness.

Case study 17.1 Naturally occurring variability

A 35-year-old man with a 10-year history of multiple site pain enrolled for the pain management programme. At preprogramme assessment he managed 250 metres on a timed 5-minute walking test. Three weeks later at postprogramme assessment he walked 400 metres in the same test: a large improvement compared with many other participants. On presenting him with the evidence of such a successful increase in functional ability he was unimpressed. 'I don't know what the fuss is about. I told you I was on one of my really bad days when you tested me at the start of the programme.'

Table 17.2 Comparison of the responsiveness of functional limitation measures in chronic low back pain following a 3 week pain management programme

Functional measure	Average pre-post change (%)	Standardised effect size[1]	Standardised response mean [2]
RMDQ total	36	1.09	0.96
ODQ total	14	0.56	0.57
Timed 20-metre speed walk	42	1.1	1.3
Step-ups in 30 seconds	43	1.2	1.3
Sit–stands in 30 seconds	48	1.3	1.2
5-minute walking distance	30	1.0	1.3

[1]Kazis et al 1989.
[2]Liang, Fossel & Larson 1990.

Validity

Measures are never in themselves valid or invalid (Ch. 9, p. 166). They are judged to be valid *for a stated purpose*. Validity can be assessed in a number of ways:

- Look at the content of the measure (e.g. items in a self-report questionnaire). Does it cover all the important points? Does it contain many irrelevant items?
- Does it show change in predictable circumstances? For example, a measure of disability should show reductions in acute cases that largely resolve by themselves.
- Do changes in the measure correlate with other observed changes in the expected way? For example, improvements in physical tests should correlate negatively with changes in reported functional limitation.

Reactivity

In their meta-analysis, Flor, Fydrich & Turk (1992) rated the outcome measures used in a number of pain management outcome studies on the basis of their reactivity—that is, their potential for patient or therapist bias, or both. They were differentiated in terms of reactivity as low (I); moderate (II) or High (III) as follows:

I   all physiological measures
     laboratory data
     blind ratings
     behavioural assessments
     medical record data
II   standardised measures with little connection with the treatment or therapist (e.g. activity diaries)
III patient self-report of improvement
     therapist improvement ratings
     instruments with an obvious relationship to treatment outcome.

Very few outcome studies had used measures of low reactivity (class I). The result is potentially biased appraisals of effectiveness.

A summary of the above points is given in Box 17.7.

> **Box 17.7** Mini-summary: Some questions you should ask about measurement quality
>
> - Was the measure designed for the use that you are intending?
>   Was it formulated on patients similar to yours?
>   Was it designed to measure changes in patients across time?
> - Have any previous studies been conducted on the quality of this measurement?
>   What were their findings (reproducibility over a clinically relevant time period, responsiveness, validity)?
>   Did they study subjects similar to your patients?
> - Has this measure been used in many other outcome studies in your field?
> - What level of reactivity is likely with this measure?
> - Does it make sense to use *this* measure in *your* setting with *your* patients?
>   Practical considerations (time, cost, facilities or equipment required)
>   Appropriateness (relevant content, acceptable to patients, floor or ceiling effects)

DESIGNING A FRAMEWORK FOR EVALUATING OUTCOME

Having considered the key 'stakeholders' in terms of outcome, the range of possible outcome domains, approaches to measurement and the properties of specific measures, it is important to consider specific practicalities and design the framework for obtaining routine, systematic, comprehensive and accurate evaluation of treatment outcome.

The following practical suggestions are influenced by experience in evaluating outcome of the Manchester and Salford's pain management programmes.

When to measure 'initial state' and 'outcome'?

This is closely linked to *what* you are evaluating. If you want to measure change in relation to a defined treatment (e.g. a 3-week pain management programme) the patients' initial state will be measured immediately prior to the programme. Before being accepted for a programme, however, patients will have discussed the programme in detail at the time of assessment and been given the opportunity to discuss their situation in detail (Ch. 12). As a result of the assessment and discussion, the patients' beliefs and attitudes, even their disability and distress, may have changed significantly. If the patients' initial state is described after this has occurred then the influence of the overall package for care may be significantly underestimated.

Measuring outcome immediately after treatment has some advantages—there is little threat of sample attrition (over and above that due to dropouts during the programme) and fewer confounding factors than with a longer follow-up period when other significant life events may have had an independent adverse effect on treatment outcome.

Immediate postprogramme assessment may give an overoptimistic picture with regard to longer term outcome. Subjects' responses in self-report questionnaires (and performance in physical tests) may be coloured by the optimism that many feel having completed a challenging programme. Such short term outcome, however, does not satisfy two essential criteria for evaluating the effectiveness of treatments for chronic pain: we cannot judge whether any of the changes have been transferred to patients' everyday lives or the skills they have acquired have any long term effect. Treatments aimed at chronic pain (with the exception of terminal cancer) can be judged by longer term follow-up. Judgements surrounding the effectiveness of spinal surgery have been based on evaluating outcome at several years' follow-up. Pain management programme outcomes have generally been based on follow-ups of between 6 and 12 months. This is probably the minimum length of follow-up required to evaluate outcome adequately.

Administering measures

Control the test environment

Care must be taken to control the environment during testing. Environmental factors influencing performance and test results include:

- the instructions given (e.g. Matheson et al 1992)
- the level of feedback and encouragement given (e.g. Guyatt et al 1984)
- the presence of other parties—especially the spouse (Paulsen & Altmaier 1995)
- the gender interaction between patients and observers (e.g. Levine & De Simone 1991)
- the time of testing—especially flexibility and strength (Ensink et al 1996).

Inadequate control over these factors can lead to erroneous conclusions about the true extent of change. An example of implementing a test protocol is given in Box 17.8. This example is just one

---

Box 17.8 A test protocol

The physical testing protocol for functional tests at Manchester and Salford Pain Centre were standardised in the following way.
1. A written manual of the exact wording of instructions for each of the tests was compiled (to minimise the effect of differences in instructions). These were designed to be as simple and straightforward for patients as possible (to minimise differences in patients' interpretation). They were therefore not to be interpreted for patients by clinicians during testing. If patients were doubtful about the instructions they were simply repeated (to minimise interaction between therapist and patient). The manual also contained guidelines on responding to pain behaviour (verbal or non-verbal) during testing. It was felt that no encouragement during testing would be given as this would be difficult to control, strongly influence patient effort and make the test more 'artificial'. Instead, during timed tests the physiotherapist issued time checks at regular intervals. Test results and any other information were recorded on standardised forms (to minimise lost data).
2. The clinical staff were then observed administering the tests on each other and were given feedback.
3. Staff were then video-recorded doing the same with a series of patients and given feedback.
4. Testing was then arranged such that a physiotherapist not involved with running the pain management programme would conduct assessments (to reduce bias). The same examiner had to be used for pre- and postprogramme and follow-up assessments (to reduce interexaminer disagreement). Spouses and other parties were not permitted to sit in on the tests (to control responses to others). After each assessment had taken place the examiner filed away the form. They were not allowed further access to it (to minimise staff bias resulting from recall). Results were not fed back to patients until after follow-up (to minimise patient bias resulting from recall).

way of formulating a protocol for testing. There are many other permutations, but a number of general considerations should be observed.

Minimise bias in outcome evaluation by using staff unconnected with the treatment

All clinicians want to believe in the effectiveness of their treatment. Patients are aware of this and do not want to 'let them down' by demonstrating no change at the end of treatment. This combination (especially during interviews and physical testing) can lead to biased appraisals of outcome. Appropriate training is required and adherence to the testing protocol must be maintained. In circumstances where it is not possible, the need to control any interaction and standardise measurement procedures becomes even more important. If more than one observer is used to administer the same test in different patients then interrater agreement must be verified.

Check patients' understanding of what is being required

If a patient does not understand the instructions for a test of muscle strength then the resulting measurement is invalid. Similarly, if a patient does not understand the questions in a self-report questionnaire or the instructions for a functional test then the results will be invalid. When subjects' responses to consistent questioning are grossly contradictory, or their written responses contradict their verbal presentation, it is important to confirm that they have understood the question and have answered appropriately. It is sometimes necessary to reiterate the written instructions on how to fill in the questionnaire. This should not extend to overinterpreting the instructions or the question. Occasionally, patients with poor literacy may need to be helped by reading the contents of self-report measures.

Getting stable baseline and outcome measures

It is not always possible to represent adequately a dynamic or changing condition such as chronic pain by a single measurement at one point in time. Twelve measurements of current pain intensity over 4 days are recommended to establish a stable baseline that might represent 'usual' pain levels in patients with chronic pain (Jensen & McFarland 1993). A single rating of current state is likely to be only an approximation of the patient's average or usual state. If possible the tests should be repeated until a representative estimate is obtained. It may be necessary to repeat physical tests to accommodate a learning effect. Intrasession repeated measures are suitable for brief measures such as range-of-movement tests. With time-consuming measures the process can become very laborious and yet may still address variability only within the particular session and not the effect of good or bad days (or weeks or months). Repeating measures over a series of days or weeks is impractical in clinical practice. Alternatively, patients may be invited to rate their average level over a defined period (Jensen 1994). When such solutions are not always feasible, a margin of normal variability should be allowed in the interpretation of the test results. This strategy is addressed in the later section of this chapter on interpreting the results.

Organisation of administrative support

It is unfortunate that many attempts to evaluate outcome falter after the stage of collecting the data. Forms are left to gather dust because of time pressures, lack of computer skills, statistical support or waning interest. If the measures have been of benefit in guiding treatment with individual patients then all the effort in collecting the data will not have gone to waste. However, because the proper administrative support has not been ensured, the opportunity to evaluate the outcome of groups of patients has been missed.

Administrative tasks such as photocopying, handing or sending out questionnaires and collecting them, computerising data, booking in patients for assessment appointments and conducting telephone follow-up surveys are an essential part of outcome evaluation. They do not require the skills of a highly paid clinician. Efficient 'system delivery' is important (Ch. 15). As many of these tasks as possible should be delegated to appropriately trained administrative workers.

The clinical process and points of sample attrition and lost data are shown in Figure 17.5.

Suitability for and enrolment in treatment

Evaluation of outcome requires a knowledge of the patients actually entering treatment, but the patients who actually receive treatment will often be a minority of all the referrals (estimated to be between one - and two-thirds by Turk & Rudy (1990)). They will will been selected non-randomly either by clinical decision making or by choosing themselves whether or not to participate in treatment (Ch. 12). The outcome results will not be generalisable to those who fail to enter treatment. It is important to have answers to the following questions:

1. How many of the patients referred to the centre actually entered the treatment?
2. Why didn't they all receive the treatment?

Four strategies can be used to address these issues:

1. take a sample of consecutive referrals (e.g. 100 or all those in a defined period such as 3 months) and follow them across time to determine how many ended up on the treatment
2. have explicit inclusion and exclusion criteria for the treatment
3. describe in detail the decision-making process
4. record briefly why decisions were made. (These are liable to be soft data such as 'unwilling to jeopardise benefits', 'requires surgical opinion', 'self-managing well' but such can be very informative and used to design more focused clinical pathways (Ch. 12.)

Dropouts

Inevitably some patients will not complete the treatment once it is begun. As in the case above, they are unlikely to be a random subset of all patients entering treatment (Carosella, Lackner & Feuerstein, 1994). If a large proportion drop out the outcome of treatment will be difficult to generalise to anything but a select group. Preventing dropouts is usually preferable to trying to account for them afterwards (Ch. 14). It is not sensible to rely on obtaining postprogramme data from dropouts but it is important to report the reason for dropping out (if known) and to include them in the results as treatment failures (Vignette 17.2).

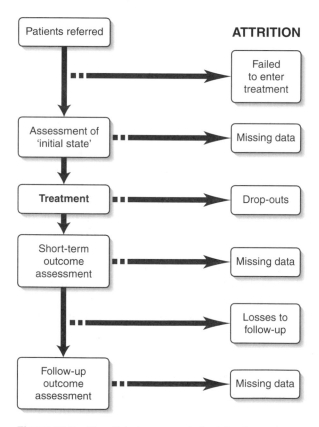

Figure 17.5 The clinical process and points of sample attrition and lost data.

Vignette 17.2

Twenty chronic low back pain patients (out of 227 = 9%) dropped out of the 3-week back pain management programme at MSPC. They gave the following reasons:
— 5 reported being unable to manage the increase in pain owing to increasing activity
— 4 developed acute health problems unrelated to their back pain
— 2 were invited to leave having made little progress and become disruptive
— 1 cited impending marital break-up
— 1 felt unable to cope with the social contact of being in a group
— 1 received a positive scan report on the morning of the pain management programme
— 1 opted to seek treatment elsewhere
— 5 gave no reason.

Effect on short term outcome
Success rate (reduction of 5 or more points on RMDQ) excluding dropouts = 126/207 = 61% Success rate including dropouts as failures = 126/227 = 56%

Losses to follow-up

It is likely that a greater proportion of the patient sample will be lost during the follow-up phase than during treatment. A large proportion of losses (traditionally greater than 20%) threaten the validity of the findings. Different centres appear to have quite different rates of losses to follow-up. Factors behind this variation probably include the length of follow-up, whether the follow-up involves attendance at the centre, distance from centre, perceived importance by staff and patients and action taken to ensure completion. In the course of running pain management programmes at Salford varied reasons have been given for non-attendance including returning to work, childcare commitments, major life events, double-booked appointments and other health problems. Not all losses are likely to be treatment failures but unless there is some evidence to suggest otherwise it is prudent to regard them as such. Their impact on outcome data can be significant, as vignette 17.3 demonstrates.

Strategies to prevent losses to follow-up include:

Vignette 17.3

Out of the 207 patients completing the BPMP, 64 (31%) failed to attend their 6-month follow-up appointment.

Effect on 6-month outcome
Success rate (reduction of 5 or more points on RMDQ) excluding dropouts and losses to follow-up
$$= 87/143 = 61\%$$
Success rate including dropouts and losses to follow-up as failures
$$= 87/227 = 38\%$$

- emphasis on follow-up and long term outcome during initial assessment and at each clinical contact thereafter (includes setting 6-month goals)
- informing patients and families of follow-up dates several months in advance
- regular telephone/postal contact.

Actions to minimise the impact of non-attendance on outcome data include:

- sending postal questionnaires with stamped addressed envelopes
- telephone follow-up including a brief classification of reason for non-attendance
- inviting non-attenders to follow-up dates later in the year.

Postal questionnaires and telephone followups suffer from the disadvantage of being quite highly reactive (i.e. patients' self-report cannot be verified and may therefore be subject to higher levels of inaccurate and biased reporting).

Missing data

Questionnaires not completed, forms that were not handed out, tests that were either not done or recorded can weaken outcome evaluation as much as dropouts or losses to follow-up. Simple check procedures are normally adequate to keep this problem to a minimum.

For an example on how to account for all patients fully in a given cohort the reader is directed to Weir et al's (1994) study flow diagram of pain clinic referrals in which the proportion of missing data and reasons for dropouts and losses are described in detail.

A summary of the above points is given in Box 17.9.

Box 17.9   Mini-summary: follow-up

- Anticipate practical problems associated with when and how to administer measures. One of the most important of these is minimising potential bias in the evaluation process
- Sample attrition due to dropouts, losses to follow-up, and missing data seriously undermine the validity of any outcome. Attempt to prevent this and take measures to minimise the impact of these
- Consider using a flow diagram to show the flow of patients and sample attrition

---

INTERPRETATION OF THE RESULTS

Non-specific reasons for change

It is tempting to attribute any changes observed between pre- and post-treatment to the treatment offered. Changes may, however, be due to a number of alternative factors and may not be attributable specifically to the content of the intervention (Bouchet et al 1996, Turner et al 1994).

Natural variation

Random measurement error and variability in the patients' condition can result in changes in measures. Error in the measurement instrument can result in the statistical artefact known as 'regression to the mean'. Furthermore, the fact that patients often consult when their symptoms are at their worst leads to a probability for their symptoms to improve over time irrespective of treatment. This phenomenon can account for significant changes in chronic pain patients (Whitney & Von Korff 1992).

Hawthorne effect

In the absence of treatment, simply measuring subjects and giving them the attention normally reserved for those receiving treatment can sometimes lead to changes in patient behaviour self-rating (Bouchet et al 1996).

Placebo response

Placebos are interventions designed to simulate medical therapy but not believed to be a specific therapy for the condition (Turner et al 1994). The response can be thought of as a non-specific aspect of treatment. Described as 'an unpopular topic' (Wall 1992) the placebo response is none the less a clinical reality and capable of effecting long-lasting subjective and objective change. Separating 'true' treatment effect from placebo response is particularly difficult when the treatment being discussed is a pain management programme. Disentangling specific from non-specific responses requires careful independently

evaluated RCTs. Clinicians in routine practice should acknowledge that at least part of the treatment response is likely to be unrelated to the specific content of their intervention. It should be recognised none the less as a potentially powerful clinical effect.

Reasons for lack of change

The most obvious reason for a lack of change following treatment is that the treatment was ineffective. Other reasons include the use of measures that are poorly responsive or contain a high degree of random error, and strategic errors in the timing of measurement so that change that occurred went undetected.

Improving the interpretation of single-cohort results

The normal practice of describing pre- and post-treatment means illustrates the changes that occur in the group of patients as a whole following treatment. Statistical tests can tell us whether the differences observed are likely to be due to chance alone. Without control observations the role of non-specific effects on treatment outcome cannot properly be evaluated. Answers to the question as to what proportion of patients made *clinically significant* improvements also requires a controlled comparison of some sort.

Reliability of change indices

A combination of pre- and post-treatment scores, an estimate of the variability in change scores, and the retest reliability coefficient of the measurement instrument cutoffs, can be computed to allow the clinician to estimate the extent to which the observed changes are likely to be a consequence of treatment rather than normal measurement variability (Hageman & Arindell 1993, Jacobson & Truax 1991, Speer 1992). This approach has been used in recent outcome studies of temporomandibular joint (TMJ) pain that did not use a control group (Rudy et al 1995). The results of this approach will be affected by the severity of individuals studied and the standard deviations of their scores (Williams, 1995a).

Defining clinically significant changes

Not all changes following treatment can be regarded as clinically significant—synonymous with qualitative patient improvement (Slater et al 1997). We need to specify the magnitude of change that is detectable and important. From Williams et al (1996) RCT of pain management programmes for chronic pain the following criteria were chosen (McQuay et al 1997, Williams 1995b):

- reduction to non-depressed level from initially depressed, by > 1 standard deviation
- > 50% gain in 10-minute walking distance
- using no analgesic or psychotropic drugs
- received no further treatment for pain.

The advantage of specifying the magnitude of change regarded as important is that it allows us to judge success on an individual basis and state the proportion of cases meeting these criteria. There is as yet no clear agreement on the best method to adopt although concerted efforts have begun to clarify solutions to this problem (Guyatt et al 1998, Slater et al 1997).

Control observations

Even with the above refinements we cannot be confident that the changes that are observed following treatment would not happen anyway. In the absence of appropriate allocation of subjects to control conditions (e.g. waiting list) other approaches must be used to compare what happens when patients do not receive treatment with when they do. One solution is to obtain baseline measures in subjects before treatment (Vignette 17.4).

Of course these measures cannot exclude the possibility of a non-specific effects but most importantly they can clarify the superiority of treatment over control conditions.

Clinically important subgroups

Expressing treatment outcome in sample averages may provide a general impression of change

---

Vignette 17.4

On referral, patients were sent the Distress and Risk Assessment Method questionnaire (Main et al 1992) as part of a patient booklet. Patients then received a multidisciplinary assessment. The measures were repeated again immediately before treatment, after treatment and at 6-month follow-up. The table below shows a comparison of the changes in depression between initial referral and pre- pain management programme (PMP) and between pre- and post-pain management programme for 121 chronic low back pain patients:

	Number of patients significantly depressed
at initial referal	62 out of 121
at pre-PMP assessment	35 out of 121
at post-PMP assessment	18 out of 121

The number of patients classed as significantly depressed halved between initial referral and attending pre-pain management programme assessment. What happened during this time to effect such a change? Patients waited several weeks whilst receiving treatment as usual and then came for a multidisciplinary assessment where a place on the pain management programme was offered (the 'control' condition).

Compare this change with that following the pain management programme. The number of significantly depressed patients is halved again. On the surface, these figures seem to suggest that regression to the mean may account for just as much change as is seen following an intensive programme. However, no measure of *clinically significant change* has been included. Nor have we made it clear over what time period these changes occur. The table below shows what happens when this is done:

	Number of significantly depressed patients who reduce their depression scores by greater than 1sd
Between initial referral and pre-PMP assessment (approx 6 months)	14 out of 62
Between pre- and post-PMP assessment (3 weeks)	25 out of 35

Over a shorter period of time a larger proportion of significantly depressed patients make clinically significant improvements than over the control period. Those whose depression has not reduced by pre- pain management programme assessment may even be more difficult to change than those whose depression has regressed as a function of time, usual management and a multidisciplinary assessment promising further help.

but by amalgamating the results for many patients we may obscure important subgroups who respond very differently to the treatment in question. 'Statistical reductionism' (Feinstein 1996) can hide a basic clinical reality—treatment is not successful for all patients. Combining results into an average does little to answer fundamental questions that are often posed by clinicians and patients alike:

- What is the chance of this treatment working for this individual?
- What kind of patients seem to benefit from this treatment?
- What kind of patients do not do well?
- Is there anything that can be done to improve the likelihood of success?

Vignette 17.5 is a simple example of how amalgamating distinct clinical subgroups can obscure a proper appraisal of treatment outcome:

in a similar way to a programme that is strongly oriented towards returning to independent activities?

Although most approaches to classifying patients have centred around biomedical factors (e.g. International Association for the Study of Pain Subcommittee on Taxonomy 1994), psychosocial, disability and pain severity factors have been most powerful in predicting long term functional limitations (e.g. Dionne et al 1997) and response to several treatments (e.g. Burton et al 1995, Main et al 1992). (The fact that many biomedical factors are crude with low reliability and are of intra- rather than interindividual significance may have contributed to this.) Multidimensional methods of classifying chronic pain patients have been validated across different pain conditions (e.g. Turk & Rudy 1992, Von Korff et al 1992). However, none have demonstrated real predictive value in determining

---

Vignette 17.5

A rehabilitation programme was set up with one of its primary targets to return individuals with chronic upper limb pain to work. After 2 years the outcome data were reviewed. Out of 300 patients, only 90 (30%) had returned to work at 1-year follow-up (an apparently fairly unimpressive result). The cohort, however, contained several distinct groups in whom the likelihood of return to work was markedly different, irrespective of treatment. The patients had included 70 who were retired, homemakers, students, or carers who had no interest in returning to full-time paid employment. Of those remaining, the length of time off work ranged from 3 months to 23 years. Some had their jobs still open, others not. Some were not in work because of non-pain-related issues or illness. The results were analysed again this time excluding

the retired, homemakers, students and carers. The results were:

	Return-to-work rate
out of work < 6 months	40 out of 50 (80%)
out of work 6–12 months	40 out of 80 (50%)
out of work > 12 months	10 out of 100 (10%)

There was a relationship between length of time out of work and return to work following treatment. By showing the results *after* stratifying for this prognostic variable (rather than combining the whole sample) a much clearer picture emerges of the likelihood of return to work for different types of patients. The implications for selecting patients for treatment and identifying those who may require alternative or additional management approaches are clarified.

Unfortunately, the issues that typically confound the interpretation of treatment outcome are rarely so straightforward. What do average changes in distress tell us about our effectiveness when some patients begin the treatment very severely depressed whereas in others it is only mild? What about two patients with comparably high levels of depression, one of whose is mainly in response to the loss of recreational activities and the other to a lack of social support? Do we expect them to respond

success (or failure) from pain management or emerged as clinically useful tools in patient selection and treatment formulation.

In the absence of accepted classifications the presence of clinically pertinent subgroups and the weaknesses in presenting simple averages to represent treatment outcome should be recognised. The use of individual and discrete criteria for successful outcome is an important step that all clinicians can take to forming hypotheses on who benefits from their treatment.

Box 17.10 Mini-summary: Patient subgroups

- The specific effect of treatment is only one possible cause of change seen when evaluating outcome. Others include natural variation, regression to the mean, the Hawthorne effect, and placebo response
- Only well-controlled trials can fully disentangle these elements. Routine prepost outcome evaluation can be clarified by using reliability of change indices, defining criteria for clinically significant change, and using available control circumstances (e.g. using patients as their own control while waiting for treatment)
- Expressing mean outcomes for groups of patients may obscure differences in response to treatment between clinically important subgroups

---

The focus in this section has been on patients. One final point should be remembered when considering clinically important subgroups and response to treatment: patient characteristics are important but the reasons for failed treatment are not found exclusively in the patient. Clinicians' skills, the appropriateness of treatment content, the timeliness and manner of its delivery, and the support of others can make the difference between success and failure. (These factors are discussed in detail earlier in the book.)

A summary of the above points is given in Box 17.10.

CONCLUSION

Careful evaluation of outcome is essential to pain management. Evaluation is important not only in negotiating about funding but also in maintaining or improving clinical standards in the light of evidence-based medicine. The identification of key stakeholders and selection of appropriate outcome variables are distinct but related tasks. Whatever the outcome, or outcomes, there are important measurement parameters to be considered. Information must be gathered in such a way as to enable the most accurate assessment to be undertaken. A variety of methods may be considered to be appropriate. The measurement instrument must be able to differentiate the population at initial presentation and be sensitive to change. The timing of assessment also is critical if an accurate appraisal of treatment outcome is to be obtained. A number of suggestions about how to minimise measurement error have been made. From the methodological point of view, missing data are a considerable problem and every effort must be made to minimise this. Careful attention also must be paid to patient attrition or 'drop-out' (whether during treatment or at follow-up) as missing information can compromise significantly both the accuracy of evaluation and the generalisability of the results. In evaluation of outcome, alternative explanations for treatment change (or lack of it) must also be considered. Post-hoc treatment subgroup analyses may be illuminating in this regard since clinically important subgroups, hitherto unrecognised, may become apparent.

KEY POINTS

- Be aware of the 'best evidence' studies in your field.
- Know that your subjective impressions can be misleading when judging the effectiveness of your treatment.
- Adopt a systematic and comprehensive approach to evaluating outcome in routine clinical practice.

- Before choosing outcome measures 'start at the end'—who's going to use the results and for what purposes?
- When deciding what to measure, be pragmatic: it is impossible and probably undesirable to cover all the areas of patient change that may be of interest; match outcome measurement with the

KEY POINTS (Cont'd)

primary objectives of your treatment (the minimum should include disability and distress); beware of playing the substitute game; consider using composite scores and patient-preference approaches.

- When deciding what measurement instruments to use: do not try to 'reinvent the wheel', there are likely to be enough existing measures to meet your needs; read around and consult your peers; strike a balance between self-report and other less reactive measurement approaches such as physical tests, behavioural observation, or blind third party ratings; don't expect to take a measure 'off the shelf' and administer it indiscriminately.

- When designing the framework: allow for at least 6- to 12-month follow-up; build into the system ways of preventing,

accounting for, or obtaining outcome data from dropouts and losses to follow-up.

- When administering measures: control the testing environment; be consistent in how tests are administered (consider the use of standard protocols); delegate clerical tasks where possible.

- When interpreting the results: acknowledge non-specific reasons for patient change; consider using reliable change indices, defining criteria for clinically significant changes, patient preference, and obtaining pseudocontrol measurements; know that expressing results in average scores for the entire group may mask important differences in response between separate subgroups.

- Use the results to inform clinical practice and improve services for patients and their families.

REFERENCES

Bergner M, Bobbitt R A, Carter W B, Gibson B S 1981 The Sickness Impact Profile: development and final revision of a health status measure. Medical Care 19:787–805

Bouchet C, Guillemin F, Briancon S 1996 Nonspecific effects in longitudinal studies: impact on quality of life measures. Journal of Clinical Epidemiology 49:15–20

Burton A K, Tillotson K M, Main C J, Hollis S 1995 Psychosocial predictors of outcome in acute and subchronic low back trouble. Spine 20:772–728

Carosella A M, Lackner J M, Feuerstein M 1994 Factors associated with early discharge from a multidisciplinary work rehabilitation program for chronic low back pain. Pain 57:69–76

Cherkin D C, Deyo R A, Street J H, Hunt M, Barlow W 1996 Pitfalls of patient education. Limited success of a program for back pain in primary care. Spine 21:345–355

Dionne C E, Koepsell T D, Von Korff M, Deyo R A, Barlow W E, Checkoway H 1997 Predicting long-term functional limitations among back pain patients in primary care settings. Journal of Clinical Epidemiology 50:31–43

Ensink F-B M, Saur P M M, Frese K, Seeger D, Hildebrandt J 1996 Lumbar range of motion: influence of time of day and individual factors on measurements. Spine 21:1339–1343

Fairbank J C T, Couper J, Davies J B, O'Brien J P 1980 The Oswestry Low Back Pain Disability Questionnaire. Physiotherapy 66:271–273

Feinstein A R 1989 Models, methods, and goals. Journal of Clinical Epidemiology 42(4):301–308

Feinstein A R 1996 Two centuries of conflict-collaboration between medicine and mathematics. Journal of Clinical Epidemiology 49:1339–1343

Fitzpatrick R, Davey C, Buxton M J, Jones D R 1998 Evaluating patient-based outcome measures for use in clinical trials. Health Technology Assessment 2(14)

Flor H, Turk D C 1988 Chronic back pain and rheumatoid arthritis: predicting pain and disability from cognitive variables. Journal of Behavioral Medicine 11:251–265

Flor H, Fydrich T, Turk D C 1992 Efficacy of multidisciplinary pain treatment centers: a meta-analytic review. Pain 49:221–230

Guyatt G H, Pugsley S O, Sullivan M J et al 1984 Effect of encouragement on walking test performance. Thorax 39:818–822

Guyatt G H, Kirschner B, Jaeschke R 1992 Measuring health status: what are the necessary measurement properties? Journal of Clinical Epidemiology 45:1341–1345

Guyatt G H, Juniper E F, Walter S D, Griffith L E, Goldstein R S 1998 Interpreting treatment effects in randomised trials. British Medical Journal 316:690–693

Hageman W J M, Arindell W A 1993 A further refinement of the reliable change (RC) index by improving the pre-post difference score: introducing RC-ID. Behavior Research Therapy 31:693–700

Harding V R, Williams A C de C, Richardson P H et al 1994 The development of a battery of measures for assessing physical functioning of chronic pain patients. Pain 58:367–375

International Association for the Study of Pain. Task Force on Taxonomy (Merskey H, Bogduk N eds) 1994 Classification of chronic pain. Descriptions of chronic pain syndromes and definitions of pain terms, 2nd edn. IASP, Seattle

Jacobson N S, Truax P 1991 Clinical significance: a statistical approach to defining meaningful change in psychotherapy research. Journal of Consulting and Clinical Psychology 59:12–19

Jensen M P 1994 Reply to Drs Dworkin and Siegfried: Hopefully, all those ratings are not necessary [letter]. Pain 58:279–280

Jensen M P 1997 Validity of self-report and observation measures. In: Jensen T S, Turner J A, Wiesenfield-Hallin Z (eds) Proceedings of the 8th world congress on pain, progress in pain management, vol 8. IASP, Seattle, pp 637–661

Jensen M P, McFarland C A 1993 Increasing the reliability and validity of pain intensity measurement in chronic pain patients. Pain 55:195–203

Kazdin A E 1982 Single case research designs, 1st edn. Oxford University Press, Oxford

Kazis LE, Anderson JJ, Meenan RF 1989 Effect sizes for interpreting changes in health status. Medical Care 27 Supplement 3: 5178-5189

Kerns R D, Turk D C, Rudy T E 1985 The West Haven–Yale Multidimensional Pain Inventory (WHYMPI). Pain 23:345–356

Kori S H, Miller R P, Todd D D 1990 Kinisophobia: a new view of chronic pain behavior. Pain Management Jan/Feb:35–43

Law M, Baptiste S, McColl M A, Opzoomer A, Polatajko H, Pollock N 1990 The Canadian Occupational Performance Measure: an outcome measure for occupational therapy. Canadian Journal of Occupational Therapy 15:82–87

Levine F M, De Simone L L 1991 The effects of experimenter gender on pain report in male and female subjects. Pain 44:69–72

Liang M H, Fossel A H, Larson M G 1990 Comparison of five health status instruments for orthopedic evaluation. Medical Care 28:632–642

McQuay H, Moore A 1998 An evidence-based resource for pain relief, 1st edn. Oxford University Press, Oxford

McQuay H J, Moore R A, Eccleston C, Morley S, de C Williams A C, 1997 Systematic review of outpatient services for chronic pain control. Health Technology Assessment 1(6).

Main C J, Waddell G 1991 A comparison of cognitive measures in low back pain: statistical structure and clinical validity at initial assessment. Pain 46:287–298

Main C J, Wood P L R, Hollis S, Spanswick C C, Waddell G 1992 The Distress and Risk Assessment Method. A simple patient classification to identify distress and evaluate the risk of poor outcome. Spine 17:42–51

Matheson L, Mooney V, Caiozzi V et al 1992 Effect of instructions on isokinetic trunk strength testing variability, reliability, absolute value, and predictive validity. Spine 17:914–921

Melzack R 1987 The Short-Form McGill Pain Questionnaire. Pain 30:191–197

Melzack R, Wall P D 1996 The challenge of pain, updated 2nd edn. Penguin, London

Morley S, Eccleston C, Williams A 1999 Systematic review and meta-analysis of randomised controlled trials of cognitive behaviour therapy and behaviour therapy for chronic pain in adults excluding headache. Pain 80: 1-13

Nicholas M K 1989 Self-efficacy and chronic pain. Paper presented to the annual conference for the British Psychological Society. St Andrews

Paulsen J S, Altmaier E M 1995 The effects of perceived versus enacted social support on the discriminative cue function of spouses for pain behaviors. Pain 60:103–110

Peat G M 1998 Functional limitation in chronic low back pain. Thesis submitted to the University of Manchester for the Degree of Doctor of Philosophy

Price C M, Prosser A 1998 Outcome assessments in pain clinics. Poster presented to the Pain Society annual scientific meeting, Leicester, 22–24 April

Roland M, Morris R 1983 A study in the natural history of back pain. Part I: development of a reliable and sensitive measure of disability in low-back pain. Spine 8:141–144

Rudy T E, Turk D C, Kubinski J A, Zaki H S 1995 Differential treatment responses of TMD patients as a function of psychological characteristics. Pain 61:103–112

Sackett D L, Rosenborg W M C, Gray J A M, Haynes R B, Richardson W S 1996 Evidence-based medicine: what it is and what it isn't. British Medical Journal 312:71–72

Slater M A, Doctor J N, Pruitt S D, Atkinson J H 1997 The clinical significance of behavioral treatment for chronic low back pain: an evaluation of effectiveness. Pain 71:257–263

Speer D C 1992 Clinically significant change: Jacobson and Truax (1991) revisited. Journal of Consulting and Clinical Psychology 60:402–408

Stratford P W, Binkley J M, Riddle D L 1996 Health status measures: strategies and analytic methods for assessing change scores. Physical Therapy 76:1109–1123

Testa M A, Simonson D C 1996 Assessment of quality-of-life outcomes. New England Journal of Medicine 334:835–840

Turk D C, Rudy T E 1990 Neglected factors in chronic pain treatment outcome studies—referral patterns, failure to enter treatment, and attrition. Pain 43:7–25

Turk D C, Rudy T E 1992 Classification logic and strategies in chronic pain. In: Turk D C, Melzack R (eds) Handbook of pain assessment. Guildford, New York, pp 409–428

Turk D C, Rudy T E, Sorkin B A 1993 Neglected topics in pain treatment outcome studies: determination of success. Pain 53:3–16

Turner J A, Deyo R A, Loeser J D, Von Korff M, Fordyce W E 1994 The importance of placebo effects in pain management and research. Journal of the American Medical Association 271:1609–1614

Von Korff M, Ormel J, Keefe F J, Dworkin S F 1992 Grading the severity of chronic pain. Pain 50:133–149

Waddell G, Newton M, Henderson I, Somerville D, Main C J 1993 A Fear-Avoidance Beliefs Questionnaire (FABQ) and the role of fear-avoidance beliefs in chronic low back pain and disability. Pain 52:157–168

Wall P D 1992 The placebo effect: an unpopular topic. Pain 51:1–3

Ware J E Jr, Sherbourne C D 1992 The MOS 36-Item Short-Form Health Survey (SF-36). I. Conceptual framework and item selection. Medical Care 30:473–481

Weir R, Browne G, Roberts J, Tunks E, Gafni A 1994 The Meaning of Illness Questionnaire: further evidence for its reliability and validity. Pain 58:377–386

Whitney C W, Von Korff M 1992 Regression to the mean in treated versus untreated chronic pain. Pain 50:281–285

Williams A C de C 1995a Pain measurement in chronic pain management. Pain Reviews 2:39–63

Williams A C de C 1995b NNTs used in decision-making in chronic pain management. Bandolier 22

Williams A C de C, Richardson P H, Nicholas M K et al 1996 Inpatient vs. outpatient pain management: results of a randomised controlled trial. Pain 66:13–22

APPENDIX: SOME QUESTIONS ABOUT YOUR TREATMENT OUTCOMES

What kind of patients do your results apply to?
— description of patient characteristics
— selection procedures

What exactly was your treatment?
— description of content
— consistency of delivery

What are the changes seen following treatment?
— have all the important outcomes been measured?
— are the measures biased in any way?
   reactive measures
   sample attrition due to dropouts, losses to follow-up, missing data

Are the changes *clinically* significant?
— how was success defined?

— is treatment better than:
   doing nothing?
   just monitoring and measuring?
   placebo?
   plausible alternative treatment?

Are the changes maintained? Over how long?
— what is the rate of relapse?

Do improvements in measurements transfer to everyday activity?

What are the harmful effects of treatment? How often do they occur?

Are there significant differences in outcome between different types of patient?

Are the changes worth the costs?

New directions in pain management

There is considerable international effort currently directed at trying to *prevent* the human and economic costs of chronic pain-associated disability. In Chapter 18, psychosocial assessment and early behavioural interventions stimulated by the New Zealand 'yellow flag' initiative are discussed. The chapter specifically addresses identification of patients 'at risk', and the nature of communication, and offers advice about management of the angry and distressed patient in health-care settings. In Chapter 19, the relevance of the principles of pain management to work rehabilitation and work retention are considered. The importance of recognising 'psychosocial hazards' as potential obstacles to recovery is highlighted and consideration is given as to how to develop programmes that blend removal of clinical obstacles to recovery (yellow flags) with reduction in perceived obstacles to work (blue flags). Finally, in Chapter 20, obstacles to recovery are considered both in terms of facets of assessment and in those of how they are addressed in clinical practice.

18

Wider applications of the principles of pain management in health-care settings

Chris J. Main   Chris C. Spanswick Paul Watson

INTRODUCTION

In earlier chapters the theoretical bases and the nature of interdisciplinary pain management have been outlined. As discussed in Chapter 6, the move towards pain management was spurred in part by the recognition that a new approach was needed to the management of chronic pain and disability. The skills and applications of pain management have been developed from and refined principally on chronic pain patients and led to the development of the biopsychosocial model of illness. The purpose of this chapter is to consider biopsychosocial management of patients in other health-care contexts and settings.

CHRONIC PAIN MANAGED IN OTHER HEALTH-CARE SITUATIONS

Although there are a significant number of referrals to pain clinics from both GPs and other hospital specialists, most patients suffering from persistent or chronic pain are referred in the first instance to other medical or surgical departments for diagnostic clarification or treatment. In addition it is well known that persistent pain is a common presentation for many chronic diseases. The management of pain is therefore an important part of the management of many clinical conditions treated within the health-care system. Although pain management programmes have been devised for patients with specific clinical syndromes such as osteoarthritis or rheumatoid arthritis, most of the focus on pain control in these situations is aimed primarily at either disease control or symptomatic relief. Indeed the management of the disease process may often be the best treatment option for treating the pain in many clinical situations. Even if the disease process cannot be halted then often controlling the disease will afford significant symptomatic relief. Pure symptom control alone is not usually considered unless disease management is not possible. If pain is severe then symptom control measures may often be instituted at the same time as diagnostic procedures or disease control measures are started. This is done with the expectation that as control of the disease process is gained the need for symptom (pain) control will diminish or disappear.

The management of chronic pain in settings other than a pain management centre is therefore aimed at treatment of disease processes or pharmacological management of pain. Commonly there are little or no resources allocated to helping patients to manage their own pain and its consequences. In specialties (e.g. diabetes, asthma) that manage chronic diseases some resources are often allocated to helping patients manage their own problems. In the UK this has historically been with the use of nurses. It has led to extension of the role of nurses in such cases, often allowing them to be responsible for patient education and to prescribe within certain limits usually driven by protocols of management. Much of the care aimed at helping patients to come to terms with their health-care problems, disease and pain is reliant upon self-help groups. These are often led by patients themselves, albeit with support from the medical, nursing and other health-care professions.

Although all of the above is entirely appropriate it does not address patients' adjustment or maladjustment to their pain problems. At best if there appear to be major problems of adjustment then education is often all that is offered. As the reader will be aware, patients' adjustment to their pain influences their pain experience and perception of their symptoms. Therefore if attention is paid to patients' ability to cope with and manage their pain then other treatments in terms

of either disease control measures or symptomatic relief may become much more effective in this group. It is for this reason that many of the pain management techniques discussed in this book apply to everyday clinical practice, especially with patients with chronic disorders that give rise to persistent pain.

THE NATURE OF THE PROBLEM PATIENT IN EVERYDAY CLINICAL PRACTICE

A number of guidelines have recently been produced for the management of patients in primary care settings. In the UK guidelines (RCGP 1996) the aforementioned diagnostic triage was accompanied by a series of recommendations concerning management with an appraisal of the strength of scientific evidence supporting a range of frequent therapeutic approaches such as drug therapy, bed rest, advice on staying active, manipulation and back exercises. Key to the management of simple backache was the giving of positive messages such as:

- there is nothing to worry about; backache is very common
- no sign of serious damage or disease; full recovery in days or weeks—but may vary
- no permanent weakness; recurrence possible—but does not mean reinjury
- activity is helpful; too much rest is not— hurting does not mean harm.

(Slightly different messages were suggested for patients with nerve root pain and possible spinal pathology.) The overall philosophy of the guidelines is clear.

As far as the actual implementation of the guidelines was concerned, it was recommended that multiple methods might be necessary. As part of the initiative, however, an evidence-based booklet was developed that could be given at the time of consultation. The Back Book (Roland et al 1996) has now been evaluated, incorporated in several research trials and translated into several languages. The booklet appears to be a useful adjunct to management of acute back pain for the majority of patients with self-limiting pain problems, who are easy to deal with and do not make extra demands upon doctors' and therapists' time and resources. In fact, most patients with chronic conditions that are painful (e.g. osteoarthritis) appear to come to terms with their pain and associated disability. They are relatively undemanding of their health-care professionals and use health-care resources to maintain the best quality of life they can within the bounds of their disease.

There appears to be a large variability in the use of health-care services in patients with similar clinical problems. A small proportion makes considerable use of health-care resources and seems much less able to cope with pain and disability. Such patients frequently present with what has commonly been called 'functional overlay'. This type of presentation is not simply a consequence of the passage of time, although it may get worse as time goes by. The patients may develop 'problems' early on in the history of their pain and may become 'chronic' in less than the statutory 3 or 6 months. They are commonly very passive and demanding, expecting treatment to be 'done' to them. They often believe that if their pain problems can be sorted out then all of their other problems will immediately resolve.

Clearly this group of patients requires a different style of management. The standard medical model of managing these patients not only does not seem to help, but may even be counterproductive. For example, escalating doses of medication or repeated sessions of physiotherapy are rarely of use.

Although it would seem that a pain management programme might be the best form of treatment for such patients, in practice such programmes are uncommon and some patients may well not be suitable for a group programme (Ch. 12). Pragmatics dictate that many such patients will have to be 'managed' by individual doctors/therapists in either primary or secondary care. In our view the principles of biopsychosocial management are equally appropriate for primary care settings. Later in this chapter there are guidelines as to how such patients may be managed by individual professionals in their own practice.

THE MOVE TO SECONDARY PREVENTION

Increasing costs of sick certification for musculoskeletal symptoms in general, and low back pain in particular, stimulated the search for new solutions to the problem of low back disability, with a particular focus of prevention of unnecessary incapacity and a redirection of effort on early management. There is serious damage or structural damage in only a small minority of patients presenting with back pain in primary care. Although it is clearly important to identify patients requiring an urgent specialist opinion, most patients do not, and therefore management delivered primarily in secondary or tertiary care settings is not only expensive and inefficient but also inappropriate. Waddell (1982) recommended an assessment strategy in the form of an initial diagnostic triage for patients presenting with back pain. This triage separated patients into simple back pain, nerve root pain or serious spinal pathology. The signs and symptoms considered to be indicative of possible spinal pathology or of the need for an urgent surgical evaluation became known as 'red flags'. These 'risk factors' for serious pathology or disease became incorporated into screening tools recommended for use in primary care by clinicians to identify those patients in whom an urgent specialist opinion was indicated. Assessment of these risk factors were included within a new set of clinical guidelines for the management of acute low back pain in the UK (CSAG 1994) and in the USA (Bigos et al 1994).

THE YELLOW FLAGS INITIATIVE

As mentioned in earlier chapters in this book, however, it is clear that chronic disability is multifactorial. Studies into predictors of outcome of treatment, and particularly into the development of chronic incapacity, have highlighted the powerful influence of psychosocial factors. These also can be conceptualised as 'flags' or risk factors. The earlier management guidelines had recommended biopsychosocial assessment once the patient had been symptomatic for 6 weeks (and indeed a similar recommendation in fact was included in the IASP Back pain in the workplace report (Fordyce 1995)) but there was little attention about how this might be delivered from a 'system' point of view. The need for a more systematic approach was recognised in New Zealand, where increasing costs of chronic non-specific low back pain became an unmanageable burden. This stimulated a new initiative designed to complement a slightly modified set of acute back pain management guidelines with a psychosocial assessment system systematically addressing the psychosocial risk factors that had been shown in the scientific literature to be predictive of chronicity (Kendall, Linton & Main 1997).

The stated purpose of assessment of yellow flags were to:

• provide a method for screening for psychosocial factors
• provide a systematic approach to assessing psychosocial factors
• suggest strategies for better management for those with back pain who appear at a higher risk of chronicity
• focus particularly on a number of key psychological factors:
  — presence of a belief that back pain is harmful or severely disabling
  — fear-avoidance behaviour patterns with reduced activity levels
  — tendency to low mood and withdrawal from social interaction
  — expectation that passive treatments rather than active participation will help.

A number of assessment strategies were recommended depending on the resources available for assessment and the clinical competence of the staff in question: structured interview prompts, a detailed guideline to clinical assessment and a screening questionnaire. They were supplemented by a guide to behavioural management. The details of these are as follows.

A Structured interview prompts (to be phrased in the assessor's own words)

• Have you had time off work in the past with back pain?
• What do you understand is the cause of your back pain?
• What are you expecting will help you?
• How are others responding to your back pain (employer, coworkers and family)?
• What are you doing to cope with back pain?
• Do you think that you will ever return to work? When?

B Detailed guideline to clinical assessment

Fuller details are given in Kendall, Linton & Main 1997 (reproduced in Waddell 1998, p. 327). The main headings are as follows.

• attitudes and beliefs about back pain
• behaviours
• compensation issues
• diagnosis and treatment
• emotions
• family
• work.

(Each of these topics has been covered in detail in earlier chapters of this book.)

C Screening questionnaire

For large scale screening, or in situations where it was neither possible nor practical to carry out the sort of clinical evaluation described above, the authors recommend the use of the Linton & Halden (1997) 24-item screening questionnaire. In their preliminary cross-validation of the questionnaire in New Zealand, Kendall, Linton & Main (1997) recommended a cut-off score of 105, which they state, produces:

• 75% correct identification of those not needing modification to ongoing management
• 86% correct identification of those who will have between 1 and 30 days off work
• 83% correct identification of those who will have more than 30 days of work.

The authors recognised the three main consequences of back problems in terms of:

- pain
- disability and limitations in function in daily living
- reduced productivity including work loss.

D   Guide to behavioural management

The guide comprises a set of 12 management guidelines to help somebody 'at risk'. They are shown in Box 18.1.

The authors finally recommend that if the problem is too complex to manage then referral should be made to a multidisciplinary team.

Overview of the yellow flags initiative

It should be noted firstly that the yellow flags (Ch. 4, p. 80) were essentially a guide to case management and were developed not only from a clinical perspective but also from an occupational perspective (and consisted of both psychological and socio-occupational risk factors). They were 'evidence based' in that their content was derived from research literature into the nature of chronicity. The suggestions regarding behavioural management relied heavily on the cognitive–behavioural approach found to be effective in pain management, and the change in emphasis from passive to active involvement in treatment derived from evidence-based medicine.

Since they were published, there has been a massive interest in early psychosocial intervention. The yellow flags initiative was an important first step (and indeed is already under revision) in the prevention of unnecessary chronicity. It was developed as an answer to a 'system' problem in a particular setting. Despite its considerable promise therefore further empirical work is needed into:

- the statistical construction and validation of screening strategies
- refinement of cognitive–behavioural management strategies appropriate for different contexts
- assessment of competencies in delivering psychosocial interventions.

IDENTIFYING THE 'AT RISK' PATIENT

The previous discussion addressed the use of screening tools to identify groups of patients with potential problems that require the allocation of specific resources, such as within a case-management system or where clinical services are organised centrally over a geographical area. Clinicians working independently, however, usually will be unlikely to have much (if any) information at their disposal prior to the

---

Box 18.1   Suggested steps to better early behavioural management of low back pain problems

1. Provide a *positive* expectation that the individual will return to work
2. Be directive in regularly scheduling reviews of progress
3. Keep the individual active and at work if at all possible
4. Acknowledge difficulties with activities of daily living, but avoid assuming that these indicate that *all* activities should be avoided
5. Help maintain *positive* cooperation between the individual, an employer, the compensation system and health-care professionals
6. Try to communicate that time off work reduces the likelihood of a successful return to work
7. Watch out for inappropriate beliefs that the individual should remain off work until totally pain free; also watch out for expectations of simple 'techno-fixes'
8. Promote self-management and self-responsibility
9. Be prepared to ask for a second opinion, provided this doesn't lead to prolonged interruption to management plan. Be prepared to say 'I don't know' rather than speculate
10. Avoid confusing reporting of symptoms with presence of emotional distress
11. Avoid suggesting working at home as a preferred option
12. Encourage people to recognise that pain can be controlled and managed

Adapted from Kendall, Linton & Main 1997 Guide to assessing psychosocial yellow flags in acute low back pain, with permission.

consultation. In such situations clinicians will need to use the principles outlined above to identify the important issues and then spend time specifically addressing them.

In reviewing the history of many patients presenting at the pain centre it has become clear that many of the 'chronic pain' patients developed substantial problems very early on. There is research evidence to show that patients who show high levels of distress early on in acute back pain are more likely to remain disabled at 12 months (Burton et al 1995). It would seem probable that had this group of patients been treated and handled in a different way at an early stage they may not have become so problematic later. Indeed, as has been mentioned in previous chapters, the subject of risks for chronicity was discussed in detail in terms of obstacles to recovery in Chapter 4. In considering a management strategy, it may be helpful to consider risk factors from a slightly different viewpoint.

Box 18.2 illustrates a number of different variables that may influence the patient's progress. Some of these factors are primarily patient characteristics and are dependent upon the patient's beliefs and attitudes. Some reflect outside influences and others are clearly dependent upon the skills and attitudes of the clinician. The later factors are dealt with in the next section of this chapter.

Without the aid of any additional information gained by questionnaire the clinician must make specific enquiries about aspects of the patient's pain and its consequences, both in terms of everyday impact and also in those of the emotional consequences. It can at times be difficult to disentangle different aspects of the patient's presenting symptomatology.

If a substantial number of the above factors are identified then it is important to initiate a treatment plan at the earliest opportunity, otherwise the patient may drift into unnecessary disability. Any intervention strategy must be derived from a set of underlying principles and informed by clear and focused assessment.

DOES EARLY INTERVENTION WORK?

There is very little systematic work on early intervention, not least because of the practical problems in arranging systematic intervention at an early stage. However, a recent prospective randomised controlled trial of CBT versus two different types of information has produced some promising results. In the study (Linton & Andersson in press), CBT led to significantly less back-pain-associated work loss than either an information package based on a back school approach or an educational leaflet (Symonds et al 1995). The results are shown in Figure 18.1.

Recent research has shown that psychosocial factors are important predictors of those who develop chronic incapacity. It is essential therefore to enquire about the psychosocial aspects of the patient's pain problem as well as to perform an

---

Box 18.2 Risk factors for developing chronic pain-associated disability problems

1. Patient characteristics
- Misunderstandings re causation ('hurt = harm')
- High levels of distress at the onset of an acute pain problem
- Catastrophising (fearing the worst)
- External locus of control (passive, expecting others to cure problem)
- Doctor and treatment shopping
- Substantial anger (at initiating cause, pain itself and medical profession)
- Fear avoidance of pain and activity

2. Outside influences
- Work, benefits
- Compensation/litigation
- Family reinforcement of illness

3. Doctor/therapist dependent
- Unclear diagnosis or mixed messages from different doctors/therapists
- Unclear explanation of pain
- Inadequate assessment or examination
- Unrealistically optimistic promises of outcome
- Reinforcing passivity of patient
- Reliance only on medication or rapid referral

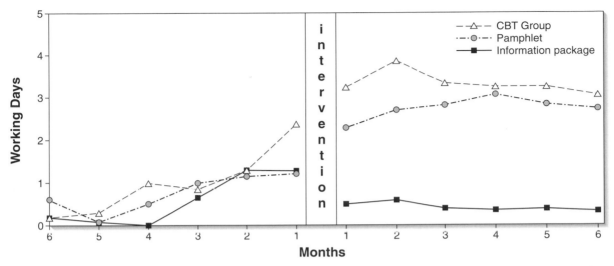

Figure 18.1   From Linton, Ryberg & Wahlstrom General principles of individual pain management in primary and secondary health-care settings, reproduced with permission.

adequate biomedical assessment. A number of recent publications have addressed the subject of miscommunications between doctors and patients (Chew-Graham 1999; Chew-Graham & May 1999). The latter identified not only a wide range of beliefs about back pain in patients attending their GP (perhaps to be expected), but also a wide variation amongst GPs themselves. However adequate assessment cannot be achieved without good communication between the doctor/therapist and the patient. The social psychology of communication has been addressed elsewhere in this book (Chs 3 and 5), but it is relevant to revisit some of the major points at this juncture in terms of the specific implications for clinical management.

Communication styles and strategies

The essence of good communication is the ability to be able to understand patients' problems from their perspective. In order to do this the doctor/therapist must gain the patient's confidence. The patient has to be convinced that the doctor/therapist takes the patient's pain seriously. Only then will patients be willing to give credence to what the doctor/therapist says to them. The converse is perhaps even more true—that is, if patients feel that the doctor/therapist is dismissive

---

Box 18.3   Important elements of communication

- Develop and apply competent listening skills
- Carefully observe the patient's behaviour
- Attend not only to *what* is said but also *how* it is said
- Attempt to understand how the patient feels
- Offer encouragement to disclose fears and feelings
- Offer reassurance that you accept the 'reality' of the patient's pain
- Correct misunderstandings or miscommunications about the consultation
- Offer appropriate challenge to negative thoughts (such as catastrophising)
- Appraise the general social and economic circumstances
- Include assessment and involvement of partner/significant other where possible

---

or not taking their pain seriously they will not be prepared to reveal sensitive information nor actively comply with treatment suggestions.

The social psychology of communication was addressed in detail in Chapter 3. A number of practical guidelines for managing the communication process are shown in Box 18.3.

In establishing a competent appraisal of a patient, the first and most important principle is to suspend judgement until all facets of the patient's difficulties have been appraised. Clinical decision making is subject to bias (Ch. 12). All clinicians are potentially subject to their own biases, which can cloud clinical judgement. They should be prepared to give the patient the benefit of the doubt and listen.

Listening skills are vital. Simply allowing patients to explain how they feel and ask questions will have a profoundly beneficial effect. Predicting what the impact of the pain may be will reinforce to patients that doctors or therapists are not out of their depth but understand their problem. This will help to establish the confidence of patients. The clinician should also check the patients' own beliefs about their pain and its causation, correcting any misconceptions at the time if necessary. A number of strategies to assist the development of an appropriate style of communication are presented in Box 18.4.

Doctors need to explain the complexity of chronic pain problems and the impact of pain. They should give reasons for enquiring not only about the pain but also what this has done to patients and how they have been coping with it. They need to observe carefully what patients say and how they say it.

It is important to empathise without colluding. It needs to be explained that the pain is real. One should also check whether others (including doctors and therapists) have implied the pain is imaginary, by enquiring what the patient has been told about the cause of their pain by others. The clinician needs to find out what treatments have been recommended or what they have been told to do or not do. It may be necessary to correct a number of misconceptions. Many patients are confused as they have received differing explanations from different professionals. It may be necessary to defuse significant anger about previous assessments and treatments. The clinician should explain potential treatment options with the expected outcome, and explain what cannot be done and why.

Enquiry about sensitive information (e.g. use of alcohol or misuse of medication) will need to be approached in a way that 'allows' the patient to disclose such information without feeling threatened (see Chs 7 to 10). Judgemental statements, questioning or even body language will not be helpful and are unlikely to reveal the truth, as the patient is then likely to become defensive.

In conclusion, the clinician should make specific enquiry about their pain: its nature, effects and how patients are coping with and managing their pain. It is helpful to predict how the pain may affect their mood (irritability, depression and anxiety), sleep, work and relationships with others. Finally, it needs to be explained that this is normal and seen in most patients with persistent pain.

Dealing with distress

Patients frequently show evidence of distress. Given the fact that most patients present primarily with the same symptom (i.e. pain), it is perhaps surprising to find that pain patients differ not only in the intensity of their distress, but also in precisely what they are distressed about. It is very important to establish clearly the specific nature of their distress. This should be appraised systematically and a distress profile obtained, which identifies the key features of their distress. It may be helpful to address the issue under the headings shown in Box 18.5.

Box 18.4 Style of communication

- Suspend judgement
- Listen and observe
- Be empathic but not collusive
- Encourage self-disclosure
- Explain what you can do
- Explain what you cannot do
- Re-establish confidence
- 'Kick-start' self-control

Box 18.5 Establishing the distress profile

- Pain
- Limitations in activity
- Sleep
- Quality of life
- Work
- Previous treatments

Box 18.6 Key strategies for the assessment and management of pain-associated distress and anger

- Give patients time
- Signal that it is permitted to be upset
- Find out gently the particular focus of their concern
- Find out *why* they are telling you
- Distinguish *pain-and disability-associated* distress from more general distress
- Identify iatrogenic *misunderstandings*
- Identify mistaken beliefs and fears
- Try to correct misunderstandings
- Identify iatrogenic *distress and anger*
- Listen and empathise
- Do not get angry yourself
- Decide what *you* can deal with and what requires someone else
- Be open about this with them
- If appropriate, offer to help them enlist additional assistance

In initiating the discussion, it may be helpful to adopt a somewhat indirect approach. Thus, rather than asking whether the patient feels depressed, for example, it may be less threatening to observe that many patients with chronic pain feel helpless and find their mood drifts down and then to enquire whether this has happened to them. Thus patients are 'permitted' to disclose feelings that they may feel very sensitive about. It enables the doctor or therapist to gain a more realistic understanding of the impact of the pain.

There are many potential reasons for anger and distress (Ch. 2). It will be necessary to elucidate the reasons so that they may be tackled. Much anger will revolve around misunderstandings about causation and unfortunately all too commonly about how patients have been treated by their previous doctors and health-care professionals.

It is a normal response to become physiologically aroused when faced with an angry patient especially when the anger appears to be directed at oneself. For clinicians to become angry or distressed themselves is not helpful. However, while it is important to empathise with patients and listen to them carefully it is also vital to remain detached from their anger or distress in order to preserve as much objectivity as possible. An overview of the most important

strategies in the assessment and management of pain-associated distress and anger is presented in Box 18.6.

A STRATEGIC APPROACH TO MANAGEMENT

The importance of physical assessment

A comprehensive history and examination must be performed. This is not only good professional practice, but will also help to convince patients that their pain problem is being taken seriously. At the end of the assessment it is important to give patients a credible explanation of their pain together with a plan for further investigation (if necessary) and treatment. It is important also to check patients' understanding of what they have just been told to ensure that they have not misunderstood what has been said or the implications of what they have been told.

The importance of active patient participation

The treatment plan must involve the patient's active participation. Realistic expectations must be given. Promise of cure should not be made unless this is a clearly achievable objective. Neither should patients simply be re-referred to another professional unless there is a clear clinical indication to do so. Furthermore the intention behind the re-referral must be made explicit to the patient. Clinicians should not make promises on behalf of other health-care professionals.

Facilitation of recovery

When immersed in the clinical complexities of a significant pain problem, it is important to strike the right balance between appropriate attention to detail and addressing the wider issues. It may be helpful initially to distinguish the patient's beliefs and coping strategies into negative or maladaptive beliefs and coping strategies on the one hand, and positive or adaptive beliefs or coping strategies on the other (as described in Ch. 2). The blend within each patient of course is much more complex, but the single-handed practitioner needs to find a way of beginning.

Minimising negative beliefs and maladaptive coping strategies

By the time patients present to pain clinics and ultimately to pain management programmes they are commonly very distressed and not coping with their pain and disability. They often develop a very negative thinking style and tend to fear the worst. Such catastrophising (Ch. 2, p. 20) is not only not helpful but has a major effect on a number of other areas including mood, activity, pain, fear, anxiety and many others. These characteristics may be present when they consult the individual practitioner. It is important to point out to patients the likely effects of persistent negative thinking and begin to help them make some changes. One could start getting them to identify what negative thoughts they have and when these occur. Many of these catastrophic reactions are based on a small number of specific irrational fears. The more common of these are illustrated in Box 18.7.

Each of these fears should be identified and then tackled if necessary by writing down the arguments against such fears for the patient to refer to later. The clinician should teach and encourage them to stop or block the negative thoughts and begin to develop some positive coping strategies, such as those described in the yellow flag behavioural management guidelines (described earlier).

Enhancing positive or adaptive beliefs and coping strategies

There are a number of simple positive strategies, which may be helpful to the patient. Most of these strategies have been outlined in the previous chapters, for instance explaining the difference between hurt and harm. The patient may need to be reassured about the future (e.g. most patients with chronic back pain do not end up in a wheelchair). The patient should also be helped to regain some control, for example by getting them to pace activities, take medication regularly rather than on a pain-contingent basis, set small achievable targets for activity and build in a reward for managing well (e.g. having a cup of their favourite coffee or listening to their favourite CD).

Many of these strategies may seem somewhat self-evident or trivial. They are not. They are vital first steps to the patients beginning to tackle the consequences of their pain, take control and re-establish normal functioning. By building confidence slowly it is possible to halt the slide into further invalidity and help patients to make positive progress either without referral to a pain centre or at least while they are waiting to be seen. A number of specific suggestions for enhancing positive beliefs and adaptive coping strategies are shown in Box 18.8.

FROM THEORY TO PRACTICE

It is possible to help patients with chronic pain and disability problems in everyday clinical

---

Box 18.7 Potential fears leading to negative thoughts and coping styles

- Fear of pain
- Fear of hurt and harm
- Fear of future disability (wheelchair)
- Fear of loss of control
- Fear of surgery
- Fear of effect on relationships
- Fear of effect on work

Box 18.8 Ways of enhancing positive beliefs and adaptive coping strategies

Get patients to:
- Identify when they are beginning to think negatively
- Identify when they are becoming tense or angry
- Take steps to stop such thoughts and begin positive relaxation
- Change what they are doing when the pain gets bad (e.g. get up and walk around a little)
- Pace physical activities
- Pick achievable goals
- Look at what they have managed to achieve
- Reward themselves when they achieve even small targets

practice, even when a full pain management programme is not available. It is essential that all clinicians learn and use the techniques of managing pain patients within normal clinical practice, not only to help the patients with chronic problems begin to self-manage, but also to prevent patients with acute pain problems from becoming chronically disabled in the first place. Much of what has been outlined is neither technically sophisticated nor particularly complex. Perhaps it can be thought of simply as good clinical practice delivered in a humane and understanding way. The three case examples (Case studies 18.1–18.3) and associated commentaries are offered to try to illustrate some of these principles.

CONCLUSION

In this chapter, an attempt has been made to translate the principles of pain management, derived mainly from tertiary care settings, into primary care settings in which the principal emphasis needs to be on secondary prevention. It has been argued throughout this textbook that the biopsychosocial framework offers a broader conceptualisation of the nature of illness than the narrower pathology-based medical model. It would be foolish to attest that all chronicity is preventable, but incorporation of the psychosocial perspective into the early management of patients appears irresistible. Effective prevention, however, requires not only reappraisal of the framework within which pain is understood, but also the development of appropriate competencies in assessment and intervention. This chapter has attempted to offer some guidance about how the problem might be approached. Much further work needs to be done.

Case study 18.1   Spondylosis pain

Background

Mrs B. was well known to her GP. She had a long history of neck pain, which had recently been made worse following a road traffic accident (the impact was at less than 15 k.p.h.). At 33 she felt older than her years having had neck pain for 10 or more years. When she had attended the emergency department she was told that the X-rays had shown spondylosis. She had been given a collar and some painkillers and sent home. She was in so much pain she could not understand why she had not been admitted and thought she must have broken something.

The pain got worse and she had to call the emergency doctor out in the middle of the night. The emergency doctor thought she was making a fuss over nothing and gave her an injection. He suggested she return to the emergency department if the pain did not settle. Mrs B. returned to the department. She was very annoyed, as it did not seem people took her seriously. She was told to visit her GP.

The consultation

The GP listened carefully to Mrs B. She empathised with her plight and reminded Mrs B. that she had had a similar episode a number of years ago that had settled in time. She explained that from Mrs B.'s history and following her careful examination of her that there was no indication of any nerve trapping or damage. The normal X-rays were reassuring that there did not appear to be any serious structural damage. That was not to deny that Mrs B.'s pain was severe. The GP explained that spondylosis was simply a medical term for describing age-related changes.

The GP then asked whether Mrs B. had any particular worries or concerns. Mrs B. then explained that she was having trouble managing her part-time job as well as looking after the house and children. She was concerned that this was not going to get better. She explained she was frightened she would not be able to cope with the pain. She had been particularly frightened by the pain on the night she had to call the emergency doctor out.

The GP arranged to review Mrs B. regularly for a short while. She explained that Mrs B. should take her painkillers and anti-inflammatory drugs on a time-contingent basis and keep active but at a reduced level for the time being. She reassured Mrs B. that although the neck hurt she was not in danger of harming herself and that she should keep mobile and plan short rest periods regularly when performing activities.

Comment

By using many of the techniques described in this chapter the GP was able to guide Mrs B. in managing her own pain offering appropriate pharmacological and moral support. The GP was able to reassure Mrs B. and encourage her to increase activity progressively.

Case study 18.2 Dealing with anger

Background
Mr J. had waited for several months for his appointment with the specialist. He was in severe pain. Despite Mr J. phoning up a number of times the specialist was unable to see him any earlier.

Mr J. was 42 and had had his back pain for 11 years. His previous surgery 6 years earlier had not been helpful. In fact Mr J. felt that it had made him worse. He had had to give up his job and now spent most of his time at home. He was unable to get out and had become progressively demoralised and fed up. Nobody seemed to listen to him or believe him.

The consultation
The first thing that the specialist noticed was Mr J.'s clear anger. The specialist gently sought the reasons for Mr J.'s anger. He discovered that Mr J. was confused as to why he was in so much pain when people were telling him there was nothing wrong. Surely there must be something wrong. He was angry with the doctors at the benefits agency who did not believe him and he did not think his GP believed him either. He felt he had been treated dismissively and had not been taken seriously.

The specialist spent a little time taking a history of Mr J.'s pain and then performed a careful examination, explaining what he was checking for as he went along. At the end of the assessment he explained carefully his own understanding of Mr J.'s pain and asked Mr J. to correct him if he had misunderstood anything. He explained it was not possible to give a precise diagnosis now (and it may not be possible even after further tests). He explained why further tests would be needed and what he was excluding. He told Mr J. his pain was very real. He reassured Mr J. that from his experience of seeing many patients with similar problems there was no reason to believe his pain would get worse although it might fluctuate quite widely.

The specialist arranged to see Mr J. again after the further tests and told Mr J. that he expected the results to show that surgery would not be helpful. He asked Mr J. to make a list of the important questions he wanted answering and bring them with him next time. The important issues were carefully charted in the notes ready for the next visit.

Comment
It is simply not possible to perform an in-depth assessment in a busy clinic. The specialist in this case tackled the most important aspect of Mr J. presentation (his anger) and thereby discovered the major fears and misconceptions lying behind them. In practice a history was taken and an examination was performed. But Mr J. was given the impression that he was understood, taken seriously and would be helped.

This first visit was simply laying the groundwork for the future. It was aimed at addressing the clinical problems and gaining the confidence of the patient. Further issues, which Mr J. was anxious about, may be discussed at the next visit while reviewing the results of the tests, interpreting them and helping planning the future.

Case study 18.3 A contraindication for further treatment

Background
Mr S. was 55 years old. He had had a history of back pain for some 25 years. He was in such pain and so disabled that he was confined to a wheelchair. He had not worked for some 30 years. He attended the clinic with his wife whom he had married 10 years ago. He had seen a large number of different specialists, none of whom were able to help him. His MRI scan of 6 years previously was essentially normal, showing only age-related changes.

The consultation
Mr S. was seen in a pain clinic. The doctor listened to his story. It became clear that Mr S. was not expecting any great cure. He seemed almost resigned to his way of life. He had a very caring partner and the family rallied around him whenever he got fed up. His son took him out in the car every week and his daughter would come round regularly with the grandchildren.

Careful examination did not demonstrate any major structural problems nor any evidence of nerve entrapment or irritation. There were no markers or important pathology (clinical red flags). There was a significant amount of illness behaviour. However, there did not appear to be a major degree of psychological distress. Mr S. did seem to be using a lot of different pain-related medications to little benefit.

The doctor explained that there was no indication to perform any further investigations. He encouraged Mr S. to take his medications on a time-contingent basis and offered help in rationalising his tablets. He agreed to review Mr S. one more time to look specifically at tablet reduction. He explained he did not think there was any likelihood of any cures for his pain. He congratulated Mrs S. on her obvious care and encouragement for her husband. The doctor emphasised the need to keep his mood up and to avoid repeated consultations.

Following a further review to help Mr S. with rationalising his medications he was discharged from the clinic with explicit advice to his GP to act simply as a moral support for Mr S. and his wife. The GP was advised not to refer again or elsewhere unless there was a clear *new* pain problem.

Case study 1.3 Cont'd

Comment
The above describes clearly a case in which it is extremely unlikely that any change will occur. The potential reinforcers of disability are so well entrenched that change is unlikely. In addition attempting to change these would potentially destroy family and marital relationships. Under these circumstances a containment exercise is all that can be offered. It is vital to give advice to the patient's GP and help prevent further unnecessary assessments and interventions.

KEY POINTS

- The principles of pain management developed in interdisciplinary pain management programmes have applications in other settings.
- The biopsychosocial model (adjustment to disease and injury) is still relevant when the focus is on biomedical treatment.
- The move to secondary prevention necessitates reappraisal of the types of assessment and decision-making processes employed by primary care and community practitioners.

- Accurate identification of patients in danger of becoming chronically incapacitated requires further research.
- Effective communication is a key component of successful early behavioural intervention.
- A new style of interview focusing specifically on pain, pain-associated distress and pain-associated incapacity needs to be developed.
- A number of key strategies for dealing with the distressed and angry patient are offered.

REFERENCES

Bigos S, Bowyer O, Braen G et al 1994 Acute low back problems in adults. Clinical practice guideline no 14. AHCPR publication no 95–0642. Agency for Health Care and Policy Research, Public Health Service, US Dept of Health and Human Services, Rockville MD

Burton A K, Tillotson K M, Main C J, Hollis S 1995 Psychosocial predictors of outcome in acute and subchronic low back trouble. Spine 20:722–728

Chew-Graham C, May C R 1999 The challenge of the back pain communication. Family Practice 16:46–49

CSAG 1994 Clinical Standards Advisory Group report on back pain. HMSO London

Fordyce W E 1995 Back pain in the workplace: management of disability in non-specific conditions. IASP, Seattle WA

Kendall N A S, Linton S J, Main C J 1997 Guide to assessing psychosocial yellow flags in acute low back pain: risk factors for long term disability and work loss. Accident Rehabilitation and Compensation Insurance Corporation of New Zealand and the National Health Committee, Wellington NZ

Linton S, Andersson T 2000 Can chronic disability be prevented? A randomised Trial of a cognitive-behavioral intervention for spinal pain patients, in press

Linton S, Halden K 1997 Risk factors and the natural course of acute and recurrent musculoskeletal pain: developing a screening instrument. In: Jensen T S, Turner J A, Wiesenfeld-Hallin Z Proceedings of the 8th world congress of pain. IASP, Seattle, WA, pp 527–536

Linton S J, Ryberg M, Wahlstrom L A 2000 Cognitive behavioral group intervention in the prevention of persistent neck and back pain: a randomized controlled trial. In press.

RCGP 1996 Clinical guidelines for the management of acute low back pain. Royal College of General Practitioners, London

Roland M, Waddell G, Klaber-Moffett J, Burton A K, Main C J, Cantrill C 1996 The back book. The Stationary Office, Norwich.

Symonds T L, Burton A K, Tillotson K M, Main C J 1995 Absence resulting from low back trouble can be reduced by psychosocial intervention at the workplace. Spine 20:2738–2745

Waddell G 1982 An approach to backache. British Journal of Hospital Medicine 23: 187–219

Waddell G 1998 The back pain revolution. Churchill Livingstone, New York

19

Pain management in occupational settings

Serena Bartys   Chris J. Main
A. K. Burton

INTRODUCTION

In earlier chapters a range of factors influencing pain and disability have been discussed. Research studies have demonstrated that disability is multifactorial and that chronic disability needs to be understood within a biopsychosocial framework. In occupational settings, interventions have been based primarily on biomedical or ergonomic principles, but investigations into predictors of outcome have shown that the specific influence of psychosocial factors may be more important than has been previously recognised. Furthermore, clinical studies into the psychosocial mechanisms associated with the development of chronic incapacity (or failure to recover after musculoskeletal injury) appear to indicate a real opportunity for the design of interventions targeted specifically at prevention. Considerable effort historically has already been directed at *primary* prevention but, as was stated in Chapter 18, given the prevalence of musculoskeletal symptoms in the population a more realistic target may be *secondary* prevention, with particular effort on the prevention of musculoskeletal symptoms becoming disabling. Rehabilitation per se is usually considered to fall within the remit of the health services, but in occupational settings there would appear to be considerable potential benefit in addressing the issue of work retention from a biopsychosocial perspective in terms specifically of obstacles to recovery. It was recommended in Chapter 4 (essentially extending the principle of pain management) that clinical and occupational perspectives should be combined. What is the evidence that such an integrated approach would be beneficial? In an attempt to amass some supporting evidence, a discussion will be offered based on a sample of some of the currently available scientific literature on attempts to reduce or prevent work loss as a result of musculoskeletal injury.

The major focus in the literature has been on the management of low back pain. Low back pain rehabilitation/prevention programmes have been well documented, and this chapter reviews the objectives and strategies of such programmes, and their outcomes. The various outcome measures of existing interventions are usually: work retention, return to work, changing beliefs about back pain and reduction in sickness absence days/costs. However, because of this variety of methods and concepts in such interventions, and a lack of defined successful outcomes, there are few substantial conclusions of what works, on whom and when (Krause, Dasinger & Neuhauser 1998).

TYPES OF INTERVENTION

Intervention/rehabilitation programmes usually comprise of one or a few elements of the following approaches:

• *Back schools* combine back pain education and strengthening exercises, and are a popular intervention technique. Back pain education can include topics related to back care: the structure and function of the spine, safe lifting, ergonomics, pain control and relaxation techniques (Brown et al 1992).

• *Exercise and physical therapy* aims to increase the individual's strength, resilience and capability through exercise. Physical therapy also aims to increase the individual's strength and mobility.

• *Functional restoration* is based on quantitative measurement of physical and functional capacity, with a psychosocial assessment of barriers to recovery. This attempts to guide a medically directed, interdisciplinary team in an individualised, intensive treatment programme

to achieve specific socioeconomic valued outcomes, namely return to work and work retention. Advocates of this approach state that it permits motivated, disabled individuals to reach their highest possible functional level (Garcy, Mayer & Gatchel 1996).

• *Modified work* recognises the individual's perceptions of function and limitation, and reorganises job duties accordingly. Types of modified work include: light duty, graded work exposure, work trial, supported employment and sheltered employment. This approach conveys a sense of understanding the psychosocial aspects of work and disability for work, as well as the physical and financial aspects (Yamamoto 1997).

Most rehabilitation programmes aiming to prevent low back pain and the ensuing disability tend to employ variants of these methods, or a combination of their essential values. Although their importance in overcoming this problem is not denied, evidence of such rehabilitation programmes to date show limited success.

A summary of the key studies underpinning the discussion on each of the types of intervention reported on for this chapter is shown in Table 19.1.

Back schools

Back schools and educational types of intervention are widely utilised in low back pain rehabilitation, and are relatively easy to carry out in a workplace or clinical setting. The outcomes in relation to the content and context of such interventions are shown in Table 19.2.

As shown in Table 19.2, demonstration of successful outcome may depend on what specific outcome is measured (i.e return to work, work retention or a reduction of injury reporting). A study by Daltroy et al (1997) showed that over 5.5 years an educational programme designed to prevent low back injury did not reduce the median cost per injury, the time off from work per injury, the rate of related musculoskeletal injuries or the rate of repeated injury after return to work; only the subject's knowledge of safe behaviour was increased by the training.

Table 19.1 Intervention/rehabilitation programmes

Back school/education	Physical therapy/exercise	Functional restoration	Modified duties
Brown et al (1992)	Friedrich et al (1998)	Hazard et al (1989)	Yassi et al (1995)
Daltroy et al (1993)	Haldorsen, Indahl &	Burke, Harms-Constas	Fitzler & Berger
Schenk, Doran	Ursin (1998)	& Aden (1994)	(1982, 1983)
& Stachura (1996)	Hochanadel &	Mayer et al (1985)	Lancourt & Kettelhut (1992)
van Poppel et al (1998)	Conrad (1993)	Oland & Tveiten (1991)	Schmidt, Oort-Marburger
Ryan, Krishna,	Jarvikoski et al (1993)	Alaranta et al (1994)	& Meijman (1995)
& Swanson (1995)	Mellin et al (1993)	Mitchell & Carmen (1990)	Loisel et al (1997)
Hurri (1989)	Torstensen et al (1998)		
Frost et al (1998)	Sinclair et al (1997)		
	Gundewall, Liljeqvist &		
	Hansson (1993)		
	Donchin et al (1990)		
	Oland & Tveiten (1991)		
	Kellett, Kellett &		
	Nordholm (1991)		
	Cherkin et al (1998)		

Table 19.2 Back school/educational interventions

Study	What was done	Where	Who to	Results
Brown et al (1992)	20- and 30-minute classes consisting of education and exercise every day for 6 weeks	At a fitness centre	Those who had reported injury	There were 16 reinjuries in back school group (23%), compared with 33 in comparison group (47%) in 6 months postintervention period
Daltroy et al (1993)	Two × 90-minute educational sessions 1 week apart + reinforcement every 6 months for 2.5 years. It was aimed at improving knowledge, attitudes and helping behaviours to prevent low back injury	In the workplace	Those who had reported injury	No significant behaviour change
Schenk et al (1996)	An educational session + 2-hour video was given with the aim to analyse the learning effects of such programmes	In the workplace	Those who had reported injury	There were significant differences demonstrated by the back school group in lifting techniques, knowledge of correct lifting techniques and body mechanics
van Poppel et al (1998)	Group 1—an educational session (lifting instructions) + lumbar support Group 2— educational sessions Group 3—lumbar support Group 4—no intervention Education consisted of three group sessions with a total duration of 5 hours	In the workplace	The total workforce	Compliance with wearing the lumbar support was 43%. There were no significant differences in back pain incidence of those with lumbar support compared with those without. This was also true for the rate of sick leave because of low back pain

Table 19.2 Cont'd

Study	What was done	Where	Who to	Results
Ryan, Krishna & Swanson (1995)	Workforce educational programme aiming at changing workplace psychosocial perceptions and encouraging early injury reporting. First aid was also taught	In the workplace	Those that had reported injury less than 1 week ago	During a period of 6 years, the median time to return to work was 10 days. The number of claims due to back pain was significantly less
Hurri (1989)	60-minute educational and exercise sessions given six times over 3 weeks	At a clinic	Those that had at least 12 months of reported injury	No effect on sickness absence
Frost et al (1998)	Eight 1-hour fitness sessions over 4 weeks, and two 90-minute back school sessions	At a hospital	Those that had been referred to a hospital	Patients in the intervention group demonstrated a mean reduction of 7.7% in the Owestry Low Back Pain Disability Index score, compared with only 2.4% in the control group

In a meta-analysis of the efficacy of back school programmes Di Fabio (1995) concluded that back schools were most efficacious when coupled with a comprehensive rehabilitation programme. Efficacy was supported for the treatment of pain and physical impairments and for education/compliance outcomes, but work, vocational and disability outcomes were not improved significantly by either the comprehensive or the primary prevention back school programmes.

Back schools and educational programmes, in aiming to teach safe behaviour and knowledge of the mechanics of the back, contain the essentials of primary prevention. Primary prevention aims to prevent injury, or reinjury and implies that back pain can be avoided, which may not be true. An episode of low back pain may be inevitable and is in itself fairly inconsequential; the problem lies with such episodes leading to low back pain disability. As Hadler (1999, p. 259) states, 'a year without at least one episode of backache is unusual for most people. Coping successfully is healthfulness'. This suggests that, in order to address the factors that may lead to disability, recovery from musculoskeletal injury needs to be understood in the context of such individuals, their lifestyle and their beliefs.

Exercise and physical therapy

Recommendation of specific exercises and engagement inactivity offers a less passive approach to rehabilitation in that active participation is required. 'Prescription' of exercise and activity is sometimes used in conjunction with specific physical therapy (such as manipulation and mobilisation). Table 19.3 lists studies including such types of interventions and their results.

Cherkin et al (1998) compared physical therapy, chiropractic manipulation and the use of an educational booklet for the treatment of patients with low back pain, and found no significant differences amongst the groups in the numbers of days of reduced activity, in missed work or in recurrences of back pain. Additionally, in a review of four types of intervention including back and aerobic exercises, Lahad et al (1994) concluded that there was limited evidence to recommend exercise to prevent low back pain in asymptomatic individuals. However, evidence exists suggesting that, when combined with other approaches, exercise may be very beneficial. For example, Lindstrom et al (1992) found that a graded activity programme coupled with a behavioural approach encouraging patients to return to work through operant

Table 19.3 Exercise and physical therapy interventions

Study	What was done	Where	Who to	Results
Friedrich et al (1998)	10 exercise sessions, plus motivation sessions	At a hospital	Those that had been referred	A reduction in` non-attendance of sessions in the short term, but no significant differences in the long term
Gundewall et al (1993)	A 20-minute workout six times per month	In the workplace	Those who had reported injury	After 13 months, one subject had been absent from work for 28 days in the training group, whereas 12 subjects had been absent 155 days from work because of low back pain in the control group. Every hour of training reduced work absence by 1.3 days, resulting in a cost–benefit ratio greater than 10
Haldorsen, Indahl & Ursin (1998)	A light mobilisation programme used with screening instruments to assess prediction of failure to return to work was implemented	At a spine clinic	Those who had an initial sick leave of 8–12 weeks	For those not returning to work within 12 months (23%), dominant variables were low Internal Health Locus of Control scores, restricted mobility and reduced work ability
Hochanadel & Conrad (1993)	A physical therapy programme	In the workplace	Those who had complained of pain/injury	Over 10 years, the programme was estimated to have saved $8.3 million in sickness costs, and it now serves 50% of employees
Jarvikoski et al (1993)	Program A was a 4-week multimodal in-patient programme. Program B consisted of a 3-day preprogramme, a 5-week home training period, and a 4-week intensive in-patient treatment programme with a 'no pain, no gain' rationale	At a clinic	Those that had been referred	60% of group B belonged to the 'positive change' group (i.e. pain, functional capacity, sickness absence, subjective state of health, depression and work status) compared with 44% of group A. The differences between the two groups were not significant
Mellin et al (1993)	A 4-week intensive physical training programme	At a hospital/clinic	Those that had been referred	There were no significant effects on return to work
Torstensen et al (1998)	Group 1—medical exercise sessions Group 2—conventional phsyiotherapy Group 3—self exercise sessions	Multicentre	Those that had been sick-listed for more than 8 weeks but less than 52 weeks	No difference was observed between groups 1 and 2 on measures of pain intensity, functional ability, patient satisfaction, return to work, number of days on sick leave and costs. However, both were significantly better than group 3. Return to work rates were equal for all groups, with 59% back in work

Table 19.3 Cont'd

Study	What was done	Where	Who to	Results
Sinclair et al (1997)	An early, active exercise and educational programme	At a clinic	Those that had reported injury in the past few weeks	Health-care costs for clinic attenders were significantly higher. Functional status, health-related quality of life, and pain measures all improved significantly for both groups
Donchin et al (1990)	Group 1—a 45 minute exercise session twice a week for 3 months Group 2—a back school programme of five sessions Group 3—a control group	In the workplace	Those who had reported an injury in the previous year	A monthly surveillance for 12 months showed a mean of 4.5 'painful months' in group 1, versus 7.3 and 7.4 months in groups 2 and 3 respectively
Kellett, Kellett & Nordholm (1991)	An aerobic exercise session once per week for 10 months	In the workplace	Those who had previous history of back pain	A greater reduction of back-pain-related sick days and back pain episodes was experienced in the intervention group compared with the control group
Oland & Tveiten (1991)	Pool traction plus general physical training	In a rehabilitiation centre	Those who had an average sick leave of 13 months	No significant influence on return to work
Cherkin et al (1998)	Physical therapy, chiropractic and an educational booklet were compared	At a physiotherapy centre	Those who had persistent pain of at least 7 days following a GP visit	There were no significant differences between the treatments on the number of days of reduced activity or missed work, or in recurrences of back pain

techniques returned patients to work 5.1 weeks earlier on average than the patients in the control groups.

A clear and direct focus on activity clearly has intuitive appeal. Outcome, however, is frequently evaluated in terms of some sort of functional criterion such as attainment of an acceptable level of functioning. In occupational settings, 'acceptability' may be defined in terms of how well an individual performs a set of tasks. Indeed rehabilitation may have been tailored to the individual in this respect. If recovery of function were determined solely by functional attainment, then results of such specifically focused rehabilitation might be more impressive. As mentioned in previous chapters, back injury claims and return to work are influenced by psychosocial as well as biomechanical factors directed primarily at work

content. Thus, aiming to increase function to perform a specific task at work as the sole criterion of success may not be adequately addressing the entirety of the problem.

Functional restoration

Mayer et al (1985) proposed functional restoration as an objective assessment of spine function, with the authors attempting to demonstrate a direct relationship between specific functional measures and subsequent back injury. Although primarily used for chronic rather than acute or subacute groups of patients, the approach deserves comment in the context of considering different approaches to occupational rehabilitation. The objectives of their functional restoration programme were 'the restoration of joint mobility, muscular strength, endurance and conditioning, as well as cardiovascular fitness leading to restoration of the ability to perform specific functional tasks such as lifting, bending, twisting, and tolerance of prolonged static positioning'. They claim that quantitative functional capacity measures can give objective evidence of patient abilities and degree of effort, and can significantly guide the clinician in administering an effective treatment programme. Table 19.4 lists the outcomes of studies on functional restoration programmes.

Mayer et al (1985) and Hazard et al (1989) have attracted methodological criticisms in their lack of proper control groups, and failure to include dropouts in the treatment groups (resulting in an overestimation of their success rates). A comprehensive review of the results of all the major studies of functional restoration was recently undertaken by Waddell (1998, p. 363), who concluded; 'Functional restoration for chronic low back pain looks promising, but there is a lack of good evidence that it does actually return patients to work'.

Functional restoration can be criticised also on conceptual grounds. Although it has the appeal of being an optimal, tailored intervention, which is designed to measure the individual's ability and capacities, an 'objective' intervention such as this does not incorporate explicitly the many important subjective factors involved in response to rehabilitation. Functional restoration makes the further claim that its focus on objectivity permits an appraisal of effort and motivation to recover. The approach has attracted interest by assessors attempting to identify malingerers.

Table 19.4 Functional restoration programmes

Study	What was done	Where	Who to	Results
Mayer et al (1985)	A functional restoration programme	At a clinic	Those who had been referred	An 85% return-to-work rate
Hazard et al (1989)	A functional restoration programme with behavioural support sessions	A back centre	Those who had at least 4 months of continuous disability	An 81% return-to-work rate
Burke, Harms-Constas & Aden (1994)	A functional restoration programme	Multicentre	Those who had been referred	The intervention group had a 62% return to work rate compared with 30% of comparison group. After 12 months, 98% of the treatment group who were working at 6 months were also working at 12 months, compared with 62% of comparison group; 38% of those in the treatment group who were not working at 6 months were back at work at 12 months, compared with 13% of comparison group
Oland & Tveiten (1991)	This was a replication of the Mayer et al (1985) study (above)	At a clinic	Those who had been referred	A 32% return-to-work rate at 6 months, and then 23% at 18 months
Alaranta et al (1994)	A randomised controlled trial of a functional restoration programme	At a clinic	Those who had back pain for more than 6 months	Strength was improved in the intervention group, as were the self-reports of disability in men for up to 12 months. There were no significant differences in the following year
Mitchell & Carmen (1990)	Functional restoration programmes were evaluated in 12 clinics and compared with control groups	Multicentre	Those who had been off work for 3–6 months	The treatment group returned to work earlier and realised substantial cost savings

Table 19.5 Modified work programmes

Study	What was done	Where	Who to	Results
Yassi et al (1995)	Prompt assessment and rehabilitation through a graded return-to-work programme	In the workplace	Those who had lost work time up to 7 weeks	A reduction of back injuries by 23%, and lost time through back injuries was reduced by 43%. The intervention was also cost beneficial
Fitzler & Berger (1982)	Light duties were given	In the workplace	Back-injured workers	A reduction in compensation claims, work days lost to injury and total costs
Fitzler & Berger (1983)	Light duties were given	In the workplace	Back-injured workers	A reduction of more than 50% in injury rates, and a reduction in workers compensation costs by sevenfold
Lancourt & Kettethut (1992)	Light duties were given	In the workplace	Back-injured workers	There was no significant effect shown
Schmidt, Oort-Marburger & Meijman (1995)	A work trial	In the workplace	Those who had had treatment of musculoskeletal injury	An improvement of return to work by a factor of 3.3
Loisel et al (1997)	Light duties were given	In the workplace	Back-injured workers	A reduction of absence by half as long

(In fact all that the 'objective' evaluation offers is a description of performance, which is determined by a wide range of subjective factors such as, for example, fears that activity may be harmful. The inferential leap therefore appears to be unwarranted.)

In conclusion, although the idea of an objective measurement that identifies clear deficits is clearly desirable, as discussed in Chapter 4, the worker's *perception* appears to be more influential than the actual work characteristics. In fact this was recognised in an early study by Magora (1973) who was one of the first to note that workers' perceptions about the nature of their jobs were critical factors in whether they recalled or reported back pain.

Modified work

A more recent approach, which takes into account the importance of context as well as content of the job, has been the modification of the actual work. Although modified work is regarded by some as a breakthrough in the job rehabilitation process, little is known about the structure, effectiveness, and efficiency of such programmes. Table 19.5 outlines the results of some such programmes.

In a systematic review of modified work and return-to-work literature, Krause, Dasinger & Neuhauser (1998) concluded that modified work programmes facilitate return to work for both temporarily and permanently disabled workers. These authors also found that injured workers who are offered modified work then return to work about twice as often as those who are not; similarly, modified work programmes cut the number of lost work days in half. A possible reason for this reported success is that the approach aims at not only reducing workers' compensation costs, but also the financial, psychological and physical strain placed on workers when a disabling injury occurs.

Modified work also aims to facilitate an early return to work, with the opinion that intervening quickly will reduce the negative, potentially disabling effects of taking time away from normal lifestyle activities such as work. The idea of intervening quickly was studied by Hazard et al (1997) who stated that a quick identification of the small number of back-injured workers who become disabled would facilitate more efficient targeting.

Other supporters of the early intervention are Yassi et al (1995), Sinclair et al (1997), Ryan, Krishna & Swanson (1995) and Galvin (1999) who all maintain that early assessment and timely rehabilitation would prevent further disability, restore optimal work capacity and reduce dependency on compensation benefits. Von Korff et al (1993) believe a critical period lies between 4 and 12 weeks after onset for an intervention to be successful, and Nachemson (1983) supports this by stating that adverse biological and psychosocial consequences compound the pain, and therefore should be addressed as soon as possible.

Conclusion

Review of the literature would suggest that there is merit in each of the approaches to rehabilitation, but the biggest challenge would appear to be the design of appropriate and effective interventions designed to prevent musculoskeletal problems becoming chronically incapacitating. In occupational contexts, the major challenge therefore is in work retention.

THE WAY FORWARD

The findings of these studies invite a number of general observations and suggest a number of more specific strategies that might be helpful in occupational settings. They are summarised in Box 19.1.

Box 19.1   General conclusions and recommendations

- Need for an integrated clinical and occupational perspective
- Appraisal of obstacles to recovery
- Type of intervention: work rehabilitation and work retention
- Implementation strategies
- Competencies
- Facilitation of return to work
- Need for systematic monitoring and evaluation of outcome

Need for an integrated clinical and occupational perspective

It is clear that some interventions are effective, but the results are frequently inconsistent, hard to interpret and the overall success rate is disappointing. There has as yet been insufficient research into which approaches are needed for which individuals in which settings. It seems clear, however, that in order to reduce unnecessary work-related incapacity it will be necessary to move both beyond the predominantly clinically focused approaches characteristic of pain management and beyond the predominantly biomechanical and ergonomic focus of occupational interventions towards a more integrated approach. As has been stated: 'The problem of musculoskeletal disorder-related work disability requires a treatment paradigm shift, including identified targets for intervention, evaluation approach, approach to treatment, and practice management' (Feuerstein & Zastowny 1999). It is clear that, although there are many general pain issues to address in any programme, there are also many non-pain related issues to be dealt with.

Appraisal of obstacles to recovery

Prior to designing an intervention, an appraisal needs to be made of obstacles to recovery. In Chapter 4, the distinction was made between *risks* of poor outcome (or chronicity) and *obstacles to recovery*. A further differentiation was suggested between clinical yellow flags (such as beliefs about pain, disability and fears that physical activity will be injurious), blue flags (addressing facets of the perception of work such as job satisfaction and the 'social climate' at work) and black flags (such as aspects of work content, working conditions and policies regarding sickness) over which the individual has no control.

Type of intervention: work rehabilitation and work retention

In an early review (Bigos & Battié 1987) it was recommended that effective early intervention should centre around:

- teaching patients about back care, including how to control symptoms through improved body mechanics
- applying these educational principles, especially to the patient's livelihood
- avoiding the debilitation that results from overusing bed rest and medication
- recommendations to increase cardiovascular fitness
- judicious use of surgery.

As can be seen, these recommendations seem to contain almost everything from education to surgery. They seem to be 'good ideas' rather than focused recommendations. In any event, concepts of cardiovascular fitness seem more appropriate in contexts of primary prevention or 'wellness programmes' rather than musculoskeletal rehabilitation as such. Surgery, furthermore, clearly falls beyond the remit of occupational services. A clearer and more specific focus is perhaps required. In arriving at a narrower focus, it might be helpful to make a distinction between work rehabilitation and work retention (although of course there can be overlap between them).

Work rehabilitation

Approaches such as functional restoration offer a strong and robust approach to work rehabilitation. However, in the best known of these programmes (Mayer & Gatchel 1998) there is a significant element of preselection, in that work either has to be available or a clear job plan negotiated. It appears furthermore that outcome of the approach appears to be facilitated by the high costs of failure. It is usually accepted that once an individual has been out of work with back pain for 2 years or more their chances of getting back to work are virtually non-existent (Frank et al 1996). However, a recent small study (Main & Watson 1995) suggests that a slightly more optimistic view can be taken. The authors developed an occupationally oriented pain management programme tailored specifically for the needs of the client group. The intervention addressed both clinical yellow flags and blue flags and the

programme was successful in returning 70% of the group into work or job training. In fact a successor to the original scheme is currently under way (funded by the UK Department of Employment under their National Disability Development Initiative) for unemployed individuals in receipt of state benefits and with back pain as the principal obstacle to work. Entrants to this scheme are referred by their local Department of Employment advisor.

This type of rehabilitation requires an initial focus on the clinical obstacles to recovery, supplemented by a specific occupational focus on re-establishing confidence, decreasing negative perceptions of work and increasing job-seeking skills.

Work retention

Work rehabilitation is costly and of uncertain benefit. A large proportion of employer costs are associated with lost productivity for employees who, although still employed, are absent from work. The identification of obstacles to recovery indicates an approach to secondary prevention applicable not only to rehabilitation but also to work retention. In addition to the obvious clinical benefits of preventing people becoming chronically incapacitated, there are clear economic benefits. Watson et al (1998) recently studied new benefit claimants for back pain on the island of Jersey. Since benefits are paid through medically certified absence from work, it was possible to quantify the costs of claimed disability extremely accurately. The study showed that the costs of second and subsequent episodes of back pain are approximately 50% higher than those of the initial episode. This suggests that there are considerable cost savings likely to accrue from secondary prevention aimed specifically at work retention. For example, van Doorn (1995) in a study of self-employed dentists, vets, doctors and physiotherapists found that, after the introduction of such an intervention, the mean cumulative duration of low back disability decreased significantly. For this early intervention programme, van Doorn found that specific low back pain, fear of becoming long term disabled and duration of low back complaints of 6 months or more were predictors of long term disability.

Conclusion

Most occupational interventions have focused either on primary prevention or on rehabilitation back to work, but perhaps there should be a redirection of effort, at least in part, towards work retention. It should be recognised further that there will need to be differences in breadth and depth of content depending on whether rehabilitation or retention is the primary emphasis.

Implementation strategies

In addition to specific objectives, it is important also to consider strategy. A number of possible strategic issues are shown in Box 19.2.

Box 19.2 Implementation strategies

- Timing of intervention
- Individual tailoring
- Liaison between clinical and occupational agencies
- Partnerships with industry

Timing of intervention

Clinicians and employers would all wish to minimise the effect of injury or incapacity. As was discussed in the last chapter, however, back pain is so frequent that perhaps it needs to be accepted that it is never going to be totally preventable. Primary prevention aims to reduce the incidence of new episodes of back pain. Most back pain gets better. Minor musculoskeletal strains are commonplace and often do not become disabling. Conditions of employment within different organisations will differ in terms of the amount of self-certification required before medical certification is required. (Indeed there are currently discussions at a national level in the UK about how the problem of unnecessary sick leave can be addressed.) The problem needs to be

considered from both a clinical and a pragmatic perspective. It is in fact very difficult to determine when individuals with back pain are beginning to appear to show signs of chronicity. Rate of recovery is influenced not only by the nature of the triggering incident (which may not always be clearly identifiable) but also by what the person actually does during the acute phase. Thus, for example, individuals may dose themselves with analgesics and struggle on, take to their beds or consult someone. Sickness registration may offer an opportunity for contact by occupational staff (although there may not be a mechanism for this) but, whatever the particular organisational requirements, contact should ideally be made with the individual as soon as is reasonably practical, before fear-avoidance patterns have started to become established and pessimism about successful return to work has started to develop.

Individual tailoring

Formulating an optimal intervention may require tailoring of treatment in order to address a diverse set of presenting problems. Feuerstein & Zastowny (1999) propose that aspects of such an intervention should include: medical management, physical conditioning, work conditioning, pain and stress management, workplace psychosocial and ergonomic consultation, and vocational counselling and placement. Clearly the breadth of intervention will depend on the severity of the dysfunction and the time since the injury. If the intervention takes place within the occupational setting, rather than in an external rehabilitation agency, it should be possible to offer a number of interventions. These might range from a relatively brief early intervention while the individual is still at work to a much more comprehensive programme focusing on re-establishing people in work who have been absent on sick leave. Occupational rehabilitation, in comparison with clinical rehabilitation, places a greater emphasis on the workplace and on specific interventions directed at workplace factors assumed to inhibit return to work. Identification of outcomes for such a programme is also crucial. For example, it may be more beneficial in the long term to aim at ongoing work retention and the prevention of disability, even for those individuals who have been returned to work. As Von Korff (1994) notes, 40% of acute sufferers are still reporting pain at a 6-month follow-up.

Liaison between health and occupational agencies

Management of acute short-lived episodes of back trouble may require no more than adequate liaison between line management and occupational health. As the episode becomes longer, the employee may be required to seek external help or initiate sick-leave certification. It is then possible for communications to break down, resulting in unnecessary sick leave. In the United States, the advent of HMOs has led to case management as an alternative to a fee-for-service system. In case management, a coordinator has the responsibility for purchasing care on behalf of the injured party. In insurance-based systems, the type of care that can be purchased may be restricted not only in terms of the body part concerned but also in terms of the type of treatment. (It is not uncommon for example to have specific psychological therapies excluded for pain problems.) The principle of coordinated care nonetheless seems intuitively sensible and certainly has the potential for reducing the iatrogenic distress consequent of miscommunication. Indeed the aforementioned yellow-flags initiative (Kendall, Linton & Main 1997) was designed specifically for a case-managed system. It seems likely that an integrated approach to work retention might be of benefit and there could be a pivotal role for occupational health in coordinating the removal of such obstacles to recovery.

Specific partnerships with industry

The need for the development of links between health and occupational agencies has been recognised. In the UK a major initiative into prevention of back pain disability was launched by HSE. The HSE has jointly funded the Department of Behavioural Medicine at Hope Hospital Salford (C. J. Main) and the Spinal Research Unit of the University of Huddersfield (A. K. Burton) to undertake a study into the implementation of biopsychosocial interventions in occupational settings as a way of enhancing work retention and reducing unnecessary disability. At the time of writing, a large workforce survey of a pharmaceutical company (SmithKline Beecham) is under way prior to the implementation of an optimal, early intervention informed by the results of the survey. It is hoped that this research will expand on the developing area of work psychology in relation to musculoskeletal disability, and will involve a new approach to treatment with particular emphasis on the aforementioned psychosocial aspects of the worker and workplace (clinical yellow and blue flags). The intervention is designed to be carried out by occupational health staff, who will be trained by a multidisciplinary research team. The training will incorporate elements of physiotherapy, medical management, psychosocial assessment techniques and ergonomic advice. The individual's lifestyle will be assessed, along with perceptions and aspects of the workplace that can be changed in order to promote a more conducive environment to well-being. Workplace factors such as job satisfaction, perceived sources of pressure, perceived physical exertion, role clarity and social support are included. These will be examined alongside self-report and presentation of symptoms in order to indicate salient psychosocial characteristics that are important in the course of recovery or initial presentation.

Competencies

Many practical challenges accompany the implementation of an integrated approach to secondary prevention in occupational settings. It is vital that the staff delivering the intervention have the necessary competencies.

As Feuerstein & Zastowny (1999) assert, 'the strategy of flexible roles is not without its difficulties'. They state that the various members of the treatment team should be able to recognise limitations of their skills and knowledge, and not to apply a 'common-sense' approach to problems. The authors propose that the 'team effectiveness model' (Tannenbaum, Beard & Salas 1992) may be useful as it has evolved from human factors research on effective teams operating under conditions that at times can characterise the occupational rehabilitation work environment.

Competencies are of course task specific. As mentioned in Chapter 16 of this book, however, delivery of interventions within a biopsychosocial framework may need the development of new skills as well as the refinement of existing skills. An essential part of systematic intervention is an adequate appraisal of the nature of the problem. (This has been explicitly recognised in a recent research project by the present authors into the delivery of psychosocial interventions by physiotherapists treating patients with acute back pain in primary care settings. A specific training protocol has been devised that included training in assessment and observational techniques as well as training to criterion in biopsychosocial management.) In occupational settings, a set of required competencies for personnel delivering occupationally oriented pain management programmes, derived from the desirable criteria for pain management programmes (Pain Society 1997) have already been accepted by staff, who vary widely in their skills and aptitudes. We consider that adequate training is an absolute prerequisite for competent intervention. The actual training required may vary in breadth and sophistication depending on the type of intervention considered appropriate, but a training-needs analysis should be undertaken as part of any systematic intervention.

Facilitation of return to work

As discussed in Chapter 4, working conditions can help or hinder return to work. Both nationally agreed conditions of employment (such as sick-leave entitlement and benefits payable in adversity) and locally agreed conditions of service can have a major influence on extent of sick leave and return to work. There is clearly a place for considering issues of social policy, but variation in individual responses to injury suggests that social policy initiatives on their own are unlikely to be more than partly successful. The IASP recently established a task force charged with the responsibility of producing a strategy to reduce the apparently increasing level of back-associated disability in employees with non-specific back pain (Fordyce 1995). In their report IASP attributed much of the problem to inappropriate medical certification and recommended, as part of their solution, that incapacity associated with non-specific low back pain that lasted beyond 6 weeks should be redefined as 'activity intolerance' and no longer be recognised as a medical problem. The task force in fact recommended multi disciplinary assessment at 6 weeks, but the proposals caused an uproar in the clinical community. Many of the sensible proposals in the report appear to have been disregarded, and it is by no means certain that any benefit has resulted from their honest endeavours. Social policy initiatives are of course political, and each society establishes its view about how the nature of injuries and injured people should be viewed. Of more specific relevance to occupationally oriented pain management are circumstances facing employees in their specific workplace.

As discussed in Chapter 4, it is important to consider aspects of the *perception* of work as potential obstacles to recovery. However, management style and the social climate in regard to injury should also be considered as they may also play a significant part in successful work retention. Establishment, for example, of a dialogue between line managers, unions and occupational health, in recognition of work retention as a shared problem, may lead to adjustments to the working context and conditions that might be of benefit in terms of work retention and reduction in sickness absence.

Need for systematic monitoring and evaluation of outcome

Finally, it is necessary to devise an appropriate index of success for any intervention. One should consider first the *context* in which the intervention is being introduced. Most adults probably spend half their time at work and therefore the potential of behaviourally targeted psychosocial interventions there, for example, may be more substantial than in many other community settings (Dishman et al 1998). It may be realistic to introduce such changes only to the workforce as a whole. Such changes, however, may be hard to evaluate. Even apparently simple outcome measures such as return to work may be difficult to assess in practice. Return to work as an outcome measure also seems to imply that, unless individuals have returned to exactly the same job in exactly the same capacity, they are not a success. This denies the benefits of modified work, for example, which promotes a supportive and encouraging environment—and whilst individuals may not be 'returned to work' in this defined sense they are *at work* none the less.

Thus instead of focusing exclusively on return to work rates a successful intervention programme should perhaps be concentrating on aspects of work retention, considering performance, focusing on blue as well as yellow flags and designing appropriate evaluations of success in reducing these potential obstacles to recovery.

CONCLUSION

In summary the principles of pain management appear highly relevant not only as an aspect of work rehabilitation but even more challengingly as an aspect of work retention. Occupational health professionals may have to develop a dual role, both as case managers, and also in carrying out specific psychosocial interventions. A new set of occupational health guidelines for the management of low back pain has recently been produced (Faculty of Occupational Medicine 2000). In their role as case managers professionals are likely to be most effective when they take a comprehensive view of the worker with a health concern. Harris (1998, p. 6–2) states that 'the cornerstone of disability management is coordination of all care through one provider' (6–2 p). This reduces the risk of conflicting and confusing advice, loss of information and barriers to communication. An additional role in targeted intervention also seems irresistible. Existing occupational guidelines (Harris 1998) advocate the use of one treatment plan used in conjunction with one set of written information. These guidelines state further, however, that the following areas must be clarified: individuals' role in their own recovery, the teaching of adequate coping skills, and the individual's

KEY POINTS

- Address the 'psychosocial hazards' in the workplace, and the interdependence of work and the individual.
- Clarify the specific obstacles to recovery and target interventions on those.
- Identify the roles of occupational health staff, both in terms of case management and in terms of possible interventions.
- Identify competencies required to undertake the tasks.

- Ensure that staff are trained to the level of competency required.
- Wherever possible, develop a genuine interdisciplinary approach.
- Define appropriate criteria for outcome of the intervention (this may be in terms of organisational as well as individual outcomes).
- Take into account the size and type of organisation and how any intervention should be optimal for those particular organisational factors.

family/support system's role in recovery; a vocational or career plan should also be implemented. The development of this important and expanded role must be based on a clear appraisal of obstacles to recovery and direction of effort specifically at those obstacles that can be overcome (the yellow and blue flags). The precise role will vary in different occupational settings and with the professional background of the staff concerned. Although competency may be far more important than specific professional affiliation, there may be considerable advantages in terms of efficacy in blending the skills of a small interdisciplinary team.

REFERENCES

Alaranta H, Rytokoski U, Rissanen A et al 1994 Intensive physical and psychosocial training program for patients with chronic low back pain: a controlled clinical trial. Spine 19:1339–1349

Bigos S J, Battié M C 1987 Acute care to prevent back disability: ten years progress. Clinical Orthopaedics and Related Research 221:121–130

Brown K C, Sirles A T, Hilyer J C, Thomas M J 1992 Cost-effectiveness of a back school intervention for municipal employees. Spine 17:1224–1228

Burke S A, Harms-Constas C K, Aden P S 1994 Return to work/work retention outcomes of a functional restoration program. Spine 19:1880–1886

Cherkin D C, Deyo R A, Battie M, Street J, Barlow W 1998 A comparison of physical therapy, chiropractic manipulation, and provision of an educational booklet for the treatment of patients with low back pain. New England Journal of Medicine 339:1021–1029

Daltroy L, Iversen M D, Larson M G et al 1993 Teaching and social support: effects on knowledge, attitudes, and behaviours to prevent low back injuries in industry. Health Education Quarterly 20:43–62

Daltroy L H, Iversen M D, Larson M G et al 1997 A controlled trial of an educational program to prevent low back injuries. New England Journal Medicine 337:322–328

Di Fabio R P 1995 Efficacy of comprehensive rehabilitation programs and back school for patients with low back pain: a meta-analysis. Physical Therapy 75(10):865–878

Dishman R K, Oldenburg B, O'Neal H, Shephard M D 1998 Worksite physical activity interventions. American Journal of Preventive Medicine 15:344–361

Donchin M, Woolf O, Kaplan L, Floman Y 1990 Secondary prevention of low-back pain: a clinical trial. Spine 15:1317–1320

Faculty of Occupational Medicine 2000 Occupational health guidelines for the management of low back pain. Faculty of Occupational Medicine, London

Feuerstein M, Zastowny T R 1999 Occupational rehabilitation: multidisciplinary management of work-related musculoskeletal pain and disability. In: Gatchel R, Turk D C (eds) Psychological approaches to pain management: a practitioner's handbook, Guildford, London pp 458–485

Fitzler S L, Berger R A 1982 Attitudinal change: the Chelsea back program. Occupational Health and Safety 51:24–26

Fitzler S L, Berger R A 1983 Chelsea back program: one year later. Occupational Health and Safety 52:52–54

Fordyce W E 1995 Back pain in the workplace: management of disability in non-specific conditions. IASP, Seattle WA

Frank J W, Brooker A S, DeMaio S E et al 1996 Disability resulting from occupational low-back pain. Spine 21:2908–2929

Friedrich M, Gittler G, Halberstadt Y, Cermak T, Hellier I 1998 Combined exercise and motivation program: effect on the compliance and level of disability of patients with chronic low back pain: a randomised controlled trial. Archives of Physical Medicine and Rehabilitation 79:475–487

Frost H, Lamb S E, Klaber-Moffett J A, Fairbank J C T, Moser J S 1998 A fitness programme for patients with chronic low back pain: 2-year follow-up of a randomised controlled trial. Pain 75:273–280

Galvin D E 1999 Employer-based disability management and rehabilitation programs. Annual Review of Rehabilitation 5:215

Garcy P, Mayer T, Gatchel R J 1996 Recurrent or new injury outcomes after return to work in chronic disabling spinal disorders: tertiary prevention efficacy of functional restoration treatment. Spine 21:952–959

Gundewall B, Liljeqvist M, Hansson T 1993 Primary prevention of back symptoms and absence from work: a prospective randomized study among hospital employees. Spine 18:587–594

Hadler N M 1999 Occupational musculoskeletal disorders, 2nd edn. Lippincott Williams & Wilkins, Philadelphia PA

Haldorsen E M H, Indahl A, Ursin H 1998 Patients with low back pain not returning to work: a 12-month follow-up study. Spine 23:1202–1208

Harris J S 1998 Occupational medicine practice guidelines: evaluation and management of common health problems and functional recovery in workers. OEM, Beverly MA

Hazard R G, Fenwick J W, Kalisch S M et al 1989 Functional restoration with behavioural support: A one-year prospective study of patients with chronic low-back pain. Spine 14:157–161

Hazard R G, Haugh L D, Reid S, McFarlane G, MacDonald L 1997 Early physician notification of patient disability risk and clinical guidelines after low back injury. Spine 22:2951–2958

Hochanadel C D, Conrad D E 1993 Evolution of an on-site industrial physical therapy program. Journal of Medicine 35:1011–1016

Hurri H 1989 The Swedish back school in chronic low back pain. II Factors predicting the outcome. Scandinavian Journal of Rehabilitation Medicine 21:41–44

Jarvikoski A, Mellin G, Estlander A et al 1993 Outcome of two multimodal back treatment programs with and without intensive physical training. Journal of Spinal Disorders 6:93–98

Kellett K M, Kellett D A, Nordholm L A 1991 Effects of an exercise program on sick leave due to back pain. Physical Therapy 71(4):283–291

Kendall N, Linton SJ, Main CJ 1997 Guide to assessing psychosocial yellow flags in acute low back pain: Risk factors for long-term disability and workloss. National Health Committee, New Zealand

Krause N, Dasinger L K, Neuhauser F 1998 Modified work and return to work: a review of the literature. Journal of Occupational Rehabilitation 8:113–139

Lahad A, Malter A, Berg A O, Deyo R 1994 The effectiveness of four interventions for the prevention of low back pain. Journal of the American Medical Association 272:1286–1291

Lancourt J, Kettelhut M 1992 Predicting return to work for lower back pain patients receiving workers compensation. Spine 17:629–640

Lindstrom I, Ohlund C, Eek C et al 1992 The effect of graded activity on patients with subacute low back pain: a randomized prospective clinical study with an operant-conditioning behavioural approach. Physical Therapy 72:279–290

Loisel P, Abenhaim L, Durand P et al 1997 A population-based, randomized clinical trial on back pain management. Spine 22:2911–2918

Magora A 1973 Investigation of the relation between low back pain and occupation. V: psychological aspects. Scandinavian Journal of Rehabilitation Medicine 5:191–196

Main C J, Watson P W 1995 Screening for patients at risk of chronic incapacity. Journal of Occupational Rehabilitation 5:207–217

Mayer T, Gatchell R 1998 Functional restoration for spinal disorders: the sports medicine approach. Lea & Febiger, Philadelphia PA

Mayer T G, Gatchel R J, Kishino N et al 1985 Objective assessment of spine function following industrial injury. Spine 10:482–494

Mellin G, Harkapaa K, Vanharanta H, Hupli M, Heinonen R, Jarvikoski A 1993 Outcome of a multimodal treatment including intensive physical training of patients with chronic low back pain. Spine 18:825–829

Mitchell R I, Carmen G M 1990 Results of a multicenter trial using an intensive active exercise program for the treatment of acute soft tissue and back injuries. Spine 15:514–521

Nachemson A 1983 Work for all: for those with low back pain as well. Clinical Orthopaedics and Related Research 179:77–85

Oland G, Tveiten G 1991 A trial of modern rehabilitation for chronic low-back pain and disability. Spine 16:457–459

Pain Society 1997 Desirable criteria for pain management programmes. Pain Society, London

Ryan W E, Krishna M K, Swanson C E 1995 A prospective study evaluating early rehabilitation in preventing back pain chronicity in mine workers. Spine 20:489–491

Schenk R J, Doran R L Stachura J J 1996 Learning effects of a back education program. Spine 21:2183–2188

Schmidt S H, Oort-Marburger D, Meijman T F 1995 Employment after rehabilitation for musucloskeletal impairments: the impact of vocational rehabilitation and working on a trial basis. Archives of Physical Medicine and Rehabilitation 76:950–954

Sinclair S J, Hogg-Johnson S, Mondloch M V, Shields S A 1997 The effectiveness of an early active intervention program for workers with soft-tissue injuries: the early claimant cohort study. Spine 22:2919–2931

Tannenbaum S I, Beard R L, Salas E 1992 Team building and its influence on team effectiveness: an examination of conceptual and empirical developments. In: Kelley K (ed) Issues, theory and research in industrial/organisational psychology. Elsevier, Amsterdam: pp 117–153

Torstensen T A, Ljunggren A E, Meen H D, Odland E, Mowinckel P, Geijerstam S 1998 Efficiency and costs of medical exercise therapy, conventional physiotherapy, and self-exercise in patients with chronic low back pain. A pragmatic, randomised, single-blinded, controlled trial with 1 year follow up. Spine 23:2616–2624

van Doorn J W C 1995 Low back disability among self-employed dentists, veterinarians, physicians and physical therapists in the Netherlands. Acta Orthopaedica Scandinavica 66 (suppl 263):1–64

van Poppel M N M, Koes B W, van der Ploeg T, Smid T, Bouter L M 1998 Lumbar supports and education for the prevention of low back pain in industry. Journal of the American Medical Association 279:1789–1794

Von Korff M 1994 Perspectives on management of back pain in primary care. In: Gebhart G F, Hammond D L, Jensen T S (eds) Progress in pain research and management, vol 2. Proceedings of the 7th world congress on pain. International Association for the Study of Pain, Seattle W A pp 97–110

Von Korff M, Deyo R A, Cherkin D, Barlow W 1993 Back pain in primary care: outcomes at one year. Spine 18(7):855–862

Waddell G 1998 The back pain revolution. Churchill Livingstone, New York

Watson P J, Main C J, Waddell G, Gales T F, Purcell-Jones G 1998 Medically certified work-loss, recurrence and costs of wage compensation for back pain: a follow-up study of the working population of Jersey. British Journal of Rheumatology 37:82–86

Yamamoto S 1997 Guidelines on worksite prevention of low back pain. Labour Standards Bureau notification no 57. Industrial Health 35:143–172

Yassi A, Tate R, Cooper J E, Snow S, Vallentyne S, Khokhar J B 1995 Early intervention for back injuries in nurses at a large Canadian tertiary care hospital: an evaluation of the effectiveness and cost benefits of a two-year pilot project. Occupational Medicine 45:209–214

20

Conclusions

Chris J. Main Chris C. Spanswick

In examining the principles behind interdisciplinary pain management and examining its role in the treatment of patients, a number of general conclusions appear to be warranted.

1. Pain management needs to be understood not so much in terms of specific techniques, but more in terms of a process of engagement. The patients' pain problems started before the first contact with the pain centre and in the vast majority of cases will continue thereafter. Patients present with widely varying clinical histories and patterns of symptoms. Interdisciplinary pain management does not offer cures, but an opportunity to clarify the nature of the patient's pain and address its impact. It is often necessary as a first step to deal with iatrogenic confusion and distress created as a consequence of previous consultations.

2. The power of pain management lies in its biopsychosocial foundations. Specialists frequently take a narrow and constricted view of the nature of pain, and miss entirely the wider picture. (In the land of the blind, the one-eyed man is king.) Pain management focuses on function and quality of life. The interdisciplinary approach permits the identification of a range of possible treatment interventions, construed in terms of obstacles to recovery.

3. The essence of the approach requires patient engagement, and active participation of the patient (which is required as part of the process), and offers a set of cognitive and behavioural strategies with which to deal with their pain in the future.

4. It appears that the lessons learned from interdisciplinary pain management are applicable in the context of secondary prevention (whether in health-care or occupational settings).

5. The delivery of effective early biopsychosocial intervention requires the establishment of adequate competencies in the staff delivering the intervention.

6. The power of social forces as potential obstacles to recovery should not be underestimated. It is necessary as a part of clinical decision making, however, first to appraise the significance of such factors, and then decide whether they can be harnessed to facilitate recovery, or whether they are likely to inhibit it. In such matters, it is important to be as open as possible with patients.

7. Finally, it appears that biopsychosocial intervention has 'come of age'. Nonetheless much remains to be done not only in terms of improving outcome but also in understanding the nature of therapeutic processes and how interventions can be refined to match the range and diversity of obstacles to recovery that are evident in many patients.

It is difficult to summarise a topic as complex and convoluted as pain management. We have attempted to conclude with a visual representation of how we understand obstacles to recovery.

Figure 20.1 illustrates the important barriers to progress. These include variables ranging from 'organic pathology' to 'social policy'. There is great temptation to concentrate only on organic pathology when assessing patients. Although it is vital to exclude serious or treatable organic pathology (clinical red flags) it is as important to assess the relative importance of the other factors that may pose barriers to progress.

Figure 20.1 also illustrates a number of other factors often considered in contemporary clinical practice. Although there has been an increasing recognition of the importance of psychosocial factors over the last decade, consideration of these is often unsystematic and ill understood. It is easy to overestimate the significance of specific factors that may have been identified (such as behavioural responses to examination, work

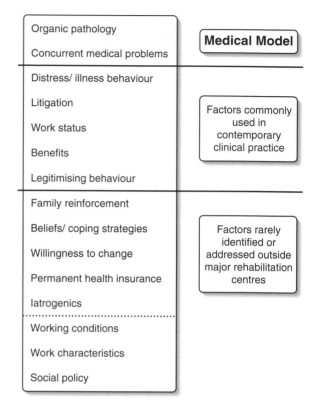

Figure 20.1 Obstacles to recovery: how they are addressed in clinical practice.

status, benefits or litigation) and fail to address other important factors. Inaccurate inferences may then be made as to the reasons why any individual patient fails to make progress, and poor clinical decision making may result.

Finally, Figure 20.1 illustrates a number of potential confounding issues, which may significantly affect the outcome of any treatment. The need for a broad-based assessment strategy is clear in order to identify all the important obstacles to recovery prior to clinical decision making, whether in terms of specific clinical objectives, or even whether to offer treatment at all.

In Figure 20.2, we offer a view of a conceptual diagram of how we understand the relationship between the biopsychosocial model of illness and obstacles to recovery. In our view the lessons learned in the development of interdisciplinary pain management offer the potential not only of 'rescuing' some of the patients who

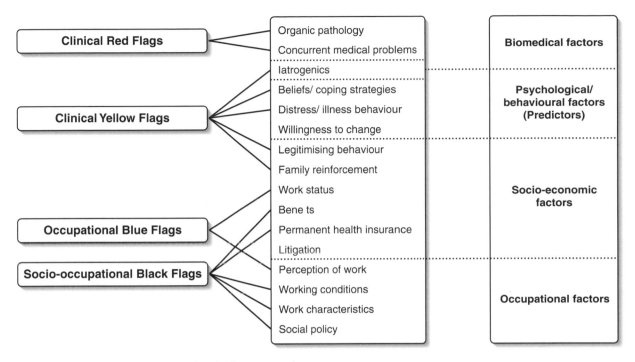

Figure 20.2 Obstacles to recovery: facets of assessment.

have become chronically incapacitated, but also of taking the principles forward into secondary prevention (whether in health-care or occupational settings). We see the latter as the main challenge for pain management at the start of the new millennium.

Index